The Physiological Basis of
Metabolic Bone Disease

Editors

Howard A. Morris, PhD, FAACB, FFSc (RCPA) is a professor of medical sciences at the University of South Australia, co-director of the Centre for Musculoskeletal Health Research, and a clinical scientist in chemical pathology at SA Pathology in Adelaide. Dr. Morris has published over 250 peer-reviewed manuscripts in the fields of metabolic bone disease, nutritional strategies for the prevention of osteoporosis, laboratory medicine, and cancer. He is the vice president of the International Federation of Clinical Chemistry and Laboratory Medicine (IFCC) and chair of the International Osteoporosis Foundation (IOF)/IFCC Working Group on Standardization of Bone Marker Assays. In 2009, he was named the American Society for Bone and Mineral Research's Louis Avioli Memorial Lecturer on the topic of "Intracrine and Paracrine Effects of Vitamin D."

Paul H. Anderson, PhD, is an associate professor of biological sciences at the University of South Australia, where he leads the Musculoskeletal Research Laboratory at the Centre for Musculoskeletal Health Research. He earned a doctorate from the School of Health Sciences at the University of Adelaide. He holds an NHRMC R.D. Wright Fellowship and is a member of the Australian and New Zealand Bone and Mineral Society (ANZBMS), the International Bone and Mineral Society (IBMS), and the American Society for Bone and Mineral Research (ASBMR). His research interests include nutritional and hormonal control of bone metabolism, with an emphasis on vitamin D endocrinology.

Dr. B.E. Christopher Nordin is a visiting professor of medicine at the University of Adelaide and also an emeritus consultant in endocrinology at the Royal Adelaide Hospital in South Australia. He has published over 500 scientific papers and edited 9 books on metabolic bone diseases during his 60-year career. He was the director of the Medical Research Council (UK) Mineral Metabolism Unit at Leeds, UK from 1964 to 1981. Dr. Nordin has been recognized worldwide for his contributions to our understanding of the pathophysiology of metabolic bone disease. He is an officer of the Order of Australia, was awarded Honorary Life Membership of the Australia and New Zealand Bone and Mineral Society and its British equivalent. He received the Frederick C. Bartter Award of the American Society of Bone and Mineral Research, the International Award for Modern Nutrition from the University of Lausanne, and a Career Recognition Award from the Vitamin D Workshop and serves on the editorial boards of several prestigious scientific journals.

Contributors

Paul H. Anderson
Musculoskeletal Health Research
Sansom Institute for Health Research
University of South Australia
Adelaide, South Australia

Arthur D. Conigrave
School of Molecular Bioscience
University of Sydney
Sydney, Australia

Rachel A. Davey
Department of Medicine
The University of Melbourne
Victoria, Australia

David M. Findlay
Centre for Orthopaedic and Trauma
    Research
University of Adelaide
Adelaide, South Australia

James C. Fleet
Department of Nutrition Science
Purdue University
West Lafayette, Indiana

J. Christopher Gallagher
Endocrine Department
Creighton University Medical School
Omaha, Nebraska

David Goltzman
Department of Medicine
McGill University and Royal Victoria
    Hospital
Montreal, Quebec, Canada

Howard A. Morris
Musculoskeletal Health Research
Sansom Institute for Health Research
University of South Australia
Adelaide, South Australia

B.E. Christopher Nordin
Endocrine and Metabolic Unit
Royal Adelaide Hospital
Adelaide, South Australia

Munro Peacock
Department of Medicine
Indiana University School of Medicine
Indianapolis, Indiana

Farzana Perwad
Division of Pediatric Nephrology
University of California San Francisco
San Francisco, California

Anthony A. Portale
Division of Pediatric Nephrology
University of California San Francisco
San Francisco, California

Richard L. Prince
Department of Endocrinology and Diabetes
Sir Charles Gairdner Hospital
Perth, Western Australia

1 Nutritional Requirements for Calcium and Vitamin D

J. Christopher Gallagher

CONTENTS

1.1 INTRODUCTION

In 2009, the Institute of Medicine (IOM) carefully reviewed the current literature and updated the dietary reference intakes (DRIs) for calcium and vitamin D for North America [1]. The committee used systematic evidence based reviews by the Agency for Healthcare Research and Quality (AHRQ) for an independent analysis of the world literature by a group of epidemiologists and statisticians [2]. After their report and a review of new studies, the IOM committee decided that the only clinical data that could be used to derive new DRIs had to be based on studies related to bone health.

DRIs are reference intakes that apply to the general, healthy population; they are not meant to serve as therapeutic guidelines. The definitions used are as follows:

Estimated average requirement (EAR)—Median requirement for a nutrient for each age and sex group

Recommended dietary allowance (RDA)—Intake that covers the needs of 97.5% of the population for each age and sex group

Tolerable upper level (TUL)—Intake (food or supplement) level above which risk begins to increase

1.2   NUTRITIONAL REQUIREMENTS FOR CALCIUM

Calcium is an essential nutrient that must be taken in the diet daily. Plasma calcium levels are maintained within narrow limits to facilitate optimal neuromuscular activities and other biological activities critical for life. The maintenance of plasma calcium homeostasis is under strict regulatory control as discussed in detail in Chapter 3. Transport of calcium by the kidneys and, in particular, the inability to reabsorb 100% of calcium from the renal glomerular filtrate is responsible for an obligatory loss of calcium in urine irrespective of the level of calcium in the diet. Calcium is also subject to obligatory losses through the skin and the gut. Skeletal calcium and phosphate act as body stores that contribute these key elements to the maintenance of plasma calcium homeostasis under specific conditions.

Humans have a clear need for adequate dietary calcium intake during growth, particularly during the modeling phase of bone growth in the pubertal stage (12 to 18 years of age) when bone mass expands by 40% to an average total skeletal calcium of 1000 g. During this period of rapid growth, the RDA for calcium is 1300 mg/d [1]. In the following years during the consolidation of adult bone mass (between the ages of 18 and 50 years), the calcium RDA is reduced to 1,000 mg/d.

Once adult bone mass is reached, what drives the calcium requirement? Because bone contains more than 99% of the calcium in the body and because net bone resorption is close to zero, we would seem to have little need for high calcium intake. However, obligatory losses of calcium through the urine, skin, and digestive juices total about 200 mg/d. If average calcium absorption is 25% of dietary consumption (as discussed in detail in Chapter 2), a total intake of 800 mg daily in subjects up to age 50 should be adequate. The current recommendations from the IOM for dietary calcium intakes are the following:

For adults 19 to 50 years of age, the EAR is 800 mg/d and the RDA is 1,000 mg/d. These levels are unchanged for males 51 to 70 years.

For females 51 to 70 years, the EAR increases to 1,000 mg/d and the RDA to 1,200 mg/d to account for the increased losses of calcium after menopause.

For both sexes after age 70, the recommendations remain at these higher levels [1].

1.3   METABOLIC BALANCE STUDIES AND MEASUREMENT OF DIETARY CALCIUM REQUIREMENTS

In terms of an overall understanding of the calcium economy, metabolic balance studies are the most instructive. Subjects are fed a controlled diet and samples of everything that they take in and all excreta are collected for measurements of calcium and phosphorus and the results are used to estimate calcium and phosphorus balances [3]. Calcium balances are used to estimate the amount of calcium needed to provide sufficient calcium for physiological requirements.

In an analysis of 212 calcium balances from the literature, Nordin [3] estimated that the mean calcium intake to equal the calcium output was 500 to 600 mg/d (9 mg/kg). However, calcium losses through the skin were ignored. More recently, a further analysis of balance studies was published from a slightly large data collection set of men whose average age was 38 years although one third were over age 65 [4]. In this case, the assumption of calcium lost in sweat added 40 mg/d to the calcium output. The estimated mean calcium intake that equaled output rose to 750 mg/d and the 95% limit was 900 mg/d.

Other calcium balance data cover younger subjects of both sexes that confirmed these EAR and RDA [5]. These data were collected under steady state conditions of calcium intakes varying between 200 and 1800 mg/d with 90% of the balances collected on calcium intakes exceeding 400 mg/d. Another data set from metabolic studies in 160 young adults aged 18 to 30 years [6] divided the results by quartiles of calcium intake. At a mean calcium intake of 435 mg/d, the calcium balance was negative at −65 mg/d; at a mean intake of 823 mg/d, calcium balance was zero; and at mean intakes of 1131 mg/d and 1550 mg/d, calcium balances were positive at 102 and 92 mg/d, respectively.

These results suggest that in the age group 20 to 30 years the mean calcium intake for neutral balance or the EAR is approximately 823 mg/d (95% confidence limits of 300 mg) and the RDA must lie between 980 and 1263 mg/d. These figures apply to young adults aged 18 to 30 years. At these ages, there is still increased calcium demand by the skeleton to consolidate the modeling phase of bone and therefore it is wiser to use the higher value of 1263 mg/d. In a recent report by the IOM, the RDA for this age group was 1200 mg/d [1].

The body can adapt to variations in dietary calcium intake through modifying calcium transport and the time for adaptation can vary from a few days to a few weeks. However, in our experience, using a technique analyzing calcium balance on a daily basis, most people seem to adapt to a new diet within 1 to 2 weeks. It is likely that adaptation in daily living probably does not occur quickly because the skeleton is available as a buffer to prevent acute physiological needs.

A rapid bone loss follows menopause but few calcium balance studies have focused on this transition in women. A study of 130 perimenopausal women, aged between 30 and 50 years has been reported but unfortunately the menopausal status was not clearly defined [7]. An average negative calcium balance in these women of −24 mg/d was such that the estimated EAR was 1241 mg/d and RDA 1316 mg/d. In a subsequent study on this group some time after they passed through the menopause, those on estrogen treatment were compared to untreated postmenopausal women. The average calcium balance in untreated postmenopausal women was −43 mg/d with EAR estimated at 1504 mg/d while for estrogen-treated women, the EAR was 990 mg/d, indicating that reduction of bone resorption reduced the EAR for calcium [8].

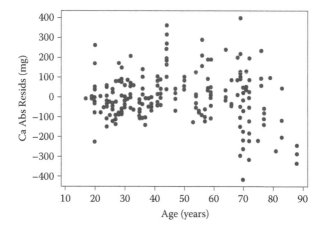

FIGURE 1.1   Calcium absorption decreases in healthy males after the age of about 60 years. From Ref. 4. With permission.

1.4   EFFECTS OF PHYSIOLOGICAL CHANGES ON INTESTINAL CALCIUM ABSORPTION

Calcium absorption decreases at the menopause. In a study published in 1989, calcium absorption decreased by about 10% of the premenopausal level when comparing estrogen-replete and estrogen-deplete women [9]. A longitudinal study of women passing through the menopause described a decrease on average of 20% in radiocalcium absorption, which assesses only the active transport of calcium between the premenopausal and postmenopausal states [10]. This fall in absorption was not associated with a fall in serum levels of the active form of vitamin D (1,25-dihydroxyvitamin D).

With increasing age, radiocalcium absorption decreases, starting at around age 65. In women, there is a 5% decrease in absorption every 10 years due to aging [9]. Calcium balance studies performed on normal men indicated a decrease in net absorption of calcium starting at about age 60 compared to younger men [4]. This is similar to the change described for the radiocalcium test [11]; see Figure 1.1.

It is likely that such decreases in intestinal calcium absorption efficiency are physiologically significant as elderly women with osteoporotic vertebral fractures often show severe malabsorption of calcium. One such series of metabolic studies demonstrated that about one third of the osteoporotic patients showed fecal calcium levels greater than calcium intake, indicating that these patients were in severe negative calcium balance [12].

1.5   EFFECTS OF DIETARY CALCIUM ON BONE LOSS, BONE MINERAL DENSITY, AND FRACTURES

At the time of the menopause, a marked increase in bone resorption occurs due to the loss of the effects of estrogen on calcium fluxes in the intestines, kidneys, and bones (see Chapter 2 for a detailed discussion). During a 5-year interval around menopause, bone mineral density (BMD) decreases in the spine and hip by about 10% [13] and total body calcium decreases by 8% [13]. Whether increasing dietary calcium can modulate this bone loss remains controversial. Perhaps a more interesting question is what level of calcium intake is required for early postmenopausal bone loss to become more rapid than average? Increasing calcium from dietary sources rather than by supplements may be safer and this largely means increasing intakes of dairy products. Since dairy products in the United States, Canada, Scandinavian countries, and other parts of the world are fortified with vitamin D, the benefit is doubled, there may be additional benefit.

Eight well-conducted randomized clinical trials studied the effects of calcium compared to placebo on bone mineral density [14–20]. Reid et al. [19] gave 1000 mg calcium daily to women (average age 58 years) in addition to a dietary calcium intake of 750 mg, thus achieving an average total intake of 1750 mg calcium daily. They showed that although bone loss continued in total body calcium, the rate of bone loss was reduced by 43% compared to placebo. There was also a significant difference in favor of calcium on spine BMD but not hip BMD.

Over 5 years, this same group showed significantly less bone loss on calcium at a total calcium intake of 1853 mg/d on spine and hip BMD compared to placebo [20]. Prince et al. [17] treated women of average age 62 years (whose baseline calcium intakes were 822 mg) with 1000 mg daily, thus achieving a total intake of 1822 mg/d. The subjects showed prevention of bone loss at the hip but not at the spine.

To summarize, these eight randomized controlled trials that utilized total calcium intakes ranging from 1000 to 2600 mg/d. Four trials demonstrated that calcium supplementation in a total of 2090 women significantly slowed the rate of bone loss at the spine by 1.7% and five trials involving a total of 2158 women showed a significant 0.84% reduction in bone loss at the hip compared to placebo. Interpretation of two studies [14,15] is confounded by the inclusion of early postmenopausal women in whom marked estrogen deficiency effects may have dominated bone loss—which is discussed further below. However, it does appear that some bone loss continues to occur with calcium supplementation although it is significantly reduced compared with placebo.

In three of these studies, total body calcium was measured [16–19] and showed decreases in loss in patients on calcium supplements compared to placebos. If one assumes a starting value for total bone calcium of 800 g, calcium losses would average 1 to 2 mg/d over 2 to 3 years with calcium supplementation. This level would be impossible to detect with calcium balance methods. We could conclude therefore from these total body measures that these women are essentially in calcium balance. However, it is plausible that total body calcium measurements may hide significant localized bone losses, rendering certain skeletal sites such as the spine and hip vulnerable for fracture. The calcium mineral at these sites would constitute only a small fraction of the total body calcium measurement. Furthermore, these sites have relatively high proportions of trabecular bone which remodels at a higher rate than cortical bone. In estimating calcium requirements, therefore, it is important to consider more than just calcium balance since this end point is unrelated to risk of fracture.

Therefore, the issue is whether higher calcium intake reduces the risk of fracture. Seven major studies included fractures as designated end points [19,23]. A total of

6242 women were studied and none of the individual studies of calcium showed significant effects on fracture. A meta-analysis by Tang et al. [24] included two smaller studies, increasing the total number of women to 6517. They found a 10% reduction in fractures (relative risk or RR of 0.90; confidence interval or CI of 0.89 to 1.00) with the optimal supplement at a level of 1200 mg/d. No statistical difference was found between the effects on fracture from calcium alone and from calcium combined with vitamin D ($P = 0.63$). Possibly there is a benefit for subgroups such as those with low calcium intakes or lower BMD but these hypotheses have not been tested.

A further meta-analysis, this time including data from 68,517 patients, reported on the effects of vitamin D alone versus vitamin D plus calcium on fracture [25]. These analyses demonstrated that calcium and vitamin D reduced the risk of all fractures by 8% ($P = 0.025$) and risk of hip fracture was reduced by 17% ($P < 0.05$). Vitamin D supplementation alone had no effect. In comparison, when estrogen was given to women of the same age, fracture risk was reduced by 35% in the Women's Health Initiative trial [26].

1.6 NUTRITIONAL REQUIREMENTS FOR VITAMIN D

The IOM committee performed an analysis using data from several vitamin D studies utilizing one or two doses of vitamin D and measured serum 25-hydroxyvitamin D (25D) to estimate what vitamin D dose was required to achieve a target serum 25D greater than 50 nmol/L (20 ng/mL). All studies were performed at latitudes above 50 degrees during winter to minimize confounding by vitamin D derived from sunlight. The simulated dose response curve demonstrated that 800 IU/d would yield a serum 25D level of 50 nmol/L (20 ng/mL) or greater [1]. This dose has since been confirmed by an independent dose response study [27].

With regard to studies limited to vitamin D administration only, seven trials in the literature involved a comparison of vitamin D supplementation in variable doses to placebo on fracture rates [28–34]. No studies showed reductions in fractures (odds ratio of 1.05). In a large trial of 2256 women aged 70 years or older, a single high dose of vitamin D (500,000 IU) annually showed a significant increase in fractures that occurred within about 3 months after dosing in 2 separate years (RR of 1.26; CI of 1.00 to 1.59).

All other published clinical trials with vitamin D used a combination regimen with calcium and studied the effects in comparison to calcium alone or to placebo. We noted considerable limitations because few of these studies included dose–response designs although a variety of doses of vitamin D and calcium were studied. In a meta-analysis and subgroup analysis, Tang et al. [24] concluded that institutionalized people showed more significant responses to calcium plus vitamin D than calcium alone (RR, 0.76; CI, 0.66 to 0.88). Doses of calcium exceeding 1200 mg/d showed more reductions in fractures [RR, 0.80; CI 0.72 to 0.89) than lower levels of supplementation [RR, 0.94; CI, 0.89 to 0.99). Vitamin D doses greater than or equal to 800 IU/d (RR, 0.84; CI 0.75 to 0.94) produced slightly better results than lower doses (RR, 0.97; CI 0.71 to 1.05).

Further evidence published from 21 clinical trials demonstrated an effect of calcium and vitamin D supplementation on BMD as a designated outcome. None of these studies included dose–response designs. The AHRQ Ottawa/Tufts meta-analysis [35] showed a small positive effect on BMD at the spine, femoral neck, and total body sites with a supplement of vitamin D3 at 800 IU/d plus ~500mg/d calcium. This effect was confirmed in the meta-analysis by Tang et al. [24] who showed significant increases in BMD of the hip (0.545) and the spine (1.2%) in favor of calcium plus vitamin D supplementation compared to placebo.

In summary, these data indicate that: (1) there is no evidence that vitamin D supplements alone reduced fractures; (2) calcium supplementation alone reduced fractures by 10%; (3) calcium plus vitamin D supplementation reduced fractures by 13%; and (4) in nursing home residents, the reduction in risk of hip fracture rose to 17% with calcium and vitamin D supplementation. The IOM report recommended an EAR for vitamin D of 400 IU/d and RDA of 600 IU/d for the general healthy population aged 1 to 70; for individuals older than 70 years, the RDA was increased to 800 IU/d.

1.7 SOURCES OF VITAMIN D

1.7.1 SUNLIGHT

Sunlight accounts for probably 80% of the vitamin D input into the body. Ultraviolet light radiation (UVB, not UVA) acts on 7-dehydrocholesterol in the skin to form pre-vitamin D and then undergoes a thermal reaction to form vitamin D. Several factors control the amount of UVB radiation reaching the deeper layers of the skin including pigmentation, latitude, season, amount of skin exposed, and use of sunscreen.

Generally the sun must rise more than 30 degrees above the horizon to avoid filtering by atmospheric pollution. For example, at 41 degrees north latitude in the U.S. Midwest, the effective months for transmittal of UV light are 6 months from the end of April to the end of October when average serum 25D levels increase from 50 to 75 nmol/L (20 to 30 ng/ml). This increase is equivalent to an oral vitamin D supplement of about 2000 IU/d [26,27]. At 55 degrees north latitude in Scotland, the seasonal increase in serum 25D was only 10 nmol/L (4 ng/mL) and at 60 degrees, effective UV light lasts only about 3 months.

1.7.2 DIET AND SUPPLEMENTS

The dietary intake of vitamin D averages about 100 to 220 IU daily based on the NHANES results and is too low to compensate for lack of sunlight [36]. The natural sources of vitamin D in the diet include many types of fatty fish, cod liver oil, and shiitake mushrooms. In the United States, fortification of milk with vitamin D is voluntary and the recommended amount is ~400 IU/L. In Canada, margarine and milk are fortified as mandated by regulation. The form of vitamin D in food supplementation is commonly vitamin D3 (cholecalciferol) although vitamin D2 (ergocalciferol) was used extensively until the year 2000.

Both forms of vitamin D behave similarly in regulation of calcium and phosphorus metabolism [37] and there thus appears no difference between them at the molecular level [38]. In rats, vitamin D2 is less toxic than vitamin D3 [39] but there are no

similar human studies. With daily supplementation of 1000 IU/d for 6 weeks, vitamin D2 and vitamin D3 produced similar serum levels of the 25-hydroxy metabolite
25D [40]. However if a weekly dose of 50,000 IU of vitamin D2 or vitamin D3 is
administered, the serum 25D3 level at 1 month is 12.5 nmol/L (5 ng/mL) higher than
25D2. If the regimen is 50,000 IU for 3 months, the 25D3 level is about 45 nmol/L
(18 ng/mL) higher than 25D2 [41], however, since final values were greater than
100 nmol/L (40 ng/ml) these differences are not clinically important.

In a study of normal older women treated with increasing doses of vitamin D
from 400 to 4800 IU/d for 1 year, the serum 25D level response was described by
a quadratic curve reaching a plateau at a level of approximately 100 to 112 nmol/L
(40 to 45 ng/mL) on a dose of 3,000 to 4,000IU/d. This demonstrated that serum
25D levels are regulated to achieve a steady state (Figure 1.2) [27]. The results also
showed that vitamin D supplementation at doses of 600 to 800/d would exceed a
serum level of 50 nmol/L (20 ng/mL) in 97.5% of the population and a dose of
400 IU/dy would exceed 50 nmol/L (20 ng/mL) in 50%. These data were confirmed
in an African American elderly population [42] and in a younger group of white
and black women [42], indicating that the response to vitamin D supplementation is
largely equivalent in both groups. One could infer from this study that a daily dose
of vitamin D does not need to exceed 4,000 IU in normal people.

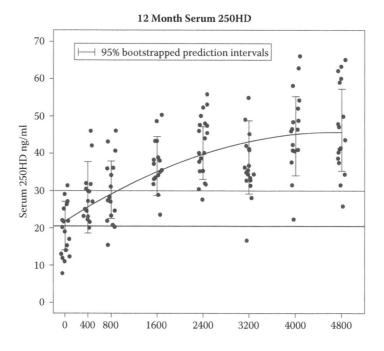

FIGURE 1.2 Dose response after 12 months of daily vitamin D dosage (international units
per day on the horizontal axis) on serum 25D levels (nanograms per milliliter units on the
vertical axis).

1.8 VITAMIN D TOXICITY

If people take larger doses of vitamin D, they may develop vitamin D intoxication. Doses between 20,000 and 40,000IU/d taken on a long-term basis can achieve serum 25D levels exceeding 500 nmol/L (200 ng/mL) and lead to hypercalcemia [43]. At such serum levels, 25D can bind directly to vitamin D receptors to stimulate biological activities simulating the effects of 1,25-dihydroxyvitamin D [44].

The IOM assessed data mostly derived from case studies of accidental occurrences in humans to define a TUL for vitamin D. The consensus of the IOM was that 20,000 IU or more would increase the risk of vitamin D intoxication and that because of safety concerns, 4,000 IU should represent the TUL [1]. This is not a recommended dose. The level may be lower in thin older people, those with impaired renal function, and individuals who take large doses of calcium supplements. The lower dose of 4,000 IU was chosen in part because of reports that serum 25 OHD 25D levels > 125 nmol/L (50 ng/ml) were associated with increased mortality rates [45–47].

1.9 SUMMARY

The total dietary calcium intake for maintaining human health remains uncertain. Until adequate safety data are available, public health bodies suggest that *total* calcium intake be limited to 1000 to 1200 mg/d. Even subjects whose total calcium intakes are 1200 mg daily can develop intermittent hypercalciuria and hypercalcemia—most likely due to the increased calcium intake [27,42]. Age-related changes in calcium and vitamin D metabolism affect vitamin D metabolism and optimum nutrition in the elderly. Vitamin D nutrition can be improved in the elderly by increasing their vitamin D intakes to 800 IU/d. There does appear to be a reduction in risk of fractures when vitamin D is given with calcium at a level of 1000 to 1200 mg daily. This combination is a simple inexpensive strategy that can reduce fractures in institutionalized people by 30%.

The dose–response curves show that 800 IU of vitamin D will achieve the target serum 25 OHD of 50 nmol/L (20 ng/mL) in most people. Therefore, there is no need for screening of serum 25D levels in normal people. For those who have medical conditions known to affect vitamin D metabolism such as treatment with anticonvulsants and corticosteroids, screening for vitamin D deficiency and insufficiency is useful.

REFERENCES

1. Ross, A.C. et al., Eds. 2011. The Institute of Medicine. *Dietary Reference Intakes for Calcium and Vitamin D*. Washington, DC, National Academies Press.
2. Chung, M. et al. 2011. Vitamin D with or without calcium supplementation for prevention of cancer and fractures: an updated meta-analysis for the U.S. Preventive Services Task Force. *Ann Intern Med*, 155(12): 827–838.
3. Nordin, B.E.. 1976. Laboratory methods: calcium balance technique. In Nordin, B.E., Ed., *Calcium Phosphate and Magnesium Metabolism*, London: Churchill Livingstone.
4. Nordin, B.E. and H.A. Morris. 2011. Recalculation of the calcium requirement of adult men. *Am J Clin Nutr*, 93(2): 442–445.

5. Hunt, C.D. and L.K. Johnson. 2007. Calcium requirements: new estimations for men and women by cross-sectional statistical analyses of calcium balance data from metabolic studies. *Am J Clin Nutr*, 86(4): 1054–1063.

6. Matkovic, V. 1991. Calcium metabolism and calcium requirements during skeletal modeling and consolidation of bone mass. *Am J Clin Nutr*, 54: 245S–260S.

7. Heaney, R.P., R.R. Recker, and P.D. Saville. 1977. Calcium balance and calcium requirements in middle-aged women. *Am J Clin Nutr*, 30(10): 1603–1611.

8. Heaney, R.P., R.R. Recker, and P.D. Saville. 1978. Menopausal changes in calcium balance performance. *J Lab Clin Med,* 92(6): 953–963.

9. Heaney, R.P. et al. 1989. Calcium absorption in women: relationships to calcium intake, estrogen status, and age. *J Bone Miner Res*, 4(4): 469–475.

10. Nordin, B.E. et al. 2004. A longitudinal study of bone-related biochemical changes at the menopause. *Clin Endocrinol (Oxf)*, 61(1): 123–130.

11. Bullamore, J.R. et al. 1970. Effect of age on calcium absorption. *Lancet*, 2(7672): 535–537.

12. Gallagher, J.C. et al. 1973. The crush fracture syndrome in postmenopausal women. *Clin Endocrinol Metabol*, 2(2): 293–315.

13. Greendale, G.A. et al. 2012. Bone mineral density loss in relation to the final menstrual period in a multiethnic cohort: results from the Study of Women's Health across the Nation (SWAN). *J Bone Miner Res*, 27(1): 111–118.

14. Dawson-Hughes, B. et al. 1990. A controlled trial of the effect of calcium supplementation on bone density in postmenopausal women. *New Engl J Med*, 323(13): 878–883.

15. Elders, P.J. et al. 1994. Long-term effect of calcium supplementation on bone loss in perimenopausal women. *J Bone Miner Res*, 9(7): 963–970.

16. Peacock, M. et al. 2000. Effect of calcium or 25 OH vitamin D3 dietary supplementation on bone loss at the hip in men and women over the age of 60. *J Clin Endocrinol Metabol*, 85(9): 3011–3019.

17. Prince, R. et al. 1995. The effects of calcium supplementation (milk powder or tablets) and exercise on bone density in postmenopausal women. *J Bone Miner Res*, 10(7): 1068–1075.

18. Prince, R.L. et al. 2006. Effects of calcium supplementation on clinical fracture and bone structure: results of a 5-year, double-blind, placebo-controlled trial in elderly women. *Arch Intern Med*, 166(8): 869–875.

19. Reid, I.R. et al. 1993. Effect of calcium supplementation on bone loss in postmenopausal women. *New Engl J Med*, 328(7): 460–464.

20. Reid, I.R. et al. 2006. Randomized controlled trial of calcium in healthy older women. *Am J Med*, 119(9): 777–785.

21. Riggs, B.L. et al. 1998. Long-term effects of calcium supplementation on serum parathyroid hormone level, bone turnover, and bone loss in elderly women. *J Bone Miner Res*, 13(2): 168–174.

22. Recker, R.R. et al. 1996. Correcting calcium nutritional deficiency prevents spine fractures in elderly women. *J Bone Miner Res*, 11(12): 1961–1966.

23. Grant, A.M. et al. 2005. Oral vitamin D3 and calcium for secondary prevention of low-trauma fractures in elderly people: a randomised placebo-controlled trial. *Lancet*, 365(9471): 1621–1628.

24. Tang, B.M. et al. 2007. Use of calcium or calcium in combination with vitamin D supplementation to prevent fractures and bone loss in people aged 50 years and older: a meta-analysis. *Lancet*, 370(9588): 657–666.

25. Dipart Group. 2010. Patient level pooled analysis of 68,500 patients from seven major vitamin D fracture trials in U.S. and Europe. *BMJ*. 340: 5463.

26. Cauley, J.A. et al. 2003. Effects of estrogen plus progestin on risk of fracture and bone mineral density: the Women's Health Initiative randomized trial. *JAMA*, 290(13): 1729–1738.

27. Gallagher, J.C. et al. 2012. Dose response to vitamin D supplementation in postmeno-pausal women: a randomized trial. *Ann Intern Med*, 156(6): 425–437.
28. Law, M. et al. 2006. Vitamin D supplementation and the prevention of fractures and falls: results of a randomised trial in elderly people in residential accommodation. *Age Ageing*, 35(5): 482–486.
29. Lips, P. et al. 1996. Vitamin D supplementation and fracture incidence in elderly per-sons: a randomized, placebo-controlled clinical trial. *Ann Intern Med*, 124(4): 400–406.
30. Lyons, R.A. et al. 2007. Preventing fractures among older people living in institutional care: a pragmatic randomised double blind placebo controlled trial of vitamin D supple-mentation. *Osteoporosis Intl*, 18(6): 811–818.
31. Meyer, H.E. et al. 2002. Can vitamin D supplementation reduce the risk of fracture in the elderly? A randomized controlled trial. *J Bone Miner Res*, 17(4): 709–715.
32. Sanders, K.M. et al. 2010. Annual high-dose oral vitamin D and falls and fractures in older women: a randomized controlled trial. *JAMA,* 303(18): 1815–1822.
33. Smith, H. et al. 2007. Effect of annual intramuscular vitamin D on fracture risk in elderly men and women: a population-based, randomized, double-blind, placebo-controlled trial. *Rheumatology*, 46(12): 1852–1857.
34. Trivedi, D.P., R. Doll, and K.T. Khaw. 2003. Effect of four monthly oral vitamin D3 (cholecalciferol) supplementations on fractures and mortality in men and women living in the community: randomised double blind controlled trial. *BMJ*, 326(7387): 469.
35. Cranney, A. et al. 2007. Effectiveness and safety of vitamin D in relation to bone health. *Evid Rep Technol Assess (Full Rep),* 158: 1–235.
36. Bailey, R.L. et al. 2010. Estimation of total usual calcium and vitamin D intakes in the United States, *J Nutr*, 140(4): 817–822.
37. Masuda, S. et al. 2006. Evidence for the activation of 1-alpha-hydroxyvitamin D2 by 25-hydroxyvitamin D-24-hydroxylase: delineation of pathways involving 1-alpha, 24-dihydroxyvitamin D2 and 1-alpha,25-dihydroxyvitamin D2. *Biochim Biophys Acta*, 1761(2): 221–234.
38. Jones G. et al. Current understanding of the molecular actions of vitamin D. *Physiol Rev*, 1998 Oct; 78(4): 1193–1231.
39. Sjoden, G. et al. 1985. One alpha-hydroxyvitamin D2 is less toxic than 1 alpha-hydroxyvitamin D3 in the rat. *Proc Soc Exp Biol Med*, 178(3): 432–436.
40. Holick M.F. et al. 2008. Vitamin D2 is as effective as vitamin D3 in maintaining circulat-ing concentrations of 25-hydroxyvitamin D, *J Clin Endorcrinol Metab*, 93(3): 677–681.
41. Heaney, R.P. et al. 2011. Vitamin D(3) is more potent than vitamin D(2) in humans. *J Clin Endocrinol Metabol,* 96(3): E447–E452.
42. Gallagher, J.C. et al. 2013. Effects of vitamin D supplementation in older African American women. *J Clin Endocrinol Metabol*, 98(3): 1137–1146.
43. Mason, R.S. and S. Posen. 1979. The relevance of 25-hydroxycalciferol measurements in the treatment of hypoparathyroidism. *Clin Endocrinol (Oxf)*, 10(3): 265–269.
44. Rowling, M.J. et al. 2007. High dietary vitamin D prevents hypocalcemia and osteoma-lacia in CYP27B1 knockout mice. *J Nutr*, 137(12): 2608–2615.
45. Melamed, M.L. et al. 2008. 25-Hydroxyvitamin D levels and the risk of mortality in the general population. *Arch Intern Med*, 168(15): 1629–1637.
46. Durup, D. et al. 2012. A reverse J-shaped association of all-cause mortality with serum 25-hydroxyvitamin D in general practice: the CopD study. *J Clin Endocrinol Metabol*, 97(8): 2644–2652.
47. Sempos, C.T. et al. 2013. Is there a reverse J-shaped association between 25-hydroxy-vitamin D and all-cause mortality? Results from the U.S. nationally representative NHANES. *J Clin Endocrinol Metabol*, 98(7): 3001–3009.

2 Physiology of Vitamin D, Calcium, and Phosphate Absorption

James C. Fleet and Munro Peacock

CONTENTS

2.1 INTRODUCTION

Whole body calcium and phosphate metabolisms are controlled by mechanisms at three organs: the intestine where calcium and phosphate enter the body from the diet, the kidney where calcium and phosphate are excreted, and the bone where calcium and phosphate are stored together as apatite crystals and serve both as mineral reservoirs and as structural components that provide strength to bone [1]. The greatest stores of calcium and phosphate reside in bone, but important smaller metabolically active stores are present both outside and inside cells. Although the density and microstructure of bone reflect the availability and utilization of calcium and phosphate in the body, homeostatic mechanisms exist to protect plasma concentrations and not bones.

A high extracellular-to-intracellular calcium ratio is used as a major signaling system to control muscle contraction, nerve transmission, and various intracellular signaling pathways. Controlling plasma and extracellular calcium within a narrow range is essential. Plasma phosphate levels are less tightly regulated and phosphate is used primarily as an intracellular molecule for energy metabolism [as adenosine triphosphate (ATP)], regulation of protein function largely through kinase-mediated phosphorylation of proteins, and as an essential molecule in structural components of cells.

Plasma calcium and phosphate levels are regulated primarily by three hormones produced in three different tissues: parathyroid hormone (PTH) produced in the parathyroid glands, fibroblast growth factor 23 (FGF23) produced in bone osteocytes, and most notably, the vitamin D metabolite, 1,25-dihydroxyvitamin D [calcitriol (1,25D)] produced in renal tubules.

In this chapter calcium, phosphate, and vitamin D will be discussed in relation to their absorption from the diet. It includes details about the regulation and absorption of calcium, phosphate, and vitamin D within a physiologic context.

2.2 VITAMIN D ABSORPTION, METABOLISM, AND MOLECULAR ACTIONS

2.2.1 Skin Synthesis and Dietary Absorption

2.2.1.1 Skin Synthesis

Vitamin D is present in the diet as cholecalciferol (D_3) and ergocalciferol (D_2). However, vitamin D is efficiently produced from 7-dehydrocholesterol when skin is exposed to ultraviolet B (UVB) light (170 to 320 nm; peak, 296 nm). Thus, in the presence of adequate sunlight exposure, there is no dietary requirement for vitamin D. However, low UVB exposure is common in countries at high latitudes and their residents have dietary requirements for vitamin D. In addition, several subpopulations have reduced skin production of vitamin D including people with deeply pigmented skin, particularly those living at high latitudes; those who use strong sunscreens; those who cover their skin for ethnic or religious reasons; and elderly and infirm housebound individuals. These groups are at risk of low vitamin D status in winter when UVB irradiation is markedly decreased [2].

2.2.1.2 Gut Absorption

The current recommendations for dietary vitamin D intake for the United States were set in 2010 by an Institute of Medicine (IOM) panel [3]. The recommended intake level for adults between the ages of 18 and 70 is 600 IU per day with no distinction made between vitamin D_3 and D_2. Fat-soluble vitamins including vitamin D have traditionally been thought to "follow the fat" during intestinal absorption (Figure 2.1). This requires association of the vitamin with bile salts for incorporation into micelles, movement of the micelles into the body, and repackaging of the vitamin into chylomicrons for transport by the lymphatic system. This model is consistent with the observations that gastrointestinal and hepatobiliary diseases leading to fat malabsorption commonly cause vitamin D deficiency in humans [4].

Administration of high oral doses of radiolabeled vitamin D to rats led to the appearance of the label within chylomicrons in the lymph [5]. Sitrin et al. [6] used lower, more physiologically relevant doses of vitamin D and perfusates high in fat and found that 33% of the dose was absorbed from the perfused jejunum and that bile acids were required for efficient absorption. Consistent with the important role of bile acids in vitamin D absorption, Watkins et al. [7] reported that the cholestyramine bile acid binder reduced vitamin D absorption and induced vitamin D deficiency in rats.

Others suggested that the majority of vitamin D absorption occurs in the portal vein [6,8]. However, this is likely an artifact that reflected leakage of vitamin D into the portal vein from unligated lymph ducts during the perfusion study since vitamin D absorption efficiency was low (14% of the dose in 24 h) and 80% of the absorbed vitamin D ended up in chylomicrons [9]. The presence of vitamin D was

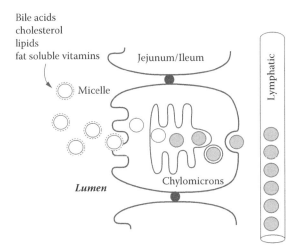

FIGURE 2.1 Model for intestinal vitamin D absorption. Vitamin D is packaged into micelles along with fats, cholesterol, and bile acids. Micelles interact with enterocytes and fat soluble compounds diffuse across the membrane. Vitamin D is repackaged with fats and cholesterol into chylomicrons that are transported into the lymphatic system for distribution throughout the body.

first observed in the lymph 2 to 4 h after oral vitamin D doses in rats [9]. This is consistent with earlier reports that vitamin D absorption occurs by passive diffusion into the lymph in the jejunum and ileum [10]. No evidence suggests any differences in the routes or mechanisms of absorption of vitamin D_2 and vitamin D_3.

Hydroxylated forms of vitamin D [25 hydroxyvitamin D (25D) and 1,25-dihydroxyvitamin D (1,25D)] are absorbed more efficiently than vitamin D [6,9]. Sitrin et al. [6] reported that for 25D, increased absorption efficiency was due to chylomicron-independent absorption—a finding consistent with Krawitt et al. [11] who found that 25D is better absorbed than vitamin D in subjects with steatorrhea. Dueland et al. [9] found that 25D is absorbed into the lymph but is associated with an alpha-globulin that is likely the vitamin D binding protein (DBP; see additional discussion below) rather than with chylomicrons. It is interesting that vitamin D absorption does not increase in rats with experimental nephrotic syndrome despite the significant loss of vitamin D metabolites in urine and reduced serum 25D levels [12]. This suggests that there are no homeostatic regulatory mechanisms to increase intestinal vitamin D absorption in times of need.

2.2.2 BRIEF OVERVIEW OF VITAMIN D METABOLISM

Vitamin D within chylomicrons is rapidly transported to the liver [9] and into the body's fat stores [13], resulting in a half-life for vitamin D in plasma of only several hours [14]. Once in the liver, vitamin D is hydroxylated on its side chain to form 25D by cytochrome P450 (CYP) enzymes like CYP2R1 and CYP27A1 [15]. This conversion is rapid, driven primarily by the level of the substrate, and is poorly inhibited by the 25D product [16]. The high capacity of the liver to produce 25D ensures that liver disease does not result in vitamin D deficiency. Rapid release of 25D from hepatocytes occurs soon after it is synthesized [17].

The 25D from the liver is transported in the circulation by the DBP [18]. The binding affinity of DBP for the vitamin D metabolites is highest for 25D. In DBP knockout mice, urinary 25D levels are higher and serum 25D levels are lower than normal [19]. Normally the 25D DBP complex in the renal filtrate is actively reabsorbed first through binding to a complex of cubulin and megalin and then internalized by receptor-mediated endocytosis [20].

Normally very little 25D is excreted in the urine, whereas urinary 25D levels are high in megalin knockout mice [20]. Because of the efficient retention of the 25D DBP complex, serum 25D has a biological half-life of 2 to 3 weeks [14,21], making serum 25D a measure of vitamin D status. A recent report from the Institute of Medicine suggested a serum 25D value of 50 nmol/L (20 ng/ml) as adequate to support optimal bone and mineral metabolism [22]. However, some argue that higher levels [greater than 80 nmol/L (32 ng/ml)] may have beneficial effects but this position is controversial [22].

Further discussion of vitamin D metabolism and modes of action is presented in Chapter 7. The chapter also covers genomic and rapid, non-genomic actions through the nuclear vitamin D receptor and a membrane receptor known as the membrane-associated rapid response steroid (MARRS) binding protein [23] that binds 1,25D with high affinity and is distinct from the classical VDR [24].

2.2.3 CONCLUSIONS

Vitamin D is a prohormone that is an important regulator of calcium and phosphate metabolism. It is synthesized in the skin by sunlight and thus is not strictly a required nutrient. When taken orally, vitamin D "follows the fat" and is absorbed in the intestine through the lymphatic system. Vitamin D from chylomicrons is delivered to the liver and rapidly converted to the 25D metabolite.

In contrast, more hydroxylated forms of vitamin D are not absorbed in chylomicrons nor are they delivered to the liver. The renal production of the active 1,25D hormonal metabolite is critical for the control of calcium and phosphate absorption and bone metabolism. However, some evidence indicates that local tissue production of 1,25D can occur and the importance of this for regulation of intestinal calcium absorption is discussed below. The molecular actions of 1,25D are mediated primarily through transcriptional events dependent upon the VDR. Loss of this ligand-activated transcription factor causes severe disruptions in calcium, phosphate, and bone metabolism. Rapid signaling events have been documented to occur through either the VDR or the MARRS and their implications for calcium and phosphate absorption are discussed below.

2.3 INTESTINAL CALCIUM ABSORPTION

2.3.1 ROLE OF INTESTINAL CALCIUM ABSORPTION IN WHOLE BODY CALCIUM METABOLISM

Whole body calcium metabolism is maintained through a balance of intake, intestinal absorption efficiency, and total calcium losses from the intestine, urine, and skin. Fecal calcium contains both unabsorbed dietary calcium and endogenous calcium lost into the intestine during absorption. This endogenous loss is 100 to 200 mg per day [25] and net calcium absorption may be negative if intake is lower than endogenous losses.

The measure of calcium absorption efficiency from the gut into the body (true or gross calcium absorption) is determined with radiotracers and pharmacokinetic analysis [26]. While the total amount of calcium absorbed increases as dietary calcium increases, the efficiency of calcium absorption is inversely proportional to intake [27]. These relationships exist because calcium crosses the intestinal barrier by both a saturable, transcellular pathway and a non-saturable, diffusion pathway [27–29] that can be modeled mathematically using a Michaelis-Menton-like equation that includes a linear component to account for the non-saturable diffusion pathway [30] (Figure 2.2).

The saturable component of calcium absorption predominates in the duodenum and jejunum and is under nutritional and physiological regulation, causing it to be increased when dietary calcium intake is low. This is an energy-dependent pathway; calcium movement into the intestinal epithelial cells is down a concentration gradient, whereas movement from cells into the blood is up a concentration gradient and requires energy [31]. The saturable pathway is absent in the ileum [32] but some animal studies have reported that saturable calcium transport may also be functional

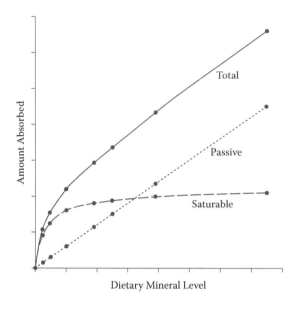

FIGURE 2.2 Calcium and phosphate absorption follow two paths. Absorption can occur via a regulated pathway that predominates at lower dietary intake levels. This pathway mediated by transporters and can be saturated. In addition, passive diffusion can occur and is directly proportional to dietary intake. As a result, at high dietary intake levels, the passive diffusion pathway predominates.

in the colon [33–35]. In contrast, passive transport occurs throughout the length of the small intestine and is directly related to luminal calcium level at 13% per hour in humans [29].

For typical levels of calcium intake (200 to 400 mg per meal), the saturable component of calcium absorption may account for as much as 60% of total calcium absorption in the proximal small intestine. However, as the calcium level in a single meal is increased, the contribution of the saturable calcium transport pathway to the total amount of calcium absorbed is reduced and the efficiency of calcium absorption falls until only the diffusional component of calcium absorption remains.

With adequate calcium intake, the proportion of calcium transported in the intestine is determined by the relative contributions of the saturable and non-saturable pathways. Calcium absorption is moderately efficient in humans, with 35% of a typical meal absorbed. Additional factors affecting the amount of calcium absorption within any given segment of the intestine include the sojourn time through the intestinal tract and the solubility of calcium within the intestinal segment (high in the duodenum and low in the ileum and lower bowel) [36] (Figure 2.3). As a result, even if calcium solubility is low and the saturable pathway is absent or very low, the total amount of calcium absorption is greatest in the ileum since transit time through this segment takes 10 times longer (or more) than the transit through the proximal intestinal segments [37,38].

The efficiency of calcium absorption is strongly influenced by physiological states including growth, pregnancy, lactation, and maturity, and habitual dietary calcium

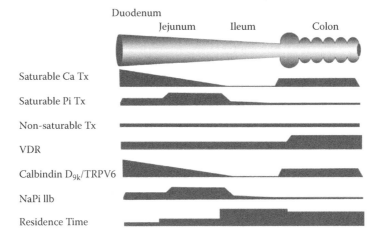

FIGURE 2.3 Depiction of relationships in the gastrointestinal tract among features that are critical for intestinal calcium or phosphate absorption. Net mineral absorption is determined by many factors; different mechanisms for mineral absorption act in different intestinal segments. The height of the black bar signifies the relative importance or abundance of a feature for a given intestinal segment. Tx = transport.

intake [1]. The fact that low habitual calcium intake increases the efficiency of intestinal absorption was shown directly by Pansu et al. [28] who found that feeding a calcium-restricted diet (0.17% versus 0.44% calcium) to rats for 5 weeks increased the efficiency of duodenal calcium absorption by increasing saturable calcium transport by 55%.

Increased efficiency of calcium absorption after consumption of a low calcium diet for 8 weeks was noted in adult humans [39,40]. It is now understood that the increased efficiency of calcium absorption resulting from habitual low calcium intake is due to adaptation mediated by increased renal production of 1,25D [41] and signaling of this hormone through the VDR [42].

Low intestinal calcium absorption efficiency can reduce bone mineral density (BMD) and increase the risk of osteoporosis. For example, physiologic limitations imposed by aging and menopause reduce calcium absorption and also blunt the positive impact of 1,25D on intestinal calcium absorption [43–48]. This may explain why low calcium absorption is more prevalent in women with osteoporosis [49] and why low calcium absorption is associated with increased hip fracture risk in post-menopausal women, especially those with low dietary calcium intakes [50].

2.3.2 Vitamin D Status and Signaling in Intestinal Calcium Absorption

Intestinal calcium absorption is dependent upon adequate vitamin D status [51,52]. The efficiency of intestinal calcium absorption is dramatically lower in vitamin D-deficient animals (reduced >75%) [32] and in dialysis patients with compromised renal function and low circulating 1,25D levels [53].

However, calcium malabsorption does not occur until vitamin D stores are severely depleted. Secondary hyperparathyroidism maintains serum 1,25D (and calcium absorption) until the deficiency is so severe (serum 25D levels below 10 nmol/L) that serum 1,25D decreases due to lack of substrate for conversion in the kidney [54]. In children with vitamin D deficiency rickets, serum 1,25D levels can be in the normal range even though serum calcium and phosphate levels are low [55,56]. However, giving vitamin D to rachitic children immediately increases serum 1,25D to supraphysiologic levels, indicating a strong compensation to correct the symptoms of vitamin D deficiency.

In animal models, the loss of active calcium absorption resulting from vitamin D deficiency is restored by either increasing vitamin D status to normal or by increasing 1,25D with injections. The effect of 1,25D on calcium absorption is on the saturable component of transport [30,32] leading to an increase in the maximal capacity of transport and reflecting the production of other transporters. Some evidence indicates that the non-saturable portion of calcium absorption in the human ileum is also vitamin D sensitive [29].

The critical role of transcellular calcium movement during calcium absorption was shown clearly using ion microscopy to follow the movement of ^{44}calcium across the chick duodenum [57]. This method showed that when vitamin D status was adequate, calcium flowed from the apical sides of enterocytes and through the epithelial cells over the course of 20 minutes. In vitamin D-deficient chicks, calcium enters the enterocytes but is trapped in the region just below the microvilli. Treating vitamin D-deficient chicks with 1,25D relieves the barrier to transcellular calcium movement [58].

The biological effects of 1,25D on absorption depend on transcriptional events mediated through the VDR. Children with inactivating mutations in the VDR gene suffer severe rickets. In VDR knockout mice, calcium absorption efficiency is reduced by 70%, causing poor growth, low serum calcium and phosphate, high serum PTH, and severe osteomalacia [59–62]. These observations suggest that the primary role of the VDR in bone metabolism is to maintain calcium absorption efficiency rather than a direct effect on bone cells. Strongly consistent with this hypothesis is that over-expression of VDR throughout the intestinal epithelium using a villin promoter-mediated VDR transgene was sufficient to completely recover the VDR knockout mouse phenotype. Duodenal calcium absorption, serum PTH and calcium, and BMD all returned to normal despite the absence of VDR in all tissues apart from the gut [42].

Some have argued that differences in intestinal VDR expression levels or modifications of functions by common gene polymorphisms may influence intestinal calcium absorption in humans. The loss of basal and vitamin D-responsive calcium absorption during aging [44,63] or after estrogen depletion [64,65] is associated with a reduction in intestinal VDR. Consistent with a role for VDR level in the regulation of intestinal calcium absorption, over-expression of VDR in the Caco-2 intestinal cell line increases 1,25D-regulated transcellular calcium transport [66] while the lower VDR levels seen in mice heterozygous for the VDR knockout allele blunt 1,25D-regulated intestinal calcium absorption efficiency [67].

Despite the number of polymorphisms in the VDR gene, only a few studies have examined their impacts on calcium absorption or the ability to adapt to dietary calcium restrictions. One such VDR gene polymorphism is the Fok I translation start site polymorphism at the transcriptional start site that produces a VDR protein shortened by three amino acids at its N-terminus and has increased transcriptional activity [68]. Two studies reported that individuals homozygous for the F allele have greater calcium absorption efficiency compared to individuals with the f allele [69,70]. Collectively these data support the hypothesis that variations in VDR level or function can influence vitamin D-regulated intestinal calcium absorption.

While it is well established that 1,25D treatment increases the efficiency of intestinal calcium absorption [32,71,72], some have suggested that calcium absorption can also increase when serum 25D levels are elevated beyond 50 nmol/L (20 ng/ml). Heaney et al. [73] reported that calcium absorption increased by 25% after 4 weeks of treatment with 50 µg 25D daily even though serum 1,25D levels did not change. This same group later pooled data from several studies and used the data to argue that increasing serum 25D levels from 50 to 86.5 nmol/L (20 to 36 ng/ml) would increase calcium absorption efficiency in post-menopausal women by 65% [74].

This proposal suggests that the enzyme necessary for the conversion of 25D to 1,25D (CYP27B1) is present in the intestine. This hypothesis is supported by detection of CYP27B1 promoter activity in the jejunum and ileum of transgenic mice expressing a 1.5 kb CYP27B1 promoter–luciferase reporter gene [75] and by detection of CYP27B1 mRNA (by RT-PCR) and protein (by IHC) in the human duodenum [76]. This concept is highly controversial and has been the subject of considerable discussion, particularly in the 2010 IOM report on dietary reference intakes for calcium and vitamin D [3].

Other data do not support this proposal. For example, serum 25D level is not associated with higher calcium absorption efficiency in school age children [77] or in adult black or white women [78]. The efficiency of intestinal calcium absorption does not change between serum 25D levels of 20 to 90 nmol/L (8 to 36 ng/ml) in post-menopausal women [54,79]. Raising serum 25D from 55 to 160 nmol/L (22 to 64 ng/ml) increased calcium absorption efficiency only modestly in women [80]. Thus, the hypothesis that improving vitamin D status beyond the level necessary for adequate renal 1,25D production can improve intestinal calcium absorption is not strongly supported by the literature.

2.3.3 MOLECULAR MODELS OF CALCIUM ABSORPTION

Several models have been proposed to explain intestinal calcium absorption. In this section we review each of these models with an emphasis on relating them to physiological data defining calcium absorption. These models are represented in Figures 2.3 and 2.4.

The facilitated diffusion model was developed based on a critical assessment of transport data from isolated brush border membrane vesicles, isolated basolateral membrane vesicles, and a variety of whole intestine transport methods in rats and chicks [81]. This model describes calcium absorption as a vitamin D-regulated process whereby uptake of calcium across the brush border membrane occurs through the apical membrane calcium channel, transient receptor potential cation channel vanilloid family member 6 (TRPV6 also known as CaT1 or ECAC2) [82]. Transcellular movement through enterocytes is mediated by the calcium binding

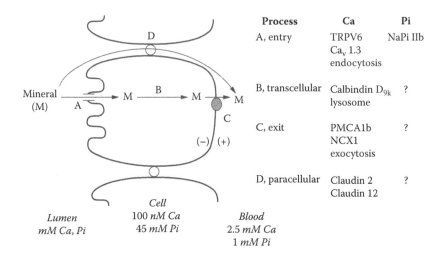

Process	Ca	Pi
A, entry	TRPV6	NaPi IIb
	Ca_v 1.3	
	endocytosis	
B, transcellular	Calbindin D_{9k}	?
	lysosome	
C, exit	PMCA1b	?
	NCX1	
	exocytosis	
D, paracellular	Claudin 2	?
	Claudin 12	

Mineral (M)

Cell
100 nM Ca
45 mM Pi

Lumen
mM Ca, Pi

Blood
2.5 mM Ca
1 mM Pi

FIGURE 2.4 Models for intestinal calcium and phosphate absorption. A general model for mineral movement across the epithelial barrier is shown with options for critical steps in the process identified. The table shows various players proposed to mediate these critical steps for calcium and phosphate.

protein calbindin D (D_{9k} in mammals, D_{28k} in chicks) [83]; and finally, energy-dependent extrusion of calcium occurs through the plasma membrane Ca ATPase, PMCA1b [84,85].

A number of studies support this model. First, the TRPV6 gene is regulated by 1,25D and its induction precedes the increase in duodenal calcium absorption [72]. In addition, TRPV6 mRNA level is reduced by 90% in the duodenum of VDR knockout mice with low intestinal calcium absorption [59,60].

Second, calbindin D protein levels directly correlate with calcium absorption over a wide range of conditions [81] and are sensitive to vitamin D status and 1,25D injections, suggesting that the calbindin D_{9k} and D_{28k} genes are vitamin D target genes [83]. In addition, disruption of calcium binding to calbindin D_{9k} with theophylline inhibits intestinal calcium absorption [86]. These data suggest that calbindins directly participate in calcium transport by acting as a ferry that permits calcium to move from the apical membrane to the basolateral membrane [57,87].

Third, extrusion of calcium from cells is energy dependent, is blocked by the ATPase inhibitor trifluoroperizine (TFP) [31], and is mediated by PMCA1b. This basolateral protein, expressed throughout the intestine, is reduced by vitamin D deficiency, and increased by vitamin D repletion or by consumption of a low calcium diet [84,85]. Some have suggested that basolateral calcium extrusion is also mediated by a sodium–calcium exchanger. However, sodium–potassium pump inhibitors that disrupt the sodium gradient necessary for sodium–calcium exchange do not reduce calcium transport across duodenal segments [31].

Recent evidence from animal models has challenged the facilitated diffusion model. For example, in TRPV6 knockout mice, intestinal calcium absorption can be increased by 1,25D [88,89] and by feeding a low calcium diet [89], strongly suggesting another vitamin D-dependent transport system separate from TRPV6. On the other hand, we recently showed that intestine-specific transgenic expression of TRPV6 dramatically increases intestinal calcium absorption which is sufficient to recover the phenotype of disrupted calcium metabolism seen in VDR knockout mice [90]. Thus, while there may be compensation by other calcium channels for the loss of TRPV6 in knockout mice, TRPV6 appears to be a bona fide mediator of intestinal calcium uptake by the brush border during absorption.

The role of calbindin D as a transcellular ferry in calcium absorption has also been challenged by several studies. While 1,25D increases calbindin D_{28k} or calbindin D_{9k} in the intestine, these increased protein levels *follow* the stimulation of calcium absorption. Calbindin D protein levels remain elevated even after calcium absorption returns to normal [72,91]. Also, neither basal nor 1,25D-induced calcium absorption is reduced in two different lines of calbindin D_{9k} knockout mice [89,92]. However, although mice with either calbindin D_{9k} or TRPV6 gene knockout mouse lines have normal duodenal calcium absorption after 1,25D treatment, the ability of the double calbindin D_{9k}/TRPV6 knockout mouse line to increase calcium absorption in response to 1,25D is reduced by 60% compared to wild type mice [89]. This result suggests that the TRPV6 and calbindin D_{9k} proteins together likely play a special role in calcium absorption and that their interaction is more complex than the current iteration of the facilitated diffusion model predicts.

Consistent with this idea, calbindin D_{9k} mRNA and protein levels are elevated in VDR knockout mice with intestine specific transgenic expression of TRPV6 [90]. This suggests that the increase in calbindin D_{9k} is a response to increased transcellular calcium flux and that it buffers the increased in intracellular calcium that accompanies the absorptive process [93].

An alternative mechanism to explain transcellular intestinal calcium absorption is the sequestration of calcium into vesicles within cells. Several groups reported that 1,25D treatment increased the number of intestinal lysosomes [94] and the release of lysosomal enzymes from enterocytes [95], suggesting that vitamin D increases the activity and cycling of lysosomes. Others have shown that calcium initially associates with endosomes in the brush border membranes of enterocytes and then accumulates in lysosomes after 1,25D treatment [96–98]. Consistent with an essential role for lysosomes in intestinal calcium absorption, disrupting lysosomal pH with agents such as quinacrine or chloroquine prevents lysosomal calcium accumulation and blocks calcium absorption [97] through a mechanism that is independent of ATP-mediated calcium extrusion [99]. Collectively these data suggest that vesicular movement may be a legitimate pathway for uptake and movement of calcium through the intestinal epithelial cells. What is unclear, however, is the mechanism by which the vesicular transport pathway is specific for calcium.

The facilitated diffusion and lysosomal models for vitamin D-mediated calcium absorption both require hours of adaptation for the effects of 1,25D to be observed. In contrast, calcium transport can occur within minutes of exposing the basolateral membranes of enterocytes to 1,25D. This rapid transport is called transcaltachia. It has been directly demonstrated only in the perfused chick duodenum where exposure to a physiologic dose of 1,25D increased calcium appearance in the serosal perfusate by 40% within 14 minutes of exposure [100]. In addition, transcaltachia occurs only in response to serosal 1,25D exposure and it is lost in vitamin D deficiency. This suggests that in absorptive epithelial cells there are membrane receptors on the basolateral surfaces whose levels or downstream components are dependent on the vitamin D-regulated activation of proteins. The exact mechanism by which calcium flows through cells during transcaltachia has not been determined with certainty, but these observations are consistent with the use of a vesicular transport model [101].

One candidate for mediating the rapid membrane-initiated actions of 1,25D is the membrane associated rapid response steroid (MARRS) binding protein. The MARRS gene knockout is embryonic lethal in mice [102] but intestine-specific MARRS knockout mice have been developed and are viable [103]. Unlike intestine-specific VDR knockout mice that have severely disrupted calcium metabolism and osteomalacia [104], no abnormal growth or bone phenotype has been reported for the intestine-specific MARRS knockout mice [103]. However, while 1,25D treatment increases calcium uptake and protein kinase A activity in normal mouse enterocytes, those isolated from intestine-specific MARRS knockout mice do not respond to 1,25D [103].

Nemere et al. [105] recently reported that calcium absorption was reduced by 20% in intestine-specific MARRS knockout mice. However, this report did not examine whether the MARRS deletion reduces bone mass and impairs vitamin D-mediated calcium absorption nor has it been demonstrated that the rapid fluxes in serum 1,25D needed for transcaltachia have been ablated. Because of these gaps in knowledge, transcaltachia has not gained full acceptance as a physiologically important mode for regulating intestinal calcium absorption.

Although most research on intestinal calcium absorption focuses on vitamin D-regulated saturable calcium transport, several studies have shown that vitamin D signaling increases diffusional, presumably paracellular, fluxes across the intestine, particularly in the jejunum and ileum [29,106,107]. These studies suggest that 1,25D induces changes in the charge selectivity of the tight junction, similar to the selectivity seen for renal magnesium and calcium uptake through the tight junction protein paracellin 1 (claudin 16) [108]. The tight junction proteins claudin 2 and claudin 12 are significantly induced by 1,25D in Caco-2 cells. Their mRNA levels fall dramatically in the jejunum of VDR knockout mice, and siRNA against these claudins reduces calcium permeability in Caco-2 cell monolayers [109]. This is a novel calcium absorption mechanism and must be further tested prior to its acceptance. Current barriers to acceptance of this hypothesis are that claudin 2 and 12 expressions are highest in the ileum [110] but are essentially absent from the duodenum where 1,25D regulates the saturable (but not diffusional) component of calcium absorption [32]. Furthermore, claudin 2 expression is highest in the undifferentiated crypt cells of the small intestine [111] whereas calcium absorption is a feature of the differentiated cells on the villi.

2.3.4   Evidence for Regulation of Calcium Absorption by Other Hormones

While most research on the regulation of calcium absorption has focused on vitamin D, other hormones have been examined as well, but to a lesser degree. Several hormones exert indirect effects on calcium absorption through their effects on the regulation of vitamin D metabolism; others may act directly on the intestine. This section provides a brief overview of the evidence linking other hormones or physiologic states, directly or indirectly, to intestinal calcium absorption.

2.3.4.1 Pregnancy and Lactation

Significant extra demands are placed on maternal calcium metabolism by fetal skeletal development during the third trimester of pregnancy and by increased calcium secretion during lactation. Maternal calcium requirements increase significantly during these periods. Serum 1,25D levels and intestinal calcium absorption are both elevated during late pregnancy [112], due in part to extrarenal, PTH-independent 1,25D production by the placenta [113]. Still, the impact of pregnancy on calcium absorption appears to have a vitamin D-independent component [114–117]. The increase in calcium absorption during pregnancy is accompanied by a greater than 10-fold increase in TRPV6 mRNA levels in both pregnant wild-type and VDR null mice [117,118]. However, the pregnancy-related factor regulating this vitamin D-independent increase in calcium absorption and TRPV6 mRNA remains unknown.

Calcium absorption is up-regulated during lactation in rodents but not in humans [119]. As during pregnancy, vitamin D-deficient rats are capable of up-regulating intestinal absorption during lactation [115,116,120]. Evidence indicates that prolactin is the factor regulating calcium absorption during lactation. Prolactin injections to vitamin D-deficient male rats increased calcium absorption 30%, leading to a significant increase in serum calcium levels [121]. The mechanism for this regulation is unclear but may include up-regulation of duodenal calbindin D_{9k} and TRPV6 mRNA levels [122].

In addition, prolactin can stimulate 1,25D production [123]. Prolactin may also stimulate calcium absorption through an L-type calcium channel in the distal jejunum and ileum. Morgan et al. [124] first observed that glucose increases intestinal calcium absorption in rat jejunum by depolarizing enterocytes. This mechanism was inconsistent with a role for TRPV6, a protein that works best under the hyperpolarizing conditions of the duodenum, but was consistent with a role for the L-type calcium channel Ca_v 1.3. Others later showed that prolactin-regulated calcium transport across Caco-2 monolayers was inhibited by L-type calcium channel inhibitors and by siRNA against Ca_v 1.3 [125,126]. Collectively, these data suggest that prolactin is capable of producing both direct and indirect effects to increase intestinal calcium absorption.

2.3.4.2 Growth Hormone and IGF-1

Growth hormone (GH) and its physiologic mediator known as insulin-like growth factor I (IGF-1) fill major roles in linear bone growth and accrual of bone mass [127–129] and may also promote intestinal calcium absorption. Some studies suggest that this effect is mediated through activation of renal CYP27B1 and the elevation of serum 1,25D levels [130]. However, GH treatment significantly increases intestinal calcium absorption and duodenal calbindin D_{9k} levels in aged rats without significantly increasing serum 1,25D levels [131].

GH treatment also prevents the loss of total intestinal VDR that occurs in ovariectomized rats [132], suggesting that GH increases cell sensitivity to 1,25D by regulating tissue VDR levels. The effect of GH on calcium absorption is most likely mediated through IGF-1 and evidence shows that this effect is independent of vitamin D signaling [60,133]. The vitamin D-independent mechanism by which the GH/IGF-1 axis regulates intestinal calcium absorption is unknown at this time.

2.3.4.3 Glucocorticoids

It is well established that glucocorticoid treatment induces bone loss and increases the risk of osteoporosis [134]. In addition, Hahn et al. [135] showed that a 14-day course of prednisone reduced calcium absorption by 31% but without a significant reduction in serum 1,25D levels. Morris et al. [136] later showed that the association between serum 1,25D and calcium absorption was blunted following corticosteroid treatment, suggesting the existence of glucocorticoid-induced intestinal resistance to vitamin D action. However, glucocorticoid treatment does not have a specific regulatory effect on VDR expression in rats [137].

The effect of glucocorticoids on calcium absorption is likely due to a non-specific effect of the hormone on intestinal "leakiness"; cortisone treatments increased bidirectional fluid movement in rat small intestine [138]. As a result, while 1,25D treatment increased mucosal-to-serosal calcium movement equally in control and cortisone-treated rat intestines, it did not reverse the increased serosal-to-mucosal calcium flux induced by cortisone, with the result that vitamin D-mediated effects on net calcium transport were reduced [139,140].

2.3.4.4 PTH, FGF23, and Thyroid Hormone

Dietary calcium deprivation increases serum PTH levels and therefore high PTH is associated with increased calcium absorption during periods of low dietary calcium intake. The effect of PTH on calcium absorption is indirect and mediated through the ability of PTH to increase serum 1,25D levels by way of induction of renal CYP27B1 expression and suppression of CYP24 expression [141,142].

Some have argued that PTH may also directly regulate intestinal calcium absorption. The PTH receptor 1 is expressed at low levels in rat intestinal epithelial cells [143] while PTH treatment activates calcium uptake through calcium channels in isolated rat enterocytes [95,144] and induces transcaltachia in isolated duodenal loops from chicks [145]. However, serum PTH levels vary significantly throughout the course of a day and we have no evidence that calcium absorption efficiency follows a similar daily rhythm.

Furthermore, in clinical states of secondary hyperparathyroidism with reduced 1,25D production such as chronic renal failure and vitamin D deficiency, calcium absorption is severely impaired despite great increases in PTH secretion, suggesting PTH alone is insufficient to regulate calcium absorption. Similarly, FGF23 may indirectly influence calcium absorption by influencing renal 1,25D production. FGF23 is a phosphatonin that controls phosphate metabolism (see below) in part by suppressing renal CYP27B1 expression and 1,25D production [146,147]. The FGF23-mediated suppression of serum 1,25D should strongly suppress intestinal calcium absorption; however, no studies have been performed to formally test this hypothesis. Several early reports showed that hypothyroidism increased [148] and hyperthyroidism reduced [149] intestinal calcium absorption. This is an indirect effect of thyroid hormones mediated by transcriptional regulation of CYP27B1 gene expression [150] that alters serum 1,25D levels [151].

2.3.4.5 Estrogen

Estrogen loss has many effects on calcium balance in post-menopausal women including reducing calcium absorption and increasing urinary calcium loss [152,153]. Despite the claim that estrogen loss reduces serum 1,25D levels in post-menopausal women [154], ovariectomy did not reduce serum 1,25D levels in rats [155]. Other data suggest that estrogen alters the intestinal responsiveness to 1,25D. In support of this concept, Gennari et al. [64] found that oophorectomy reduced 1,25D-induced intestinal calcium absorption in young women and that this effect could be reversed by estrogen repletion.

Several studies suggest that the loss of intestinal vitamin D responsiveness in the absence of estrogen is due to reduced VDR levels [65,132,156], although this hypothesis is not universally accepted [157]. Because functional estrogen receptors (ERs) have been detected in rat small intestinal cells [158], it is plausible that estrogen may directly regulate intestinal calcium absorption. Consistent with this hypothesis, intestinal calcium absorption in rats can be increased with estradiol benzoate treatment, and can be blocked by the ICI 182780 pure ER antagonist [159].

Duodenal expression of TRPV6 is increased by estradiol treatment in ovariectomized rats, reduced 55% in ERα-null mice, and increased by estradiol treatment even in CYP27B1- or VDR-null mice. This suggests that the intestinal effects of estrogen are vitamin D-independent [122,160]. However, no current evidence indicates that ERα directly stimulates TRPV6 transcription by binding to the TRPV6 promoter.

2.3.4.6 Androgens

Loss of androgens in men reduces BMD [161,162] by disrupting osteoblast function [163] but little is known about the impact of testosterone on calcium absorption or vitamin D metabolism. In prepubertal boys, testosterone therapy increased intestinal calcium absorption by 61% [164] but this was accompanied by higher serum IGF-1 levels associated with increased intestinal calcium absorption.

As men age, calcium absorption decreases and is associated with a decline in serum levels of dehydroepiandrosterone sulfate (DHEAS)—the sulfated form of the DHEA testosterone prohormone [165]. However, the change in calcium absorption was independent of changes in serum 1,25D, suggesting that the effects of androgens on calcium absorption were independent of vitamin D metabolism. This report is consistent with the observation that serum vitamin D metabolite levels are unaltered by changes in testosterone that accompany puberty [166].

2.3.5 CONCLUSIONS ABOUT INTESTINAL CALCIUM ABSORPTION

Optimizing calcium intake and the efficiency of intestinal calcium absorption are critical for growth of the fetal skeleton, for attaining peak bone mass during childhood and adolescence, for maintaining adult bone mass, and for reducing bone loss after menopause and as a result of aging. The primary regulator of intestinal calcium absorption is the vitamin D metabolite 1,25D acting through the VDR in enterocytes to regulate gene expression.

This 1,25D-VDR complex mediates transcriptional regulation, leading to increased levels of one or more transporters that mediate saturable, transcellular calcium transport from the gut lumen to blood. Because serum 1,25D levels are elevated by habitually low dietary calcium intake and low dietary calcium intake is common in the general population, the saturable, vitamin D-regulated component of intestinal calcium absorption plays a major role in maintaining the efficiency of calcium absorption in most individuals.

Neither local gut production of 1,25D as a result of high serum 25OHD levels nor rapid signaling mechanisms through enterocyte membrane VDR or the MARRS protein are strongly supported as physiologically relevant mechanisms for intestinal calcium absorption. Other hormones, particularly those involved with pregnancy, lactation and growth, may also influence calcium absorption efficiency directly while several hormones also affect calcium absorption indirectly by regulating renal production of 1,25D and/or intestinal VDR levels.

The exact mechanisms by which calcium is transported across the enterocyte remain unknown. Each model we used to explain calcium transport (i.e., facilitated diffusion, vesicular transport, transcaltachia, regulated paracellular movement) presents gaps in knowledge that must be resolved through additional research.

2.4 INTESTINAL PHOSPHATE ABSORPTION

Phosphorus in the diet is categorized as inorganic and organic. The latter type is less readily absorbed because of the need to digest the element to phosphate before absorption. In developed societies, dietary phosphate follows protein consumption and is always sufficient except in very special groups such as premature babies. Indeed the clinical problem is excess dietary phosphate intake.

Phosphate absorption is highly efficient, with 60 to 70% of an intestinal load absorbed from a typical diet. Clinically, phosphate absorption is a major concern in chronic kidney disease, where serum phosphate increases as renal excretion becomes progressively impaired and accompanying disruption of the serum phosphate hormonal regulators, FGF23 and PTH occurs [167]. Under these conditions, phosphate binders are used to limit phosphate bioavailability for absorption and reduce the serum phosphate concentration [168].

Rats [169,170] and humans [171] efficiently absorb phosphate from the jejunum and duodenum; in mice, the highest efficiency of absorption is in the ileum [172,173] (Figure 2.3). As with calcium, phosphate transport occurs through both saturable and non-saturable pathways [171,174] (Figure 2.2). However, unlike calcium, at dietary phosphate levels typical for a Western diet, the active component of transport is saturated and the bulk of phosphate absorption is via the non-saturable, paracellular route. While whole body calcium homeostasis is controlled by both the efficiency of calcium absorption and renal excretion, phosphate metabolism is controlled largely through renal phosphate excretion. Nonetheless, phosphate absorption is regulated and understanding the underlying mechanisms is essential for managing mineral nutrition and various diseases.

2.4.1 Sodium Dependence and Mediation of Intestinal Phosphate Absorption via Na Phosphate IIb Transporter

Eto et al. [175] estimated that more than 50% of intestinal phosphate transport in the rat jejunum is sodium-dependent and is therefore dependent on the sodium gradient established by the sodium–potassium ATPase. While the rat jejunum contains many phosphate transporters (Pit1, Pit2, BNPi, and NaPi IIb) [176], studies using knock-out mouse models show that 90% of sodium-dependent and 50% of total phosphate transport is mediated by the transporter NaPi IIb (gene name: SLC34A2) [177]; see Figures 2.3 and 2.4.

NaPi IIb is part of a family of membrane-spanning sodium-dependent phosphate transporters that includes the renal phosphate transporters NaPi IIa and IIc [178]. NaPi IIb is a glycoprotein located on the apical brush border membranes of epithelial cells in the intestine whose Na phosphate-co-transport is electrogenic ($3 Na^+:1 PO^{4-}$) [179]. Consistent with the importance of NaPi IIb in phosphate absorption, NaPi IIb mRNA levels fall as rats mature and this is reflected by a 70% decline in phosphate uptake into jejunal brush border membrane vesicles [179].

The regulation of intestinal phosphate uptake is mediated in part by interaction of the PDZ domain protein NHERF1 with the C-terminus of NaPi IIb; this may control the stability or apical localization of the transporter [180]. This redistribution occurs when phosphate status is high and the need to absorb phosphate from the diet is reduced. In contrast to the apical membrane uptake of phosphate, the mechanisms mediating the intracellular movement and basolateral export of phosphate from intestinal cells are not known. However, since the internal concentration of phosphate is high relative to the serum level (Figure 2.4), movement across the basolateral membrane is likely down this chemical gradient through a specialized channel.

2.4.2 Major Physiologic Regulator of Intestinal Phosphate Absorption: Habitual Dietary Phosphate Intake

Habitual dietary phosphate intake directly influences phosphate absorption efficiency [174,176]. In pig jejunum, the rate of phosphate transport is 90% higher when dietary phosphorus is reduced by 40% [181]. However, the strength of this adaptation may be limited to certain segments of the intestine and this varies with species. In rats, 7 days of dietary phosphate restriction increased phosphate transport in jejunal brush border membrane vesicles but not duodenal brush border membrane vesicles [173]. In mice, dietary phosphate restriction had a greater effect on phosphate transport in ileum brush border membrane vesicles compared to those from the jejunum [170]. The adaptation of intestinal phosphate transport due to changes in dietary phosphate is accompanied by alterations in NaPi IIb mRNA and protein levels [170, 173]. However, the mechanism for diet-induced regulation of phosphate transport and NaPi IIb levels is unclear.

Because dietary phosphate restriction increases renal CYP27B1 expression and serum 1,25D levels [182] it has been assumed that phosphate transport is largely regulated by 1,25D. It has long been known that vitamin D deficiency reduces the efficiency of intestinal phosphate absorption [183] and that vitamin D repletion or

1,25D treatment restores phosphate absorption to normal [169, 184-187]. Davis et al. [171] showed that 1,25D increases jejunal phosphate absorption in subjects with chronic renal failure, a condition in which low serum 1,25D is present. The effect of 1,25D treatment in these patients and in vitamin D-deficient rats is on the saturable component of phosphate transport [171,176] and due to increased levels of NaPi IIb protein in the brush border membrane [172].

However, while these data suggest that 1,25D is a direct regulator of NaPi IIb gene expression and phosphate absorption, other data do not support such a straight-forward interpretation. For example, a classical VDR response element has not been identified in the NaPi IIb promoter [179]. The ability of 1,25D to increase NaPi IIb mRNA is present in 2-week old mice with immature intestines but is lost in 12-week old mice [179]. Also, while intestinal phosphate transport in brush border membrane vesicles is reduced by 30 to 70% in VDR knockout mice, it is accompanied by a reduction in NaPi IIb protein but not mRNA [188,189].

This suggests that the VDR acts through post-transcriptional effects on either new protein production from existing message or through the redistribution of existing protein to the apical membrane. Surprisingly, dietary phosphate restriction can also increase intestinal phosphate absorption even in vitamin D deficient, VDR knockout, and CYP27B1 null mice [189, 190] suggesting that a component of the regulation of phosphate absorption by dietary phosphate restriction is vitamin D independent.

Evidence indicates that 1,25D rapidly (within minutes) stimulates phosphate uptake into perfused chick intestines and isolated enterocytes of chicks and mice [191,192]. The rapid effect of 1,25D on phosphate uptake is lost upon treatment of chick enterocytes with a ribozyme against MARRS and in enterocytes from mice with intestine-specific MARRS knockouts [192,193]. In chick enterocytes, the actions of 1,25D on phosphate uptake depend on activation of protein kinase C while protein kinase A is involved in the mouse intestine [192,194]. However, the action of 1,25D through MARRS on phosphate uptake has not been linked to the NaPi IIb phosphate transporter or any other transporter. In addition, rapid fluxes of 1,25D in the circulation or locally have not been reported. As a result, the physiologic relevance of rapid phosphate transport remains unclear.

Dietary phosphate also affects the secretion of a set of molecules referred to collectively as phosphatonins. They are regulators of renal phosphate reabsorption and include matrix extracellular phosphoglycoprotein (MEPE), secreted frizzled-related protein 4 (sFRP-4), dentin matrix protein 1 (DMP1), fibroblast growth factor 7 (FGF7), and the most studied phosphatonin called fibroblast growth factor 23 (FGF23) [195]. As discussed in Chapter 6, FGF23 and other phosphatonins inhibit renal phosphate reabsorption and their serum levels are directly related to dietary phosphate intake and serum phosphate levels [196,197]. However, their role in the regulation of intestinal phosphate absorption is less clear.

FGF23 binds to FGF receptors 1c, 3c, and 4 and requires the klotho co-receptor to signal through FGF receptors [198,199]. Although the receptors for FGF23 (R1c, R3c, and R4) are present in the intestine, the klotho co-receptor is not [200]. As a result, although injections of FGF23 and MEPE inhibit intestinal phosphate absorption in mice [201,202], the lack of klotho expression in the intestine suggests that FGF23 works indirectly on the intestine to alter phosphate absorption.

This is consistent with the fact that FGF23 regulates serum 1,25D levels by suppressing renal CYP27B1 activity and expression [146,147]. Furthermore FGF23-mediated suppression of jejunal phosphate absorption is lost in VDR-null mice [202]. Thus, low dietary phosphate increases intestinal phosphate transport efficiency through increased serum 1,25D by direct stimulation of renal CYP27B1 activity and by releasing the FGF23-mediated inhibition of renal CYP27B1 expression.

2.4.3 REGULATION OF INTESTINAL PHOSPHATE ABSORPTION: CONCLUSIONS

High dietary phosphate intake is common and the efficiency of phosphate absorption is generally over 60%. Thus, intestinal phosphate absorption is less important for maintaining phosphate balance than calcium absorption is for maintaining calcium balance. Nevertheless, phosphate absorption efficiency is inversely related to habitual dietary intake, demonstrating that the regulation of phosphate absorption is an important mechanism in controlling phosphate metabolism.

It is clear under normal conditions that the saturable portion of intestinal phosphate absorption depends upon adequate vitamin D status. However, the mechanism for regulation by 1,25D is unclear. The central pathway in phosphate absorption is the apical membrane sodium–phosphate co-transporter NaPi IIb. However, while 1,25D changes the level of the NaPi IIb protein at the membrane, it does not strongly regulate the NaPi IIb gene; if it does so at all, regulation appears indirect, through a still unidentified factor.

More importantly, the body has the ability to adapt to low phosphate diets even in the absence of VDR or CYP27B1. This suggests that a major regulator of phosphate absorption is vitamin D-independent and that critical regulators of intestinal phosphate absorption are yet to be discovered. While phosphatonins are essential regulators of renal phosphate excretion, their role in the intestine is less clear but the likely candidate is their ability to modulate renal vitamin D metabolism.

ACKNOWLEDGMENTS

This work was supported by National Institutes of Health Award DK054111 to JCF.

REFERENCES

1. Fleet JC. 2006. Molecular regulation of calcium metabolism. In Weaver, CM and RP Heaney, Eds., *Calcium in Human Health.* Humana Press: Totowa, NJ. pp. 163–190.
2. Holick MF. 2003. Vitamin D: A millenium perspective. *J Cell Biochem* 88: 296–307.
3. Ross AC et al. 2011. The 2011 report on dietary reference intakes for calcium and vitamin D from the Institute of Medicine: what clinicians need to know. *J Clin Endocrinol Metabol* 96: 53–58.
4. Sitrin M et al. 1978. Vitamin D deficiency and bone disease in gastrointestinal disorders. *Arch Intern Med* 138: 886–888.
5. Schachter D et al. 1964. Metabolism of vitamin D. I. Preparation of radioactive vitamin D and its intestinal absorption in the rat. *J Clin Invest* 43: 787–796.
6. Sitrin MD et al. 1982. Comparison of vitamin D and 25-hydroxyvitamin D absorption in the rat. *Am J Physiol* 242: G326–G332.

7. Watkins DW et al. 1985. Alterations in calcium, magnesium, iron, and zinc metabolism by dietary cholestyramine. *Digest Dis Sci* 30: 477–482.

8. Maislos M et al. 1981. Intestinal absorption of vitamin D sterols: differential absorption into lymph and portal blood in the rat. *Gastroenterology* 80: 1528–1534.

9. Dueland S et al. 1983. Absorption, distribution, and transport of vitamin D3 and 25-hydroxyvitamin D3 in the rat. *Am J Physiol* 245: E463–E467.

10. Hollander D. 1981. Intestinal absorption of vitamins A, E, D, and K. *J Lab Clin Med* 97: 449–462.

11. Krawitt EL and Chastenay BF. 1980. The 25-hydroxy vitamin D absorption test in patients with gastrointestinal disorders. *Calcif Tiss Intl* 32: 183–187.

12. Khamiseh G et al. 1991. Vitamin D absorption, plasma concentration and urinary excretion of 25-hydroxyvitamin D in nephrotic syndrome. *Proc Soc Exp Biol Med* 196: 210–213.

13. Brouwer DA et al. 1998. Rat adipose tissue rapidly accumulates and slowly releases an orally administered high vitamin D dose. *Br J Nutr* 79: 527–532.

14. Smith JE and Goodman DS. 1971. The turnover and transport of vitamin D and of a polar metabolite with the properties of 25-hydroxycholecalciferol in human plasma. *J Clin Invest* 50: 2159–2167.

15. Christakos S et al. 2010. Vitamin D: metabolism. *Endocrinol Metabol Clin North Am* 39: 243–253.

16. Vieth R and Fraser D. 1979. Kinetic behavior of 25-hydroxyvitamin D-1-hydroxylase and –24-hydroxylase in rat kidney mitochondria. *J Biol Chem* 254: 12455-12460.

17. Davies M et al. 1980. Comparative absorption of vitamin D3 and 25-hydroxyvitamin D3 in intestinal disease. *Gut* 21: 287–292.

18. White P and Cooke N. 2000. The multifunctional properties and characteristics of vitamin D-binding protein. *Trends Endocrinol Metabol* 11: 320–327.

19. Safadi FF, et al. 1999. Ostopathy and resistance to vitamin D toxicity in mice null for vitamin D binding protein. *J Clin Invest* 103: 239–251.

20. Leheste JR, et al. 2003. Hypocalcemia and osteopathy in mice with kidney-specific megalin gene defect. *FASEB J* 17: 247–249.

21. Haddad JG, Jr. and Rojanasathit S. 1976. Acute administration of 25-hydroxycholecalciferol in man. *J Clin Endocrinol Metabol* 42: 284–290.

22. Rosen CJ et al. 2012. IOM committee members respond to Endocrine Society vitamin D guideline. *J Clin Endocrinol Metabol* 97: 1146–1152.

23. Farach-Carson MC and Nemere I. 2003. Membrane receptors for vitamin D steroid hormones: potential new drug targets. *Curr Drug Targets* 4: 67–76.

24. Nemere I et al. 2004. Identification and characterization of 1,25D(3)-membrane-associated rapid response, steroid (1,25D(3)-MARRS) binding protein. *J Steroid Biochem Mol Biol* 89–90: 281–285.

25. Heaney RP and Skillman TG. 1964. Secretion and excretion of calcium by the human gastrointestinal tract. *J Lab Clin Med* 64: 29–41.

26. Heaney RP. 2003. Quantifying human calcium absorption using pharmacokinetic methods. *J Nutr* 133: 1224–1226.

27. Heaney RP et al. 1975. Calcium absorption as a function of calcium intake. *J Lab Clin Med* 85: 881–890.

28. Pansu D et al. 1981. Effect of Ca intake on saturable and nonsaturable components of duodenal Ca transport. *Am J Physiol* 240: 32–37.

29. Sheikh MS et al. 1990. In vivo intestinal absorption of calcium in humans. *Miner Electrolyte Metabol* 16: 130–146.

30. Giuliano AR and Wood RJ. 1991. Vitamin D-regulated calcium transport in Caco-2 cells: unique in vitro model. *Am J Physiol* 260: G207–G212.

31. Favus MJ et al. 1983. Effects of trifluoperazine, ouabain, and ethacrynic acid on intestinal calcium. *Am J Physiol* 244: G111–G115.
32. Pansu D et al. 1983. Duodenal and ileal calcium absorption in the rat and effects of vitamin D. *Am J Physiol* 244: G695–G700.
33. Favus MJ et al. 1981. Kinetic characteristics of calcium absorption and secretion by rat colon. *Am J Physiol* 240: G350–G354.
34. Grinstead WC et al. 1984. Effect of 1,25-dihydroxyvitamin D3 on calcium absorption in the colons of healthy humans. *Am J Physiol* 247: G189–G192.
35. Karbach U and Feldmeier H. 1993. The cecum is the site with the highest calcium absorption in rat intestine. *Dig Dis Sci* 38: 1815–1824.
36. Fordtran JS and Locklear TW. 1966. Ionic constituents and osmolality of gastric and small intestinal fluids after eating. *Am J Dig Dis* 11: 503–521.
37. Marcus CS and Lengemann FW. 1962. Absorption of Ca 45 and Sr 85 from solid and liquid food at various levels of the alimentary tract of the rat. *J Nutr* 77: 155–160.
38. Duflos C et al. 1995. Calcium solubility, intestinal sojourn time, and paracellular permeability codetermine passive calcium absorption in rats. *J Nutr* 125: 2348–2355.
39. Norman DA et al. 1981. Jejunal and ileal adaptation to alterations in dietary calcium: changes in calcium and magnesium absorption and pathogenetic role of parathyroid hormone and 1,25-dihydroxyvitamin D. *J Clin Invest* 67: 1599–1603.
40. Dawson-Hughes B et al. 1988. Effect of lowering dietary calcium intake on fractional whole body calcium retention. *J Clin Endocrinol Metabol* 67: 62–68.
41. Favus MJ et al. 1974. Effects of dietary calcium restriction and chronic thyroparathyroidectomy on the metabolism of (3H)25-hydroxyvitamin D3 and the active transport of calcium by rat intestine. *J Clin Invest* 53: 1139–1148.
42. Xue Y and Fleet JC. 2009. Intestinal vitamin D receptor is required for normal calcium and bone metabolism in mice. *Gastroenterology* 136: 1317–1312.
43. Alevizaki CC et al. 1973. Progressive decrease of true intestinal calcium absorption with age in normal man. *J Nucl Med* 14: 760–762.
44. Bullamore JR et al. 1970. Effect of age on calcium absorption. *Lancet* 2: 535–537.
45. Kinyamu HK et al. 1997. Serum vitamin D metabolites and calcium absorption in normal young and elderly free-living women and in women living in nursing homes. *Am J Clin Nutr* 66: 454.
46. Need AG et al. 2004. The effects of age and other variables on serum parathyroid hormone in postmenopausal women attending an osteoporosis center. *J Clin Endocrinol Metabol* 89: 1646–1649.
47. Wood RJ et al. 1998. Intestinal calcium absorption in the aged rat: evidence of intestinal resistance to 1,25(OH)$_2$ vitamin D. *Endocrinology* 139: 3843–3848.
48. Agnusdei D et al. 1998. Age-related decline of bone mass and intestinal calcium absorption in normal males. *Calcif Tiss Intl* 63: 197–201.
49. Nordin BE et al. 2004. Radiocalcium absorption is reduced in post-menopausal women with vertebral and most types of peripheral fractures. *Osteoporosis Intl* 15: 27–31.
50. Ensrud KE et al. 2000. Low fractional calcium absorption increases the risk for hip fracture in women with low calcium intake. *Ann Intern Med* 132: 345–353.
51. Nicolaysen R. 1937. Studies upon the mode of action of vitamin D. III: influence of vitamin D on the absorption of calcium and phosphorus in the rat. *Biochem J* 37: 122–129.
52. Gershoff SN and Hegsted DM. 1956. Effect of vitamin D and Ca:P ratios on chick gastrointestinal tract. *Am J Physiol* 187: 203–206.
53. Sheikh MS et al. 1988. Role of vitamin D-dependent and vitamin D-independent mechanisms in absorption of food calcium. *J Clin Invest* 81: 126–132.
54. Need AG and Nordin BE. 2008. Misconceptions: vitamin D insufficiency causes malabsorption of calcium. *Bone* 42: 1021–1024.

55. Kruse K. 1995. Pathophysiology of calcium metabolism in children with vitamin D deficiency rickets. *J Pediatr* 126: 736–741.

56. Markestad T et al. 1984. Plasma concentrations of vitamin D metabolites before and during treatment of vitamin D deficiency rickets in children. *Acta Paediatr Scand* 73: 225–231.

57. Chandra S et al. 1990. Ion microscopic imaging of calcium transport in the intestinal tissue of vitamin D-deficient and vitamin D-replete chickens: a 44Ca stable isotope study. *Proc Natl Acad Sci USA* 87: 5715–5719.

58. Fullmer CS et al. 1996. Ion microscopic imaging of calcium during 1,25 dihydroxyvitamin D-mediated intestinal absorption. *Histochem Cell Biol* 106: 215–222.

59. Van Cromphaut SJ et al. 2001. Duodenal calcium absorption in vitamin D receptor knockout mice: functional and molecular aspects. *Proc Natl Acad Sci USA* 98: 13324–13329.

60. Song Y et al. 2003. Vitamin D receptor (VDR) knockout mice reveal VDR-independent regulation of intestinal calcium absorption and ECaC2 and calbindin D9k mRNA. *J Nutr* 133: 374–380.

61. Haussler MR and Norman AW. 1969. Chromosomal receptor for a vitamin D metabolite. *Proc Natl Acad Sci USA* 62: 155–162.

62. Haussler MR et al. 1998. The nuclear vitamin D receptor: biological and molecular regulatory properties revealed. *J Bone Miner Res* 13: 325–349.

63. Nordin BE et al. 2004. Effect of age on calcium absorption in postmenopausal women. *Am J Clin Nutr* 80: 998–1002.

64. Gennari C et al. 1990. Estrogen preserves a normal intestinal responsiveness to 1,25-dihydroxyvitamin D3 in oophorectomized women. *J Clin Endocrinol Metabol* 71: 1288–1293.

65. Liel Y et al. 1999. Estrogen increases 1,25-dihydroxyvitamin D receptors expression and bioresponse in the rat duodenal mucosa. *Endocrinology* 140: 280–285.

66. Shao A et al. 2001. Increased vitamin D receptor level enhances 1,25-dihydroxyvitamin D3-mediated gene expression and calcium transport in Caco-2 cells. *J Bone Miner Res* 16: 615–624.

67. Song Y and Fleet JC. 2007. Intestinal resistance to 1,25 dihydroxyvitamin D in mice heterozygous for the vitamin D receptor knockout allele. *Endocrinology* 148: 1396–1402.

68. Jurutka PW et al. 2000. The polymorphic N terminus in human vitamin D receptor isoforms influences transcriptional activity by modulating interaction with transcription factor IIB. *Mol Endocrinol* 14: 401–420.

69. Ames SK et al. 1999. Vitamin D receptor gene Fok1 polymorphism predicts calcium absorption and bone mineral density in children. *J Bone Miner Res* 14: 740–746.

70. Huang ZW et al. 2006. Relationship between the absorption of dietary calcium and the Fok I polymorphism of VDR gene in young women. *Zhong Yu Fang Yi Xue Za Zhi* 40: 75–78.

71. Boyle IT et al. 1971. Regulation by calcium of in vivo synthesis of 1,25-dihydroxycholecalciferol and 21,25-dihydroxycholecalciferol. *Proc Natl Acad Sci USA* 68: 2131–2134.

72. Song Y et al. 2003. Calcium transporter 1 and epithelial calcium channel messenger ribonucleic acid are differentially regulated by 1,25 dihydroxyvitamin D3 in the intestine and kidney of mice. *Endocrinology* 144: 3885–3894.

73. Heaney RP et al. 1997. Calcium absorptive effects of vitamin D and its major metabolites. *J Clin Endocrinol Metabol* 82: 4111–4116.

74. Heaney RP et al. 2003. Calcium absorption varies within the reference range for serum 25-hydroxyvitamin D. *Journal of the American College of Nutrition.* 22: 142–146.

75. Anderson PH et al. 2008. Co-expression of CYP27B1 enzyme with the 1.5-kb CYP27B1 promoter–luciferase transgene in the mouse. *Mol Cell Endocrinol* 285: 1–9.

76. Balesaria S et al. 2009. Human duodenum responses to vitamin D metabolites of TRPV6 and other genes involved in calcium absorption. *Am J Physiol Gastrointest Liver Physiol* 297: G1193–G1197.

77. Abrams SA et al. 2009. Higher serum 25-hydroxyvitamin D levels in school-age children are inconsistently associated with increased calcium absorption. *J Clin Endocrinol Metabol* 94: 2421–2427.

78. Aloia JF et al. 2010. Serum vitamin D metabolites and intestinal calcium absorption efficiency in women. *Am J Clin Nutr* 92: 835–840.

79. Need AG et al. 2008. Vitamin D metabolites and calcium absorption in severe vitamin D deficiency. *J Bone Miner Res* 23: 1859–1863.

80. Hansen KE et al. 2008. Vitamin D insufficiency: disease or no disease? *J Bone Miner Res* 23: 1052–1060.

81. Bronner F et al. 1986. An analysis of intestinal calcium transport across the rat intestine. *Am J Physiol* 250: G561–G569.

82. Peng JB et al. 1999. Molecular cloning and characterization of a channel-like transporter mediated intestinal calcium absorption. *J Biol Chem* 274: 22739–22746.

83. Christakos S et al. 1992. Molecular aspects of the calbindins. *J Nutr* 122: 678–682.

84. Wasserman RH et al. 1992. Vitamin-D and mineral deficiencies increase the plasma membrane calcium pump of chicken intestine. *Gastroenterology* 102: 886–894.

85. Cai Q et al. 1993. Vitamin D and adaptation to dietary calcium and phosphate deficiencies increase intestinal plasma membrane calcium pump gene expression. *Proc Natl Acad Sci USA* 90: 1345–1349.

86. Pansu D et al. 1988. Theophylline inhibits active Ca transport in rat intestine by inhibiting Ca binding by CaBP. *Progr Clin Biol Res* 252: 115–120.

87. Feher JJ et al. 1992. Role of facilitated diffusion of calcium by calbindin in intestinal calcium absorption. *Am J Physiol* 262: C517–C526.

88. Kutuzova GD et al. 2008. TRPV6 is not required for 1-alpha,25-dihydroxyvitamin D3-induced intestinal calcium absorption in vivo. *Proc Natl Acad Sci USA* 105: 19655–19659.

89. Benn BS et al. 2008. Active intestinal calcium transport in the absence of transient receptor potential vanilloid type 6 and calbindin-D9k. *Endocrinology* 149: 3196–3205.

90. Cui M et al. 2012. Villin promoter-mediated transgenic expression of transient receptor potential cation channel, subfamily V, member 6 (TRPV6) increases intestinal calcium absorption in wild-type and vitamin D receptor knockout mice. *J Bone Miner Res* 27: 2097–2107.

91. Spencer R et al. 1978. The relationship between vitamin D-stimulated calcium transport and intestinal calcium-binding protein in the chicken. *Biochem J* 170: 93–101.

92. Akhter S et al. 2007. Calbindin D9k is not required for 1,25-dihydroxyvitamin D3-mediated Ca^{2+} absorption in small intestine. *Arch Biochem Biophys* 460: 227–232.

93. Schroder B et al. 1996. Role of calbindin-D9k in buffering cytosolc free Ca^{2+} ions in pig duodenal enterocytes. *J Physiol* 492: 715–722.

94. Davis WL and Jones RG. 1982. Lysosomal proliferation in rachitic avian intestinal absorptive cells following 1,25-dihydroxycholecalciferol. *Tiss Cell* 14: 585–595.

95. Nemere I and Szego CM. 1981. Early actions of parathyroid hormone and 1,25-dihydroxycholecalciferol on isolated epithelial cells from rat intestine 2. Analyses of additivity, contribution of calcium, and modulatory influence of indomethacin. *Endocrinology* 109: 2180–2187.

96. Warner RR and Coleman JR. 1975. Electron probe analysis of calcium transport by small intestine. *J Cell Biol* 64: 54–74.

97. Nemere I et al. 1986. 1, 25 dihydroxyvitamin D3-mediated intestinal calcium transport: biochemical identification of lysozomes containing calcium and calcium-binding protein (calbindin-D28k). *J Biol Chem* 261: 16106–16114.

98. Nemere I and Norman AW. 1988. 1,25-Dihydroxyvitamin D3-mediated vesicular transport of calcium in intestine: time course studies. *Endocrinology* 122: 2962–2969.

99. Favus MJ et al. 1989. Effects of quinacrine on calcium active transport by rat intestinal epithelium. *Am J Physiol* 257: G818–G822.

100. Nemere I et al. 1984. Calcium transport in perfused duodena from normal chicks: enhancement within 14 minutes of exposure to 1,25 dihydroxyvitamin D3. *Endocrinology* 115: 1476–1483.

101. Nemere I and Norman AW. 1990. Transcaltachia, vesicular calcium transport, and microtubule-associated calbindin-D28K: emerging views of 1,25-dihydroxyvitamin D3-mediated intestinal calcium absorption. *Miner Electrolyte Metabol* 16: 109–114.

102. Garbi N et al. 2006. Impaired assembly of the major histocompatibility complex class I peptide-loading complex in mice deficient in the oxidoreductase ERp57. *Nat Immunol* 7: 93–102.

103. Nemere I et al. 2010. Intestinal cell calcium uptake and the targeted knockout of the 1,25D3-MARRS (membrane-associated, rapid response steroid-binding) receptor/PDIA3/Erp57. *J Biol Chem* 285: 31859–31866.

104. Lieben L et al. 2012. Normocalcemia is maintained in mice under conditions of calcium malabsorption by vitamin D-induced inhibition of bone mineralization. *J Clin Invest* 122: 1803–18015.

105. Nemere I et al. 2012. Role of the 1,25D3-MARRS receptor in the 1,25(OH)2D3-stimulated uptake of calcium and phosphate in intestinal cells. *Steroids* 77: 897–902.

106. Karbach U. 1992. Paracellular calcium transport across the small intestine. *J Nutr* 122: 672–677.

107. Tudpor K et al. 2008. 1,25-dihydroxyvitamin d(3) rapidly stimulates the solvent drag-induced paracellular calcium transport in the duodenum of female rats. *J Physiol Sci* 58: 297–307.

108. Simon DB et al. 1999. Paracellin-1, a renal tight junction protein required for paracellular Mg^{2+} resorption. *Science* 285: 103–106.

109. Fujita H et al. 2008. Tight junction proteins claudin-2 and -12 are critical for vitamin D-dependent Ca^{2+} absorption between enterocytes. *Mol Biol Cell* 19: 1912–1921.

110. Fujita H et al. 2006. Differential expression and subcellular localization of claudin-7, –8, –12, –13, and –15 along the mouse intestine. *J Histochem Cytochem* 54: 933–944.

111. Rahner C et al. 2001. Heterogeneity in expression and subcellular localization of claudins 2, 3, 4, and 5 in the rat liver, pancreas, and gut. *Gastroenterology* 120: 411–422.

112. Ritchie LD et al. 1998. A longitudinal study of calcium homeostasis during human pregnancy and lactation and after resumption of menses. *Am J Clin Nutr* 67: 693–701.

113. Breslau NA and Zerwekh JE. 1986. Relationship of estrogen and pregnancy to calcium homeostasis in pseudohypoparathyroidism. *J Clin Endocrinol Metabol* 62: 45–51.

114. Quan-Sheng D and Miller SC. 1989. Calciotrophic hormone levels and calcium absorption during pregnancy in rats. *Am J Physiol* 257: E118–E123.

115. Halloran BP and DeLuca HF. 1980. Calcium transport in small intestine during pregnancy and lactation. *Am J Physiol* 239: E64–E68.

116. Brommage R et al. 1990. Vitamin D-independent intestinal calcium and phosphorus absorption during reproduction. *Am J Physiol* 259: 631–638.

117. Fudge NJ and Kovacs CS. 2010. Pregnancy up-regulates intestinal calcium absorption and skeletal mineralization independently of the vitamin D receptor. *Endocrinology* 151: 886–895.

118. Van Cromphaut SJ et al. 2003. Intestinal calcium transporter genes are upregulated by estrogens and the reproductive cycle through vitamin D receptor-independent mechanisms. *J Bone Miner Res* 18: 1725–1736.

119. Kent GN et al. 1991. The efficiency of intestinal calcium absorption is increased in late pregnancy but not in established lactation. *Calcif Tiss Intl* 48: 293–295.
120. Boass A et al. 1981. Calcium metabolism during lactation: enhanced intestinal calcium absorption in vitamin D-deprived, hypocalcemic rats. *Endocrinology* 109: 900–907.
121. Pahuja DN and DeLuca HF. 1981. Stimulation of intestinal calcium transport and bone calcium mobilization by prolactin in vitamin-D-deficient rats. *Science* 214: 1038–1039.
122. Bouillon R et al. 2003. Intestinal calcium absorption: molecular vitamin D-mediated mechanisms. *J Cell Biochem* 88: 332–339.
123. Robinson CJ et al. 1982. Role of prolactin in vitamin D metabolism and calcium absorption during lactation in the rat. *J Endocrinol* 94: 443–453.
124. Morgan EL et al. 2007. Apical GLUT2 and Cav1.3: regulation of rat intestinal glucose and calcium absorption. *J Physiol* 580: 593–604.
125. Thongon N et al. 2009. Enhancement of calcium transport in Caco-2 monolayer through PKCzeta-dependent Cav1.3-mediated transcellular and rectifying paracellular pathways by prolactin. *Am J Physiol Cell Physiol* 296: C1373–C1382.
126. Nakkrasae LI et al. 2010. Transepithelial calcium transport in prolactin-exposed intestine-like Caco-2 monolayer after combinatorial knockdown of TRPV5, TRPV6 and Ca(v)1.3. *J Physiol Sci* 60: 9–17.
127. Mora S et al. 1999. Serum levels of insulin-like growth factor I and the density, volume, and cross-sectional area of cortical bone in children. *J Clin Endocrinol Metabol* 84: 2780–2783.
128. Boot AM et al. 1997. Changes in bone mineral density, body composition, and lipid metabolism during growth hormone (GH) treatment in children with GH deficiency. *J Clin Endocrinol Metabol* 82: 2423–2428.
129. Rudman D et al. 1990. Effects of human growth hormone in men over 60 years old. *New Engl J Med* 323: 1–6.
130. Zoidis E et al. 2002. IGF-I and GH stimulate Phex mRNA expression in lungs and bones and 1,25-dihydroxyvitamin D(3) production in hypophysectomized rats. *Eur J Endocrinol* 146: 97–105.
131. Fleet JC et al. 1994. Growth hormone and parathyroid hormone stimulate intestinal calcium absorption in aged female rats. *Endocrinology* 134: 1755–1760.
132. Chen C et al. 1997. Modulation of intestinal vitamin D receptor by ovariectomy, estrogen and growth hormone. *Mech Ageing Dev* 99: 109–122.
133. Fatayerji D et al. 2000. The role of insulin-like growth factor I in age-related changes in calcium homeostasis in men. *J Clin Endocrinol Metabol* 85: 4657–4662.
134. Weinstein RS. 2012. Glucocorticoid-induced osteoporosis and osteonecrosis. *Endocrinol Metabol Clin North Am* 41: 595–611.
135. Hahn TJ et al. 1981. Effects off short term glucocorticoid administration on intestinal calcium absorption and circulating vitamin D metabolite concentrations in man. *J Clin Endocrinol Metabol* 52: 111–115.
136. Morris HA et al. 1990. Malabsorption of calcium in corticosteroid-induced osteoporosis. *Calcif Tiss Intl* 46: 305–308.
137. Lee S et al. 1991. Effect of glucocorticoids and 1,25-dihydroxyvitamin D3 on the developmental expression of the rat intestinal vitamin D receptor gene. *Endocrinology* 129: 396–401.
138. Yeh JK and Aloia JF. 1986. Influence of glucocorticoids on calcium absorption in different segments of the rat intestine. *Calcif Tiss Intl* 38: 282–288.
139. Favus MJ et al. 1973. Effects of 1,25-dihydroxycholecalciferol on intestinal calcium transport in cortisone-treated rats. *J Clin Invest* 52: 1680–1685.
140. Yeh JK and Aloia JF. 1984. Effect of hypophysectomy and 1,25-dihydroxyvitamin D on duodenal calcium absorption. *Endocrinology* 114: 1711–1717.

141. Zierold C et al. 2003. Regulation of 25-hydroxyvitamin D3-24-hydroxylase mRNA by 1,25-dihydroxyvitamin D3 and parathyroid hormone. *J Cell Biochem* 88: 234–237.
142. Armbrecht HJ et al. 2003. Hormonal regulation of 25-hydroxyvitamin D3-1-alpha-hydroxylase and 24- hydroxylase gene transcription in opossum kidney cells. *Arch Biochem Biophys* 409: 298–304.
143. Gentili C et al. 2003. Characterization of PTH/PTHrP receptor in rat duodenum: effects of ageing. *J Cell Biochem* 88: 1157–1167.
144. Picotto G et al. 1997. Parathyroid hormone stimulates calcium influx and the cAMP messenger system in rat enterocytes. *Am J Physiol Cell Physiol* 42: C1349–C1353.
145. Nemere I and Norman AW. 1986. Parathyroid hormone stimulates calcium transport in perfused duodena from normal chicks: comparison with the rapid (transcaltachic) effect of 1,25-dihydroxyvitamin D3. *Endocrinology* 119: 1406–1408.
146. Shimada T et al. 2001. Cloning and characterization of FGF23 as a causative factor of tumor-induced osteomalacia. *Proc Natl Acad Sci USA* 98: 6500–6505.
147. Perwad F et al. 2007. Fibroblast growth factor 23 impairs phosphorus and vitamin D metabolism in vivo and suppresses 25-hydroxyvitamin D-1alpha-hydroxylase expression in vitro. *Am J Physiol Renal Physiol* 293: F1577–F1583.
148. Lekkerkerker JF et al. 1971. Enhancement of calcium absorption in hypothyroidism: observations with a new method measuring calcium absorption. *Isr J Med Sci* 7: 399–400.
149. Haldimann B et al. 1980. Intestinal calcium absorption in patients with hyperthyroidism. *J Clin Endocrinol Metabol* 51: 995–997.
150. Kozai M et al. 2013. Thyroid hormones decrease plasma 1-alpha,25-dihydroxyvitamin D levels through transcriptional repression of the renal 25-hydroxyvitamin D3 1-alpha-hydroxylase gene (CYP27B1). *Endocrinology* 154: 609–622.
151. Bouillon R et al. 1980. Influence of thyroid function on the serum concentration of 1,25-dihydroxyvitamin D3. *J Clin Endocrinol Metabol* 51: 793–797.
152. Heaney RP et al. 1978. Menopausal changes in calcium balance performance. *J Lab Clin Med* 92: 953–963.
153. Riggs BL et al. 2002. Sex steroids and the construction and conservation of the adult skeleton. *Endocr Rev* 23: 279–302.
154. Gallagher JC et al. 1980. Effect of estrogen on calcium absorption and serum vitamin D metabolites in postmenopausal osteoporosis. *J Clin Endocrinol Metabol* 51: 1359–1364.
155. Pavlovitch H et al. 1980. Lack of effect on ovariectomy on the metabolism of vitamin D and intestinal calcium-binding protein in female rats. *J Endocrinol* 86: 419–424.
156. Arjmandi BH et al. 1994. In vivo effect of 17a-estradiol on intestinal calcium absorption in rats. *Bone Miner* 26: 181–189.
157. Colin EM et al. 1999. Evidence for involvement of 17-beta-estradiol in intestinal calcium absorption independent of 1,25-dihydroxyvitamin D3 level in the rat. *J Bone Miner Res* 14: 57–64.
158. Thomas ML et al. 1993. The presence of functional estrogen receptors in intestinal epithelial cells. *Endocrinology* 132: 426–430.
159. Ten Bolscher M et al. 1999. Estrogen regulation of intestinal calcium absorption in the intact and ovariectomized adult rat. *J Bone Miner Res* 14: 1197–1202.
160. van Abel M et al. 2003. Regulation of the epithelial Ca^{2+} channels in small intestine as studied by quantitative mRNA detection. *Am J Physiol Gastroint Liver Physiol* 285: G78–G85.
161. Orwoll ES and Klein RF. 1995. Osteoporosis in men. *Endocr Rev* 16: 87–116.
162. Finkelstein JS et al. 1996. A longitudinal evaluation of bone mineral density in adult men with histories of delayed puberty. *J Clin Endocrinol Metabol* 81: 1152–1155.
163. Colvard DS et al. 1989. Identification of androgen receptors in normal human osteoblast-like cells. *Proc Natl Acad Sci USA* 86: 854–857.

164. Mauras N et al. 1994. Calcium and protein kinetics in prepubertal boys: positive effects of testosterone. *J Clin Invest* 93: 1014–1019.
165. Chen RY et al. 2008. Relationship between calcium absorption and plasma dehydroepiandrosterone sulphate (DHEAS) in healthy males. *Clin Endocrinol* 69: 864–869.
166. Krabbe S et al. 1986. Serum levels of vitamin D metabolites and testosterone in male puberty. *J Clin Endocrinol Metabol* 62: 503–507.
167. Wahl P and Wolf M. 2012. FGF23 in chronic kidney disease. *Adv Exp Med Biol* 728: 107–125.
168. Navaneethan SD et al. 2011. Phosphate binders for preventing and treating bone disease in chronic kidney disease patients. *Cochrane Database Syst Rev* Feb 16: CD006023.
169. Harrison HE and Harrison HC. 1961. Intestinal transport of phosphate: action of vitamin D, calcium, and potassium. *Am J Physiol* 201: 1007–1012.
170. Giral H et al. 2009. Regulation of rat intestinal Na-dependent phosphate transporters by dietary phosphate. *Am J Physiol Renal Physiol* 297: F1466–F1475.
171. Davis GR et al. 1983. Absorption of phosphate in the jejunum of patients with chronic renal failure before and after correction of vitamin D deficiency. *Gastroenterology* 85: 908–916.
172. Marks J et al. 2006. Intestinal phosphate absorption and the effect of vitamin D: a comparison of rats with mice. *Exp Physiol* 91: 531–537.
173. Radanovic T et al. 2005. Regulation of intestinal phosphate transport I. Segmental expression and adaptation to low P(i) diet of the type IIb Na(+)–P(i) cotransporter in mouse small intestine. *Am J Physiol Gastrointest Liver Physiol* 288: G496–G500.
174. Rizzoli R et al. 1977. Role of 1,25-dihydroxyvitamin D3 on intestinal phosphate absorption in rats with a normal vitamin D supply. *J Clin Invest* 60: 639–647.
175. Eto N et al. 2006. NaPi-mediated transcellular permeation is the dominant route in intestinal inorganic phosphate absorption in rats. *Drug Metabol Pharmacokinet* 21: 217–221.
176. Katai K et al. 1999. Regulation of intestinal Na+-dependent phosphate co-transporters by a low-phosphate diet and 1,25-dihydroxyvitamin D3. *Biochem J* 343: 705–712.
177. Sabbagh Y et al. 2009. Intestinal npt2b plays a major role in phosphate absorption and homeostasis. *J Am Soc Nephrol* 20: 2348–2358.
178. Murer H et al. 2004. The sodium phosphate cotransporter family SLC34. *Pflugers Arch* 447: 763–767.
179. Xu H et al. 2002. Age-dependent regulation of rat intestinal type IIb sodium-phosphate cotransporter by 1,25-(OH)(2) vitamin D(3). *Am J Physiol Cell Physiol* 282: C487–C493.
180. Giral H et al. 2012. NHE3 regulatory factor 1 (NHERF1) modulates intestinal sodium-dependent phosphate transporter (NaPi-2b) expression in apical microvilli. *J Biol Chem* 287: 35047–35056.
181. Saddoris KL et al. 2010. Sodium-dependent phosphate uptake in the jejunum is post-transcriptionally regulated in pigs fed a low-phosphorus diet and is independent of dietary calcium concentration. *J Nutr* 140: 731–736.
182. Yoshida T et al. 2001. Dietary phosphorus deprivation induces 25-hydroxyvitamin D(3) 1-alpha-hydroxylase gene expression. *Endocrinology* 142: 1720–1726.
183. Bauer W and Marble A. 1932. Studies on the mode of action of irradiated ergosterol II. Effect on the calcium and phosphorus metabolism of individuals with calcium deficiency diseases. *J Clin Invest* 11: 21–35.
184. Carlsson A. 1954. The effect of vitamin D on the absorption of inorganic phosphate. *Acta Physiol Scand* 31: 301–307.
185. Tanaka Y and DeLuca HF. 1974. Role of 1,25-dihydroxyvitamin D3 in maintaining serum phosphorus and curing rickets. *Proc Natl Acad Sci USA* 71: 1040–1044.
186. Chen TC et al. 1974. Role of vitamin D metabolites in phosphate transport of rat intestine. *J Nutr* 104: 1056–1060.

187. Rizzoli R et al. 1977. Role of 1,25-dihydroxyvitamin D3 (1,25-(OH)2D3) on intestinal inorganic phosphate (Pi) absorption in rats with normal vitamin D supply. *Calcif Tiss Res* 22: 561–562.

188. Segawa H et al. 2004. Intestinal Na-P(i) cotransporter adaptation to dietary P(i) content in vitamin D receptor null mice. *Am J Physiol Renal Physiol* 287: F39–F47.

189. Capuano P et al. 2005. Intestinal and renal adaptation to a low-Pi diet of type II NaPi cotransporters in vitamin D receptor- and 1-alpha-OHase-deficient mice. *Am J Physiol Cell Physiol* 288: C429–C434.

190. Lee DB et al. 1986. Intestinal phosphate absorption: influence of vitamin D and non-vitamin D factors. *Am J Physiol* 250: G369–G373.

191. Nemere I. 1996. Apparent nonnuclear regulation of intestinal phosphate transport: effects of 1,25-dihydroxyvitamin D3,24,25-dihydroxyvitamin D3, and 25-hydroxyvitamin D3. *Endocrinology* 137: 2254–2261.

192. Nemere I et al. 2012. Intestinal cell phosphate uptake and the targeted knockout of the 1,25D(3)-MARRS receptor/PDIA3/ERp57. *Endocrinology* 153: 1609–1615.

193. Nemere I et al. 2004. Ribozyme knockdown functionally links a 1,25(OH)2D3 membrane binding protein (1,25D3-MARRS) and phosphate uptake in intestinal cells. *Proc Natl Acad Sci USA* 101: 7392–7397.

194. Tunsophon S and Nemere I. 2010. Protein kinase C isotypes in signal transduction for the 1,25D3-MARRS receptor (ERp57/PDIA3) in steroid hormone-stimulated phosphate uptake. *Steroids* 75: 307–313.

195. Marks J et al. 2010. Phosphate homeostasis and the renal-gastrointestinal axis. *Am J Physiol Renal Physiol* 299: F285–F296.

196. Ferrari SL et al. 2005. Fibroblast growth factor-23 relationship to dietary phosphate and renal phosphate handling in healthy young men. *J Clin Endocrinol Metabol* 90: 1519–1524.

197. Perwad F et al. 2005. Dietary and serum phosphorus regulate fibroblast growth factor 23 expression and 1,25-dihydroxyvitamin D metabolism in mice. *Endocrinology* 146: 5358–5364.

198. Razzaque MS. 2009. The FGF23-Klotho axis: endocrine regulation of phosphate homeostasis. *Nat Rev Endocrinol* 5: 611–619.

199. Bergwitz C and Juppner H. 2009. Disorders of phosphate homeostasis and tissue mineralisation. *Endocr Dev* 16: 133–156.

200. Khuituan P et al. 2012. Fibroblast growth factor-23 abolishes 1,25-dihydroxyvitamin D(3)-enhanced duodenal calcium transport in male mice. *Am J Physiol Endocrinol Metabol* 302: E903–E913.

201. Marks J et al. 2008. Matrix extracellular phosphoglycoprotein inhibits phosphate transport. *J Am Soc Nephrol* 19: 2313–2320.

202. Miyamoto K et al. 2005. Inhibition of intestinal sodium-dependent inorganic phosphate transport by fibroblast growth factor 23. *Ther Aphor Dial* 9: 331–335.

3 Plasma and Extracellular Fluid Calcium Homeostasis in Relation to Metabolic Bone Disease: Role of Kidneys

Richard L. Prince

CONTENTS

3.1   INTRODUCTION

This chapter addresses the physiological processes by which the skeletal system contributes to maintenance of extracellular calcium homeostasis through a dual role as both the recipient of calcium ions to maintain skeletal function and the source of calcium ions. These processes can either consolidate or reduce bone mineral status. The chapter will review (1) the mechanisms that control calcium flow into and out of the extracellular fluid; (2) how these systems are regulated to protect the extracellular fluid from excessive changes in calcium concentration; (3) the role of the kidneys in this regulation; (4) how the kidneys can protect from and also cause bone disease and how such outcomes may be managed.

Extracellular calcium homeostasis and its regulation were first studied at the turn of the 20th century, a time when the concepts of homeostasis and hormonal regulation were still under development. Calcium homeostasis remains a complex and important component of human health. Indeed, in the past 10 years, we have seen an explosion of new knowledge in this area that needs to be integrated into a functional holistic concept to allow scientists and clinicians to solve the new challenges of the 21st century.

It is also important to identify what this chapter will not include, namely the role of calcium ions in intracellular processes except to the extent that transcellular transport involves the intracellular compartment. Thus, calcium and its many roles in cell division, apoptosis, and regulation of cell function via intracellular calcium sensors will not be covered. For a review of these topics, see Reference [1]. This chapter will also not discuss the role of calcium transport among cells by way of gap junctions [2].

3.1.1 Extracellular Calcium Homeostasis

The functional mechanisms by which extracellular ionized calcium fills its diverse roles are characterized by the concept of homeostasis. This concept, first described by Claude Bernard in the 1860s, is encapsulated in the famous aphorism, "La fixité du milieu intérieur est la condition d'une vie libre et indépendante (the constancy of the internal environment is the condition for a free and independent life). This concept became central to the field of physiology through the work of Walter Cannon who developed the *homeostasis* term in 1926. In recent years, the concept expanded from organs to cells and is now called cell physiology. This new dimension encapsulates regulation of transmembrane calcium transport handled via a variety of ion transporters and pumps that are the functional components of the physiological regulation of organs and their cellular constituents. These concepts are explained in this chapter.

3.1.2 Cellular Function

In the short term, the constancy of extracellular calcium concentration is important for many cellular processes but is particularly vital for nerve and muscle action as it is the source for conducting the action potential along nerves and for the coupling of excitation and contraction in striated and cardiac muscle.

3.1.3 Bone

It is important to emphasize the two functions of calcium in the skeleton. The first is biomechanical—aiding locomotion by providing a rigid scaffold for muscle function. The second is physiological—acting as a reservoir for calcium to defend the extracellular calcium concentration during times of dietary calcium deficit. The tension between the requirements of maintaining both extracellular calcium concentration and bone structure sets the scene for the importance of calcium homeostasis in the prevention and treatment of many metabolic bone diseases. The critical concept of cell physiology is that extracellular calcium concentration is kept constant from minute to minute by regulation of the flow of calcium into and out of tissues and other body compartments.

3.2 OVERVIEW OF ORGAN LEVEL REGULATION OF CALCIUM HOMEOSTASIS

At tissue level, the principal organs involved in extracellular calcium homeostasis are bone, intestine, kidney and, to a lesser extent, skin. These structures are the sites of the principal flow of calcium into and out of the extracellular spaces (Figure 3.1). Calcium is continually cycling in and out of the bloodstream to bathe these organs. In the kidneys, 98% of the calcium filtered at the glomeruli is reabsorbed, approximating 150 mmol/d. In bone, 5 to 10 mmol/d of calcium cycles into and out of the skeleton. Calcium in the bowel is secreted into the lumen as part of the secretion from the

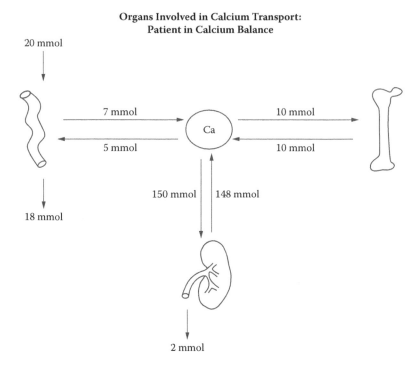

FIGURE 3.1 Overview of calcium transport to and from organs controlling extracellular calcium homeostasis.

exocrine pancreas, bile, and intestinal enterocytes at a rate of about 4 mmol/d. Food contributes about 20 mmol/d of calcium to the intestine and approximately 7 mmol of calcium is absorbed and reabsorbed in the gut daily.

Thus, calcium is in a state of continuous flux into and out of the organs involved in extracellular calcium homeostasis. Calcium also continually moves into and out of all the cells of the body. Thus, the critical issue in the control of this system is to regulate the relative transport activity of the various organs and cells to maintain a constant internal cellular calcium environment.

3.3   OVERVIEW OF CELL LEVEL REGULATION OF EXTRACELLULAR CALCIUM HOMEOSTASIS

Knowledge of the cell physiology of calcium transport is helpful for understanding the physiology and pathology of calcium metabolism. Two principal mechanisms are involved: transcellular and tight junction paracellular calcium transport. These calcium transport mechanisms are present in many tissues but specifically exist in the intestines, kidneys, and bones—the principal organs defending extracellular calcium. The similarities and differences among the calcium transport mechanisms in these tissues allow some generalizations in this complex area. The physiological

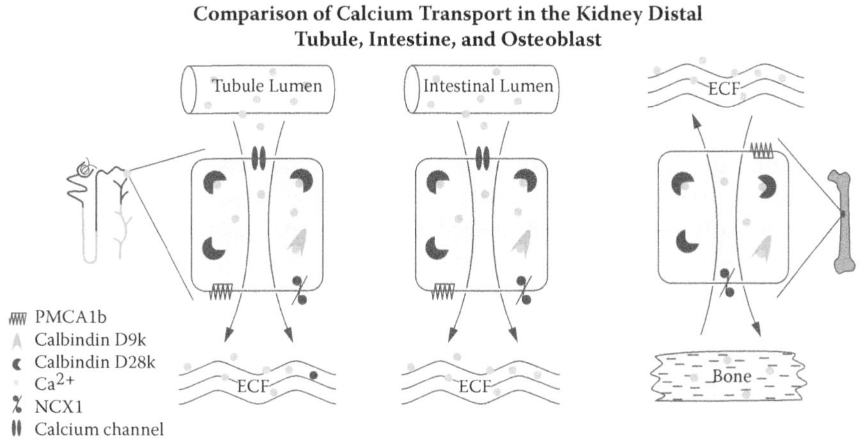

FIGURE 3.2 Overview of calcium transport proteins in three organs regulating extracellular calcium homeostasis.

basis of these particular mechanisms is meeting the changing needs of the whole organism in order to competently adapt to periods of calcium deprivation.

Paracellular transport of calcium via tight junctions plays a major role in calcium transport in many tissues. Nine isoforms of the claudin protein class involved in this autoregulation have been identified to date [3]. The transcellular transport of calcium is similar in the intestine, kidney and, to a lesser extent, in bone. It involves three cellular components that combine to provide an integrated regulated system for calcium transport into the extracellular compartment and thus subserve calcium homeostasis (Figure 3.2). A basic knowledge of these systems facilitates understanding of the pathophysiology of metabolic bone disease.

Calcium enters a cell across the apical plasma membrane mediated through discrete calcium channels [4] characterized at the gene, mRNA, and protein levels as transient receptor potential vallenoid channels 5 (TRPV5) [5] and TRPV6 [6]. Subsequently, two intracellular calcium binding (calbindin) proteins act to expedite transcellular calcium movement and prompt delivery to the opposing basolateral membrane [7]. Finally, calcium efflux at the basolateral membrane occurs via two transport mechanisms of plasma membrane calcium ATPase (PMCA). PMCA1 and PMCA4 are relevant to homeostatic calcium transport [8]. The sodium/calcium Na^{1}/Ca^{2+} exchanger (NCX) of which NCX1 and NCX2 are components also contributes to homeostatic calcium transport [9].

3.3.1 CLAUDINS

The claudins constitute a group of proteins that play integral parts in paracellular calcium transport as part of the structures called tight junctions. As noted previously, these proteins are important components of ion transport in epithelial membranes of many tissues. In the kidney, they have been identified in the thick ascending limb of the loop of Henle that is a major site of regulated calcium reabsorption. At this site, claudins 14, 16, and 19 are thought to be expressed [10].

3.3.2 TRANSIENT RECEPTOR POTENTIAL (TRP) CATION CHANNELS

These epithelial calcium channels are now classified as members of the Trp family found on chromosome 7. The two members are TrpV5 (previously named ECaC1) and TrpV6 (previously known as ECaC2). TrpV5 is a 729-amino acid protein localized to the apical membranes of enterocytes and distal renal tubule cells [5]. TrpV6 is a 727-amino acid protein [6]. They both consist of six transmembrane domains with the putative calcium transport region occurring between transmembrane domains 5 and 6.

Both combine in tetramers to facilitate calcium transport and both bind calbindins and possibly calmodulin [11]. TrpV5 in rats is expressed at higher concentration in the kidneys while TrpV6 is more highly expressed in the intestines. Evidence indicates that co-expression occurs in the same cell and that both may co-expressed in the same calcium channel structure [12].

3.3.3 CALBINDINS

Calbindin-D_{28K} is a 28-kD cytoplasmic protein of approximately 261 amino acid residues. It is a member of the EF-hand loop helix proteins that bind calcium with high affinity. Each molecule has six high affinity calcium binding sites although only four are active [13]. The distribution of calbindin-D_{28K} is widespread in mammalian tissues. In addition to expression in classical transport tissues, including the distal convoluted tubule and collecting ducts of the kidneys, the intestinal enterocytes in some species, and the osteoblasts, calbindin-D_{28K} expression has also been found in neurons, pancreatic islet cells, and testes.

Calbindin-D_{9K} is another member of the high affinity calcium binding proteins containing two EF-hand structures. It has little sequence homology with calbindin-D_{28K} and consists of about 79 amino acid residues with two high affinity calcium binding sites [13]. The tissue distribution of calbindin-D_{9K} is similar to that of calbindin-D_{28K} except that D_{9K} is more highly expressed in the intestines.

Both calcium transporters exist within the cytosols of epithelial cells lining the distal kidney tubules [14]. While hypercalciuria develops in calbindin D_{28K} knockout mice, circulating serum calcium levels are maintained because both D_{28K} and D_{9K} play roles in renal calcium transport [15]. Chronic metabolic acidosis has also been noted to increase calbindin D_{28K} expression in rat kidney distal tubules [16].

3.3.4 PLASMA MEMBRANE CALCIUM ATPASES

At least four different genes code for the calcium efflux pump (PMCA1 through PMCA4) and post-transcriptional modification of each gene transcript produces distinct and uniquely different isoforms that create a great diversity of functional consequences [17,18]. PMCAs are members of the P-type ATPase family; they are calmodulin-dependent and form phosphorylated intermediates. Calmodulin affinity chromatography was the first method utilized to separate and purify a

PMCA [18]. A PMCA consists of a single 130- to 140-kD polypeptide chain with some 75% amino acid homology between each isoform. The homologous amino acid residues are restricted to several highly conserved regions within the protein [19]. The site of ATP binding and the site of phosphorylation represent two of these highly conserved regions.

PMCA is expressed on the basolateral membranes of the kidney distal tubules in conjunction with NCX [14,20]. The availability of isogene-specific antibodies to PMCA confirmed results of earlier immunohistochemical studies with the detection of PMCA1 and PMCA4 (but not PMCA2 and PMCA3) isogenes in human kidneys using polyclonal antibodies specific for each of the four isogenes [21]. This finding was verified using crude microsomal preparations from human kidney and monoclonal antibodies to PMCA1, PMCA4a, and PMCA4b [22].

3.3.5 Sodium–Calcium Exchanger (NCX)

The NCX [9] has three isoforms. It is a secondary active transport protein that uses the electrochemical gradient produced by sodium ATPase activity to move large amounts of calcium across basolateral membranes [23]. Only NCX1 has been identified in kidney and intestine tissues although other NCXs are abundant in other tissues that handle large fluxes of calcium across their membranes such as contractile and neuronal cells and the regulation of calcium transport across bone cells.

NCX1 is localized to the basolateral membranes of avian osteoblasts [24,25] and its inhibition has been shown to impair mineralization of bone formed by cultured primary osteoblasts, suggesting an important role for this protein in the mineralization process [25]. It is a 970-amino acid protein with a primary structure that contains 11 transmembrane spanning regions and a large cytoplasmic loop between transmembrane segments 6 and 7. The orientation of NCX is determined by the predominance of two inwardly directed electrochemical gradients generated by plasma membrane sodium and calcium pumps. NCX1 is expressed on the basolateral membranes of kidney distal tubules [20,26,27]. Stimulation of the Na^+-H^+ antiporter in the distal kidney tubules by calbindin D_{28K} reduces intracellular sodium and may consequently increase calcium transport, highlighting one mechanism that may explain how calbindin D_{28K} may influence NCX1 activity in these cells [28].

3.4 OVERVIEW OF HORMONAL REGULATION OF CALCIUM FLOWS BETWEEN ORGANS

Three organs (intestine, kidney, and bone) are involved intimately in extracellular calcium regulation. Clearly, endocrine hormonal regulation plays a leading role in coordinating their responses to calcium excesses or deficiencies. In this system, calcium acts as an agonist for the calcium sensing receptor (CaSR) expressed in the parathyroid glands, kidney, and bone. CaSRs are found on the surfaces of parathyroid cells, along both the apical (luminal) and basolateral (capillary) surfaces of the renal proximal tubules, and on the surfaces of mature osteoclasts [29] as discussed in the following sections and in Chapter 4.

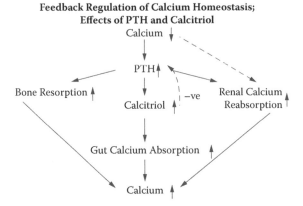

FIGURE 3.3 Mechanisms by which PTH and calcitriol regulate extracellular calcium homeostasis.

These organs, especially the parathyroid gland, provide an additional signal to the kidney and bone to correct calcium fluxes. Calcium ions act as short loop regulators of their own concentrations to initiate actions of the more sophisticated hormonal systems of parathyroid hormone (PTH) and calcitriol (1,25-dihydroxyvitamin D) that play major roles in regulating extracellular calcium concentrations (Figure 3.3). These hormones respond to the many physiological stresses under which plasma calcium homeostasis must be maintained. For example if dietary calcium intake is reduced, the coordinated action of PTH and calcitriol increases absorption of calcium from the bowel, urine, and bone compartments to correct the extracellular deficit [30].

This regulatory system includes feedback regulation between PTH and calcitriol and coordinated action in the kidney and bone (and not in the intestine). To this paradigm must be added another set of circulating regulatory factors that also affect bone structure and function: the estrogen, progesterone, and androgen gonadal hormones.

It is best to consider these hormones primarily as regulators of calcium balance. As discussed earlier, bone is the principal site of calcium storage and thus whole body calcium balance. Gonadal hormones may be considered conservators of the skeletal stores of calcium because deficiency causes losses of the stores. To maintain the skeletal stores, the movements of calcium across intestinal and renal epithelia are regulated directly by gonadal hormones. If this co-regulation, which is capable of increasing bone calcium stores, is not coordinated, variation may occur in extracellular calcium concentrations activating the PTH–calcitriol system to maintain plasma calcium homeostasis. In this way, the dual requirements of calcium as a critical component of the skeletal system and a regulator of intracellular function are seamlessly linked.

The next regulatory factor to be integrated into this overview is fibroblast growth factor 23 (FGF23)–klotho system considered a part of the phosphatonin system that regulates extracellular phosphate homeostasis [31]. Variations in phosphate metabolism and concentration may affect extracellular calcium metabolism via a variety of mechanisms, one of which is the extracellular calcium–phosphate product. This calculated variable has been shown to be of clinical interest only related to the very high phosphate levels encountered in renal failure.

3.4.1 PARATHYROID HORMONE (PTH)

PTH is regulated by the concentration of calcium in the extracellular fluid via a G protein-linked calcium receptor in the membranes of parathyroid hormone cells. This calcium sensing receptor (CaSR) is discussed in detail in Chapter 5. It plays the lead sensing and activation role in correcting plasma calcium deficits [32] and participates in feedback regulation by calcitriol to inhibit PTH production under certain circumstances. PTH corrects low extracellular calcium concentrations by increasing calcium inflow into extracellular spaces directly from calcium excreted into the renal tubules and calcium stored in the skeleton. It is also an important regulator of calcitriol formation in the kidneys that plays a major role in increasing intestinal calcium absorption from the diet. The coordinated increase in calcium influx corrects extracellular calcium concentrations, causing a reduction in PTH secretion and a reduction in the relative fluxes from the three separate compartments in the intestine, kidney, and bone.

3.4.2 CALCITRIOL

Calcitriol is the biologically active metabolite of the vitamin D as described in Chapter 7. The simplest concept that integrates these regulators is that calcitriol with PTH is a major defender of extracellular calcium concentrations to prevent hypocalcemia. Calcitriol directly regulates plasma calcium levels via the renal CaSR, which is critical in patients with hypoparathyroidism. Extracellular phosphate also regulates renal calcitriol production. The recent elucidation of the FGF23–klotho system adds a further level of sophistication to our understanding but does not alter the fundamental paradigm outlined above.

3.4.3 CALCITONIN

Calcitonin secretion (discussed in Chapter 8) is up-regulated in hypercalcemia, which stimulates renal excretion of calcium and inhibits bone resorption. It is interesting that a total thyroidectomy in a human, which removes the primary source of circulating calcitonin, does not appear to produce a demonstrable effect on calcium homeostasis.

3.4.4 GONADAL HORMONES

Some evidence demonstrates the effects of the principal gonadal hormones on bone and calcium homeostasis. Estrogen has been the most studied and therefore will be the focus of this section. Estrogen deficiency plays a central role in the development of post-menopausal osteoporosis and also in male hypogonadism-induced osteoporosis. However, it is not usually considered to be involved in extracellular calcium homeostasis. Indeed, the effects of estrogen deficiency on extracellular calcium are so subtle that the events should be compared to the activities of a "thief in the night" (1 Thessalonians 5:20).

Estrogen exerts direct actions on calcium handling by the intestine, kidney, and bone. However, with estrogen deficiency, only occasionally is a measurable change in plasma calcium concentration detected–a somewhat crude measure of physiological disturbance. Under these circumstances, the rate of flux of calcium into and out of the bone, kidney tubules, and bowel lumen can determine circulating concentrations of PTH and calcitriol indirectly [33]. If calcium fluxes are considered measures of physiological effects, estrogen carries far more importance for human disease than PTH and calcitriol since estrogen deficiency is the primary cause of increased bone loss after menopause and exacerbates low peak bone mass and age-related bone loss.

It is argued by many that the loss of the beneficial effects of estrogen on renal calcium reabsorption and intestinal calcium absorption plays a major role in the pathogenesis of post-menopausal osteoporosis [34]. Estrogen deficiency appears to be involved in the release of calcium from specific skeletal sites, particularly those with trabecular bone. It is possible that the physiological basis of estrogen deficiency and skeletal calcium mobilization relates to the supply of calcium for lactation [35,36].

3.4.5 Fibroblast Growth Factor 23 (FGF23) and Klotho Protein

The FGF23 hormone is formed by osteocytes and acts on the kidneys to promote phosphate loss in the urine and reduced intestinal phosphate absorption by impairing renal calcitriol synthesis as discussed in detail in Chapter 6. These effects are to an extent mediated by the klotho membrane protein synthesized in distal tubules [31] although we now have evidence of a circulating form of klotho.

This system is usually considered separately from those involved in extracellular calcium regulation as currently the main evidence is for regulation of extracellular phosphate [37]. The reason for its inclusion in this section on the hormonal control of calcium flow is to alert readers to the close interrelation between the calcium and phosphate regulatory systems such that alterations in the levels of one ion may indirectly modulate the levels of the other.

3.5 PHYSIOLOGY OF REGULATION OF CALCIUM TRANSPORT IN NEPHRON

It is clear that the kidney is a vital organ for regulating extracellular calcium in humans, but the exact mechanisms by which regulation occurs have proved difficult to characterize, possibly because of the complexities of the interacting systems. It has been essential to undertake work in non-primate species, particularly in genetically modified mouse lines. In view of species differences, comparison to human kidney physiology is difficult. Also the nutritional and hormonal factors in experimental situations are not always specified in animal experiments and this makes extrapolation difficult.

Developing a coherent overview of the complex hormonal, nutritional, and metabolic factors that regulate human renal calcium homeostasis presents a daunting and complex task. It is also important to recognize that renal calcium handling may be regulated directly by extracellular ionized calcium concentrations via signaling by CaSRs at various locations along the renal tubules. Thus, the early concept of renal auto-regulation has a physiological basis.

At the most basic level, the kidneys filter approximately 100 to 200 mmol of calcium per day and about 98% is reabsorbed. Because of the high rate at which calcium cycles across the renal tubular membranes, it is possible for subtle variations in the rate of reabsorption to exert profound effects on the extracellular calcium balance. Approximately 65% of calcium reabsorption occurs in the proximal tubules [38]. The process is largely passive, voltage-dependent, and associated with active reabsorption of sodium, glucose, and other solutes. A further 20% is resorbed via paracellular routes in the thick ascending limb of the loop of Henle. In terms of extracellular homeostasis, the distal tubules including the connecting tubules are the main renal sites for homeostatic fine control of calcium reabsorption as discussed in the next section. For a more detailed review, see Boros et al. [39].

3.5.1 CALCIUM

The calcium sensing receptor (CaSR) is the principal mechanism by which extracellular calcium ions are detected. The CaSR connects the concentration of ionized calcium to a variety of mechanisms designed to maintain calcium homeostasis. The receptor acts at three locations along the renal tubule: the proximal tubule, the thick ascending limb of the loop of Henle, and the inner medullary collecting duct (IMCD).

Various intracellular signaling mechanisms have been identified [40]. In the proximal tubule, activation of the receptor inhibits the synthesis of calcitriol, thus reducing intestinal calcium absorption [41]. In the cortical thick ascending limb of the loop of Henle, the CaSR contributes to inhibition of renal tubular calcium reabsorption [42]. Both mechanisms play important roles in extracellular calcium regulation along with the PTH–calcitriol system. This intrarenal calcium regulating system, although using the same receptor, is a separate mechanism that acts via a physiological transduction pathway separate from that of the PTH–calcitriol system [43].

3.5.2 HORMONAL REGULATION OF RENAL CALCIUM TRANSPORT

3.5.2.1 Parathyroid Hormone

PTH stimulates activity in the distal tubule transepithelial calcium transport system that includes the apical membrane channel (TRPV5), cytosolic binding proteins (calbindins), and basolateral transporters (and NTX1) [44]. The effector system utilizes the basolateral membrane PTH receptor G protein system and intracellular signaling via cAMP and protein kinase A to alter the phosphorylation state of the TRPV5 releasing calmodulin and stimulating a cascade of signaling molecules. The direct effects of PTH on the distal tubule epithelial cells synergize with its stimulation of proximal tubule calcitriol production that exerts endocrine effects on distal tubules via the vitamin D receptor to stimulate the production of the key TRPV5, calbindin, and NCX1 calcium transport proteins.

3.5.2.2 Calcitriol

Rates of gene transcription and levels of protein expression for calbindin D_{28K} and $D_{9K,}$ NCX1 and 2, and PMCA1b are all up-regulated by calcitriol in the distal tubule epithelial cells and intestinal enterocytes [45]. While several isoforms of PMCA exist within the kidney, only one (PMCA1b) appears to be hormonally responsive. PMCA1b is regulated by calcitriol in rabbit and bovine distal kidney tubule cells [46–48] and this effect probably accounts for increased calcium reabsorption demonstrable in calcitriol-treated vitamin D-deficient rabbits [49]. The mechanism for activation of PMCA probably involves calbindin D_{28K} and calbindin D_{9K}, both of which are up-regulated by calcitriol in chicks [50], rats [51], and mice [52], probably by transcriptional regulation [53].

3.5.2.3 Estrogen

Estrogen deficiency has been associated with increased bone loss in post-menopausal females since the 1940s. In the 1960s, the role of renal calcium loss at menopause was reported [54] and later supported by a study of renal calcium handling in pre- and post-menopausal women [55]. These data showed that estrogen was associated with increased renal tubular calcium reabsorption. Indeed, renal calcium excretion increases at menopause and remains elevated into old age [30] (Figure 3.4a).

Interestingly post-menopausal women with high circulating endogenous estrogen levels reveal renal calcium excretion about 40% lower than women with low circulating estrogen independent of PTH levels [56]. Increased renal calcium excretion by post-menopausal women can be corrected by estrogen replacement as shown by a randomized placebo control trial [57]. Estrogen specifically increases reabsorption of tubular calcium into the extracellular compartment (Figure 3.4b). A PTH infusion study of post-menopausal women before and after estrogen replacement confirmed that both estrogen and PTH reduce renal calcium excretion by increasing renal calcium reabsorption, which is reduced further when both are administered [58].

Both estrogen receptors (α and β) have been localized to the kidneys in humans and other species. They are expressed in the proximal and distal tubules and presumably serve as the bases for estrogen's actions in the kidneys [59]. In animals and cell lines, estrogen increases expression of TRPV5 [60], calbindin D_{28K} [61], and distal kidney tubule PMCA [62]. These data are consistent with the concept that the role of estrogen in maintaining skeletal mineral mass depends in part on stimulation of renal calcium reabsorption using similar molecular machinery to that regulated by calcitriol.

3.5.3 NUTRITIONAL FACTORS AFFECTING RENAL CALCIUM EXCRETION

Three dietary constituents in addition to calcium have been shown to increase renal calcium excretion. These are sodium chloride, protein, and food acid. The overall effect on skeletal calcium depends on the ability of the intestine to increase calcium absorption in response to these nutrients and thus maintain calcium balance without requiring increased bone resorption.

3.5.3.1 Sodium Chloride

Sodium competes with calcium for reabsorption in the proximal and distal tubules as demonstrated by the association of sodium excretion and calcium excretion [63]. These data appear to be specific for sodium chloride; other sodium salts such as the

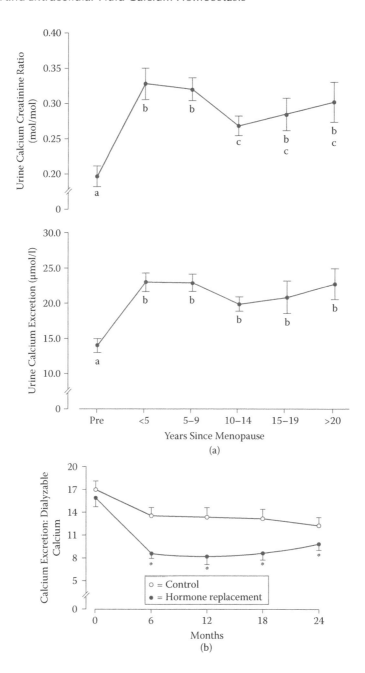

FIGURE 3.4 (a) Effect of years since menopause on renal calcium excretion expressed per mol urine creatinine or per liter glomerular filtrate. Data show that low estrogen state present 5 years after menopause is associated with a 50% increase in urine calcium. (b) Effects of estrogen replacement on urine calcium excretion factored for calcium load filtered at glomeruli over 2 years of a randomized controlled trial of estrogen compared to placebo in post-menopausal women. *Source:* Reference 57 with permission.

bicarbonate and citrate do not increase renal calcium excretion [64,65]. In a 2-year prospective epidemiological study of the effects of sodium intake on bone mass in elderly post-menopausal women, higher sodium intake was associated with a greater degree of bone loss [66]. In the same cohort, high calcium intake prevented bone loss and the interaction of both minerals predicted changes in bone mass better than either element alone.

3.5.3.2   Dietary Protein

Dietary protein intake increases renal calcium excretion [67,68]. The protein effect may increase glomerular filtration rate but the effect appears related to excretion of fixed organic acid as a result of protein metabolism, particularly of sulfur-containing amino acids. Certainly the effect can be reversed by increasing alkali intake at the same time [69]. In population studies of the effects of dietary intake on the risk of developing renal calculi, no excess risk of protein intakes over 76 g/d compared to intakes under 42 g/d was noted [70]. Evidence indicates that a protein supplement will improve bone density and clinical outcomes after hip fracture in old age [71]. Certainly a positive association between protein intake and IGF1 levels [72] and protein intake and bone mass was noted in post-menopausal women [73]. However, results of a 2-year randomized controlled trial of protein supplementation demonstrated no beneficial effects in participants who already had high protein intakes [74].

3.5.3.3   Food Acid

The effect of alkali in reducing renal calcium excretion is well described and has been attributed to effects on bone resorption and renal calcium excretion [75,76]. The primary effect is uncertain and indeed it is likely that effects on bones and kidneys may be linked as a method of buffering excess food acid. However, these data have been extended to the concept that food acid in general and proteins containing acidic amino acids in particular adversely affect calcium balance and exacerbate the losses of bone minerals.

This theory has been studied extensively [77]. Although food acid as determined by the acid ash content in a diet can increase urine calcium excretion, the relation is weak and small [78]. Extrapolating these data to an effect on bone calcium and structure ignores the overall regulation of calcium metabolism, particularly the increase in intestinal calcium absorption that accompanies increased urine calcium excretion [79]. For these reasons, no relation between food acid and bone loss has been documented in a long-term trial [80].

3.6   CONTRIBUTION OF RENAL CALCIUM DYSREGULATION TO METABOLIC BONE DISEASE

3.6.1   Kidneys and Development of Osteoporosis

Bone is a two-phase structure consisting of osteoid and hydroxyapatite (a hydrated crystal of calcium and phosphate). Osteoporosis is a reduction of the bone within the bone and abnormal calcium homeostasis may play a key role in the etiology of reduction of the bone mineral within the bone organ and increase the loss of osteoid.

Indeed, as outlined below, the kidney and intestine may be important factors in the causation of several types of osteoporosis including ovarian and testicular failure, age-related osteoporosis, intestinal malabsorption, and hypercalciuria. These disorders put an individual at great risk of fracture, especially in the presence of a low peak bone mass, which is strongly related to genetic factors [81].

Genetic variation also impacts the calcium homeostatic system. One example is variation in the gene for the vitamin D receptor gene that has been associated with reduced intestinal calcium absorption [82] and may consequently predispose an individual to osteoporosis.

3.6.2 CALCIUM REGULATION

A further important concept is an internal calcium-related skeletal economy that has dual regulatory tasks of defending extracellular calcium homeostasis and defending bone structure in the face of calcium deficiency. Calcium is preferentially resorbed from specific regions of the skeleton. For example, a loss of endocortical bone, which is less important for resisting bending forces, is resorbed in preference to more critical mechanical structures. The mechanisms by which such skeletal regions are identified as susceptible to preferential resorption may be based on mechano-stimulatory activities by osteocytes.

The functional role of the kidney in the development of osteoporosis depends on the exact nature of the pathological process. A conceptual basis incorporating two homeostatic systems involved in renal calcium homeostasis is helpful. One is directed to maintaining extracellular calcium homeostasis while the other is directed to maintaining skeletal anatomy.

3.7 OSTEOPOROSIS TYPES AND ETIOLOGIES

3.7.1 OVARIAN AND TESTICULAR FAILURE

Although testicular failure in males clearly is associated with bone loss and increased risk of fracture, the exact role of androgenic steroids such as testosterone and androstenedione in the pathophysiology of the disorder in humans remains uncertain. This is because both androgens are precursors for estradiol and estriol as a result of the action of aromatase. Thus, it is difficult to be certain of the effects of the androgen as a direct effector on bone and calcium metabolism and its indirect effects via estrogen in any one individual. The principal focus of this section will be on estrogen mechanisms as they have been well researched.

The concept that estrogen deficiency plays a major role in bone loss was first identified by Fuller Albright at Massachusetts General Hospital in the 1940s. The major effect of estrogen deficiency was considered a reduction in osteoid formation. In the 1960s, Nordin published a review largely based on animal data supporting the concept that the principal effect of estrogen deficiency is impairment of calcium balance and this defect causes osteoporosis [83].

Later the effects of the loss of estrogen were identified at the intestine as a reduction of calcium absorption and at the kidney as an increase of urine calcium

Role of Estrogen in Post-Menopausal Bone Loss

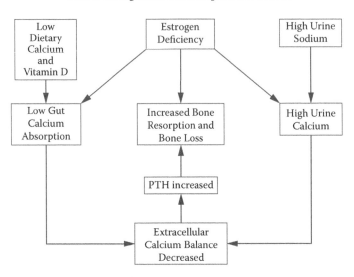

FIGURE 3.5 Overview of physiology of estrogen action on three organs regulating extracellular calcium homeostasis.

excretion [84]. The recent identification of direct estrogen stimulation of the major calcium transport mechanisms across the renal and intestinal epithelium identifies the physiological basis for these effects of estrogen that are independent of its effects on the skeleton (Figure 3.5).

The identification of the signal transduction pathway by which the relative intestinal calcium malabsorption and renal calcium loss stimulate bone loss has been controversial because no change in circulating PTH has been identified [85,86]. Data, however, support the concept that PTH stimulation of bone resorption is increased in the presence of low estrogen.

Thus, the uncertainty about the primary organs involved in estrogen deficiency osteoporosis is resolved because estrogen is a primary hormonal regulator of skeletal bone mass by increasing calcium absorption in the intestine and reabsorption in the kidney. The result is increased calcium entry to the extracellular compartment and its availability for deposition in the skeleton. The plasma calcium concentration is not as important as the flow of calcium across membranes into and out of the skeleton, intestine, and kidney. Such flows are independent of the extracellular calcium concentration.

The therapeutic implication of this view of the pathogenesis of hypogonadal osteoporosis is that negative calcium balance is a cause of the disorder and thus is amenable to treatments directed to increase the supply of calcium to the extracellular space or inhibit the loss of calcium from the body. Thus, dietary calcium supplementation may be sufficient to prevent or reduce bone loss in some patients. However, this intervention may need to be supplemented by direct pharmacological inhibition of osteoclast activity using bisphosphonates or denosumab, for example or, where appropriate, estrogen.

3.7.2 AGE-RELATED OSTEOPOROSIS

Evidence from a large number of randomized, placebo-controlled trials have convincingly demonstrated that calcium supplementation in women over the age of 65 substantially reduces and may completely prevent bone loss [87]. The size of the effect is sufficient to reduce clinical appendicular fracture rates by about 20% [87]. Such data demonstrate that in these women and also in early post-menopausal women, correction of the negative calcium balance is important for preventing resorption of bone.

3.7.2.1 Secondary Hyperparathyroidism

One difference that occurs with increasing age is an increase in PTH, which is not a feature of bone loss closer to menopause [86]. The importance of decreasing renal function during aging age needs consideration. The effect of more severe degrees of renal dysfunction on bone is discussed in Section 3.5. At a community level, a gradual decline in renal function develops only in rare cases into renal osteodystrophy. The effects of a reduction in renal function on calcium homeostasis begin at an estimated glomerular filtration rate of 60 ml/min—the cut-off between stages 2 and 3 of the recent classification of chronic kidney disease (CKD). Studies of patients with this degree of CKD have shown that calcitriol production may be impaired, possibly as a result of an increase in serum FGF23 to a level sufficient to inhibit synthesis of calcitriol or possibly due to loss of renal cells [88,89].

3.7.2.2 Vitamin D Deficiency

The exact role of vitamin D deficiency in the pathogenesis of osteoporosis has been a subject of some contention, primarily because of uncertainty as to whether a patient has osteomalacia or osteoporosis. The differential diagnosis requires bone biopsy after two administrations of fluorescent bone labels to determine the mineralization lag time that is substantially increased in osteomalacia. Furthermore, a decrease in vitamin D status with age due to thinning of the skin contributes to a rise in PTH levels in the elderly [90].

Since vitamin D deficiency plays a role in both bone disorders, it can be reasonably argued that age-related osteoporosis is first treated with a combination of calcium and vitamin D [33]. Finally, the assessment of other dietary factors including excessive salt and protein should be included in the examination as salt and protein increase urine calcium loss and will exacerbate bone loss if combined with malabsorptive conditions such as celiac disease or low calcium intake.

3.7.2.3 Kidneys and Development of Osteomalacias

While osteoporosis is defined as "too little bone of normal appearance" under light microscopy, osteomalacia involves excessive uncalcified osteoid due to a delay in osteoid mineralization. The two principal systemic disorders producing this appearance are calcium and phosphate deficiencies for which severe vitamin D deficiency may be a cause. Evidence also indicates that calcium deficiency alone, without the effects of vitamin D deficiency, can result in clinical rickets in rapidly growing children [91].

In the adult skeleton although excessive osteoid production may arise from severe vitamin D deficiency, it is now relatively rare. What is far more common in the adult population is secondary hyperparathyroidism presenting as osteoporosis [92]. The kidney is the major organ regulating extracellular phosphate homeostasis and abnormalities in renal phosphate handling cause osteomalacia. This is another example of the link between renal calcium and phosphate handling and metabolic bone disease.

3.7.2.4   Kidneys in Primary Hyperparathyroidism and Familial Hypocalciuric Hypercalcemia

The main bone phenotype of primary hyperparathyroidism is osteoporosis characterized as both trabecular and cortical losses of bone mass [93,94]. Histological studies demonstrated that the major difference from other causes of osteoporosis is a high rate of bone formation and increased osteoid volume [94]. The biochemical bases of hypercalcemia are increased relative calcium resorptive activity at the kidney and increased bone turnover [95]. There is also evidence of increased calcium absorptive activity at the intestine due to increased levels of calcitriol with increased 24-hour urine excretion [95]. All these activities raise the level of extracellular calcium required to suppress PTH action arising from the increased parathyroid mass due to an enlarged single adenoma or four-gland hyperplasia.

Familial hypocalciuric hypercalcemia (FHH) has a strong relationship to renal pathology. The primary abnormality is in the calcium sensing receptor expressed both in the parathyroid gland and the kidney which demonstrates impaired calcium signaling interpreted by intracellular mechanisms in both organs as low extracellular calcium. In the parathyroid gland, the result is increased PTH secretion; in the kidney, reduced calcitriol synthesis and reduced reabsorption of tubular calcium in the thick ascending limb of the loop of Henle were noted. The combination of these responses produces the biochemical abnormalities of hypercalcemia and hypocalciuria. Despite the raised PTH levels, FHH patients demonstrate increased bone mass at appendicular sites compared to patients with primary hyperparathyroidism. This demonstrates the important modulation of parathyroid action on bone in this disorder [95].

3.7.2.5   Kidneys in Hypoparathyroidism and Hypocalcemia

The major consequence of hypoparathyroidism due to a genetic mutation (DiGeorge syndrome), surgical procedure, or autoimmune dysfunction at the parathyroid gland is hypocalcemia with abnormal neuromuscular function as its major manifestation. The kidneys contribute to the pathogenesis of low serum calcium through impaired renal tubular calcium reabsorption, resulting in increased urine calcium excretion relative to the circulating plasma calcium concentration. This occurs as a result of the reduction of PTH-dependent renal calcium reabsorption.

Both trabecular and cortical bone mass are increased [96,97]. The abnormalities in bone turnover causing this phenotype have been explored by histomorphometry [98]. In essence, the data show both reduced bone formation and reduced bone resorption. The net result of reduced bone turnover favors an increase in bone mass. This is distinct from hyperparathyroidism that involves increased bone turnover with net bone loss. Hypoparathyroidism is significant as an example of dissociation of extracellular calcium homeostasis and the regulation of skeletal structure, which is influenced and regulated by intrinsic mechanical and cell biology factors and hormonal status.

A second large group of disorders, first described by Fuller Albright and colleagues, is pseudo-hypoparathyroidism characterized as the classical end-organ resistance endocrine disorder due to mutations in the G proteins that connect the PTH receptor with the intracellular signalling cascade of the specific adenylate cyclase responsible for the synthesis of cyclic AMP (cAMP). This mutation abolishes cAMP signalling. For an excellent detailed review of these disorders and their modern management, see Bilezikian et al. [99].

When investigating patients with familial hypocalcemia, one factor that should be considered is severe autosomal-dominant hypocalcemia although it does not have a major skeletal phenotype. This condition arises from a mutation in the calcium sensing receptor that causes a constitutive gain of function resulting in hypocalcemia, principally due to reduced renal tubular reabsorption of calcium [42].

3.7.2.6 Renal Osteodystrophy: CKD Mineral and Bone Disorder (CKD-MBD)

At an eGFR level of 30 ml per minute or less, the loss of functioning nephrons causes the loss of important renal mechanisms including phosphate excretion and calcitriol production. In recent years, attempts have been made to systematize the terminology and therapy of chronic renal disease.

One attempt was the position statement of the group known as Kidney Disease: Improving Global Outcomes (KDIGO) [100]. They defined CKD-MBD as "a constellation of bone disorders present or exacerbated by chronic kidney disease that leads to bone fragility and fractures, abnormal mineral metabolism, and extraskeletal manifestations." For those interested in the complexities of the histological appearances of bone reported for renal osteodystrophy, a detailed classification [101] was simplified into a classification of bone formation rate, mineralization of osteoid, and bone volume [100]. This new classification codifies and expands the older terms.

Osteomalacic disease is a condition involving delayed mineralization of bone with normal or low bone volumes. Adynamic bone disease has low turnover with normal mineralization and low or normal bone volume; some consider it the nephrological equivalent of age-related osteoporosis. Another category is hyperparathyroid bone disease which can be sufficiently severe to produce marrow fibrosis, giving the appearance of osteitis fibrosa in which turnover is increased and bone volume is high without evidence of a mineralization defect. The final category is mixed uremic osteodystrophy defined as high turnover, abnormal mineralization, and normal bone volume.

These conditions are linked loosely to calcium and phosphate metabolic disorders. The osteomalacic disorder is associated with vitamin D deficiency, calcium deficiency, acidosis, or excessive aluminium deposition, any one of which can impair the deposition of hydroxyapatite on preformed osteoids. The adynamic picture is not associated with major abnormalities in biochemistry; indeed some consider that it is associated with excessive suppression of PTH which is considered anabolic in this situation. The hyperparathyroid appearance is the result of secondary hyperparathyroidism due to hypocalcemia arising from decreased intestinal calcium absorption and precipitation of calcium on vessel walls if the calcium-phosphate product level is high. The condition is treated with vitamin D and calcitriol together with calcium, often as calcium carbonate that acts as an intestinal phosphate binder.

3.7.3   RENAL TUBULAR DISEASES

3.7.3.1   Hypercalciurias

Hypercalciuria is defined as excessive inappropriate calcium excretion causing pathology in the renal tract or, less commonly, in the skeleton based on evidence related to low bone mass [102]. It should be considered when 24-hour urine calcium exceeds 6.2 mmol in women and 7.5 mmol in men. Diagnostically, hypercalciurias are classified as two types. In the first, excessive inappropriate calcium excretion is due to abnormalities in the various transporters involved in calcium reabsorption; this is termed primary or renal hypercalciuria and is characterized classically by high fasting urine calcium excretion and elevated PTH. Alternatively, hypercalciuria may be an appropriate physiological response to excessive intestinal calcium absorption, often due to inappropriate renal calcitriol production associated with hypophosphatemia—a condition known as absorptive hypercalciuria [103].

Consumption of foods high in protein and salt increase calcium excretion and can cause bone disease if not offset by increased intestinal calcium absorption. For example, high urine sodium can cause increased urine calcium excretion associated with low bone mass in post-menopausal women [66]. Fasting hypercalciuria can result in a negative calcium balance and consequent bone loss. The descriptions of several specific genetic abnormalities of renal calcium transport mechanisms have improved our understanding of the cellular physiology of calcium transport. These include mutations in three of the claudin genes (14, 16, and 19) presenting with hypercalciuria and nephrocalcinosis rather than bone disease.

3.7.3.2   Hypophosphatemias

A large number of congenital disorders resulting in hypophosphatemia have their genesis in abnormal excessive renal phosphate excretion. They all exert major effects on bone by causing serious osteomalacic lesions. They rate a comment in this section because excessive phosphate therapy may result in transient hypocalcemia with consequent hyperparathyroidism that exacerbates phosphate wasting [104]. These conditions are discussed in detail in Chapter 6.

REFERENCES

1. Jaskova K et al. 2012. Calcium transporters and their role in the development of neuronal disease and neuronal damage. *Gen Physiol Biophys* 31: 375–382.
2. Orellana JA et al. 2012. Regulation of intercellular calcium signaling through calcium interactions with connexin-based channels. *Adv Exp Med Biol* 740: 777–794.
3. Bleich M et al. 2012. Calcium regulation of tight junction permeability. *Ann NY Acad Sci* 1258: 93–99.
4. Hofmann F et al. 1994. Molecular basis for Ca^{2+} channel diversity. *Annu Rev Neurosci* 17: 399–418.
5. Hoenderop JG et al. 1999. Molecular identification of the apical Ca^{2+} channel in 1,25-dihydroxyvitamin D3-responsive epithelia. *J Biol Chem* 274: 8375–8378.

6. Anon. 2006. Fatalities and injuries from falls among older adults: United States, 1993-2003 and 2001–2005. *MMWR* 55: 1221–1224.
7. Christakos S et al. 1992. Molecular aspects of the calbindins. *J Nutr* 122: 678–682.
8. Carafoli E et al. 1996. The plasma membrane calcium pump: recent developments and future perspectives. *Experientia*. 52: 1091–1100.
9. Dominguez JH et al. 1992. The renal sodium–calcium exchanger. *J Lab Clin Med* 119: 640–649.
10. Hou J. 2012. New light on the role of claudins in the kidney. *Organogenesis* 8: 1–9.
11. Lambers TT et al. 2004. Regulation of the mouse epithelial Ca2(+) channel TRPV6 by the Ca^{2+} sensor calmodulin. *J Biol Chem* 279: 28855–28861.
12. Hoenderop JG et al. 2003. Homo- and hetero-tetrameric architecture of the epithelial Ca^{2+} channels TRPV5 and TRPV6. *EMBO J* 22: 776–785.
13. Christakos S et al. 1989. Vitamin D-dependent calcium binding proteins: chemistry, distribution, functional considerations, and molecular biology. *Endocr Rev* 10: 3–26.
14. Borke JL et al. 1988. Co-localization of erythrocyte Ca^{++}–Mg^{++} ATPase and vitamin D-dependent 28-kDa calcium binding protein. *Kidney Intl* 34: 262–267.
15. Zheng W et al. 2004. Critical role of calbindin-D28k in calcium homeostasis revealed by mice lacking both vitamin D receptor and calbindin-D28k. *J Biol Chem* 279: 52406–52413.
16. Rizzo M et al. 2000. Effect of chronic metabolic acidosis on calbindin expression along the rat distal tubule. *J Am Soc Nephrol* 11: 203–210.
17. Strehler EE and Zacharias DA. 2001. Role of alternative splicing in generating isoform diversity among plasma membrane calcium pumps. *Physiol Rev* 81: 21–50.
18. Niggli V et al. 1979. Purification of the (Ca^{2+}–Mg^{2+}) ATPase from human erythrocyte membranes using a calmodulin affinity column. *J Biol Chem* 254: 9955–9958.
19. Carafoli E. 1994. Biogenesis: plasma membrane calcium ATPase: 15 years of work on the purified enzyme. *FASEB J* 8: 993–1002.
20. Magyar CE et al. 2002. Plasma membrane Ca^{2+} ATPase and NCX1 Na+/Ca^{2+} exchanger expression in distal convoluted tubule cells. *Am J Physiol Renal Physiol* 283: F29–F40.
21. Stauffer TP et al. 1995. Tissue distribution of the four gene products of the plasma membrane Ca^{2+} pump: a study using specific antibodies. *J Biol Chem* 270: 12184–12190.
22. Caride AJ et al. 1996. Detection of isoform 4 of the plasma membrane calcium pump in human tissues by using isoform-specific monoclonal antibodies. *Biochem J* 316 (Pt 1): 353–359.
23. Blaustein MP and Lederer WJ. 1999. Sodium–calcium exchange: its physiological implications. *Physiol Rev* 79: 763–854.
24. Stains JP and Gay CV. 1998. Asymmetric distribution of functional sodium–calcium exchanger in primary osteoblasts. *J Bone Miner Res* 13: 1862–1869.
25. Stains JP and Gay CV. 2001. Inhibition of Na+/Ca^{2+} exchange with KB-R7943 or bepridil diminished mineral deposition by osteoblasts. *J Bone Miner Res* 16: 1434–1443.
26. Bourdeau JE et al. 1993. Immunocytochemical localization of sodium–calcium exchanger in canine nephron. *J Am Soc Nephrol* 4: 105–110.
27. Reilly RF et al. 1993. Immunolocalization of the Na+/Ca^{2+} exchanger in rabbit kidney. *Am J Physiol* 265: F327–F332.
28. Brunette MG et al. 1999. Effect of calbindin D28K on sodium transport by the luminal membrane of the rabbit nephron. *Mol Cell Endocrinol* 152: 161–168.
29. Thakker RV. 2004. Diseases associated with the extracellular calcium-sensing receptor. *Cell Calcium* 35: 275–282.
30. Prince RL et al. 1990. The effects of the menopause on calcitriol and parathyroid hormone: responses to a low dietary calcium stress test. *J Clin Endocrinol Metabol* 70: 1119–1123.

31. Razzaque MS. 2009. The FGF23–klotho axis: endocrine regulation of phosphate homeostasis. *Nat Rev Endocrinol* 5: 611–619.
32. Brown EM and MacLeod RJ. 2001. Extracellular calcium sensing and extracellular calcium signaling. *Physiol Rev* 81: 239–297.
33. Prince RL. 1994. Counterpoint: estrogen effects on calcitropic hormones and calcium homeostasis. *Endocr Rev* 15: 301–309.
34. Nordin BE. 1997. Calcium and osteoporosis. *Nutrition* 13: 664–686.
35. Kalkwarf HJ et al. 1997. The effect of calcium supplementation on bone density during lactation and after weaning. *New Engl J Med* 337: 523–528.
36. Laskey MA et al. 2011. Proximal femur structural geometry changes during and following lactation. *Bone* 48: 755–759.
37. Martin A et al. 2012. Regulation and function of the FGF23–klotho endocrine pathways. *Physiol Rev* 92: 131–155.
38. Suki WN. 1979. Calcium transport in the nephron. *Am J Physiol* 237: F1–F6.
39. Boros S et al. 2009. Active Ca^{2+} reabsorption in the connecting tubule. *Pflugers Arch* 458: 99–109.
40. Chakravarti B et al. 2012. Signaling through the extracellular calcium-sensing receptor (CaSR). *Adv Exp Med Biol* 740: 103–142.
41. Maiti A and Beckman MJ. 2007. Extracellular calcium is a direct effecter of VDR levels in proximal tubule epithelial cells that counterbalances effects of PTH on renal vitamin D metabolism. *J Steroid Biochem Mol Biol* 103: 504–508.
42. Vargas-Poussou R et al. 2002. Functional characterization of a calcium-sensing receptor mutation in severe autosomal dominant hypocalcemia with a Bartter-like syndrome. *J Am Soc Nephrol* 13: 2259–2266.
43. Toka HR et al. 2012. Deficiency of the calcium-sensing receptor in the kidney causes parathyroid hormone-independent hypocalciuria. *J Am Soc Nephrol* 23: 1879–1890.
44. van Abel M et al. 2005. Coordinated control of renal Ca^{2+} transport proteins by parathyroid hormone. *Kidney Intl* 68: 1708–1721.
45. Song Y et al. 2003. Calcium transporter 1 and epithelial calcium channel messenger ribonucleic acid are differentially regulated by 1,25 dihydroxyvitamin D3 in the intestine and kidney of mice. *Endocrinology* 144: 3885–3894.
46. Bindels RJ et al. 1991. Active Ca^{2+} transport in primary cultures of rabbit kidney CCD: stimulation by 1,25-dihydroxyvitamin D3 and PTH. *Am J Physiol* 261: F799–F807.
47. Glendenning P et al. 2000. Calcitriol upregulates expression and activity of the 1b isoform of the plasma membrane calcium pump in immortalized distal kidney tubular cells. *Arch Biochem Biophys* 380: 126–132.
48. Glendenning P et al. 2000. The promoter region of the human PMCA1 gene mediates transcriptional downregulation by 1,25-dihydroxyvitamin D(3). *Biochem Biophys Res Commun* 277: 722–728.
49. Bouhtiauy I et al. 1993. Effect of vitamin D depletion on calcium transport by the luminal and basolateral membranes of the proximal and distal nephrons. *Endocrinology* 132: 115–120.
50. Hall AK and Norman AW. 1990. Regulation of calbindin D28K gene expression by 1,25-dihydroxyvitamin D3 in chick kidney. *J Bone Miner Res* 5: 325–330.
51. Huang YC and Christakos S. 1988. Modulation of rat calbindin D28 gene expression by 1,25-dihydroxyvitamin D3 and dietary alteration. *Mol Endocrinol* 2: 928–935.
52. Li H and Christakos S. 1991. Differential regulation by 1,25-dihydroxyvitamin D3 of calbindin-D9k and calbindin-D28k gene expression in mouse kidney. *Endocrinology* 128: 2844–2852.
53. Gill RK and Christakos S. 1993. Identification of sequence elements in mouse calbindin D28k gene that confer 1,25-dihydroxyvitamin D3- and butyrate-inducible responses. *Proc Natl Acad Sci USA* 90: 2984–2988.

54. Young MM and Nordin BE. 1969. The effect of the natural and artificial menopause on bone density and fracture. *Proc R Soc Med* 62: 242.
55. Nordin BE et al. 1991. Evidence for a renal calcium leak in post-menopausal women. *J Clin Endocrinol Metabol* 72: 401–407.
56. Dick IM et al. 2005. Effects of endogenous estrogen on renal calcium and phosphate handling in elderly women. *Am J Physiol Endocrinol Metabol* 288: E430–E435.
57. Prince RL et al. 1991. Prevention of post-menopausal osteoporosis: A comparative study of exercise, calcium supplementation, and hormone-replacement therapy. *New Engl J Med* 325: 1189–1195.
58. McKane WR et al. 1995. Mechanism of renal calcium conservation with estrogen replacement therapy in women in early post-menopause: a clinical research center study. *J Clin Endocrinol Metabol* 80: 3458–3464.
59. Sabolic I et al. 2007. Gender differences in kidney function. *Pflugers Arch* 455: 397–429.
60. Van Abel M et al. 2002. 1,25-dihydroxyvitamin D(3)-independent stimulatory effect of estrogen on the expression of ECaC1 in the kidney. *J Am Soc Nephrol* 13: 2102–2109.
61. Criddle RA et al. 1997. Estrogen responsiveness of renal calbindin-D28k gene expression in rat kidney. *J Cell Biochem* 65: 340–348.
62. Dick IM et al. 2003. Estrogen and androgen regulation of plasma membrane calcium pump activity in immortalized distal tubule kidney cells. *Mol Cell Endocrinol* 212: 11–18.
63. Massey LK and Whiting SJ. 1996. Dietary salt, urinary calcium, and bone loss. *J Bone Miner Res* 11: 731–736.
64. Sakhaee K et al. 1983. Contrasting effects of potassium citrate and sodium citrate therapies on urinary chemistries and crystallization of stone-forming salts. *Kidney Intl* 24: 348–352.
65. Lemann J, Jr. et al. 1989. Potassium bicarbonate, but not sodium bicarbonate, reduces urinary calcium excretion and improves calcium balance in healthy men. *Kidney Intl* 35: 688–695.
66. Devine A et al. 1995. A longitudinal study of the effect of sodium and calcium intakes on regional bone density in post-menopausal women. *Am J Clin Nutr* 62: 740–745.
67. Hegsted MS et al. 1981. Urinary calcium and calcium balance in young men as affected by level of protein and phosphorus intake. *J Nutr* 111: 553–562.
68. Schuette SA et al. 1981. Renal acid, urinary cyclic AMP, and hydroxyproline excretion as affected by level of protein, sulfur amino acid, and phosphorus intake. *J Nutr* 111: 2106–2116.
69. Lutz J. 1984. Calcium balance and acid-base status of women as affected by increased protein intake and by sodium bicarbonate ingestion. *Am J Clin Nutr* 39: 281–288.
70. Curhan GC et al. 1993. A prospective study of dietary calcium and other nutrients and the risk of symptomatic kidney stones. *New Engl J Med* 328: 833–838.
71. Schurch MA et al. 1998. Protein supplements increase serum insulin-like growth factor-I levels and attenuate proximal femur bone loss in patients with recent hip fracture: A randomized, double-blind, placebo-controlled trial. *Ann Intern Med* 128: 801–809.
72. Devine A et al. 1998. Effects of zinc and other nutritional factors on insulin-like growth factor 1 and insulin-like growth factor binding proteins in post-menopausal women. *Am J Clin Nutr* 68: 200–206.
73. Devine A et al. 2005. Protein consumption is an important predictor of lower limb bone mass in elderly women. *Am J Clin Nutr* 81: 1423–1428.
74. Zhu K et al. 2011. The effects of a two-year randomized, controlled trial of whey protein supplementation on bone structure, IGF-1, and urinary calcium excretion in older post-menopausal women. *J Bone Miner Res* 26: 2298–2306.
75. Barzel US. 1995. The skeleton as an ion exchange system: implications for the role of acid-base imbalance in the genesis of osteoporosis. *J Bone Miner Res* 10: 1431–1436.

76. Sebastian A et al. 1994. Improved mineral balance and skeletal metabolism in post-menopausal women treated with potassium bicarbonate. *New Engl J Med* 330: 1776–1781.

77. Fenton TR et al. 2011. Causal assessment of dietary acid load and bone disease: a systematic review and meta-analysis applying Hill's epidemiologic criteria for causality. *Nutr J* 10: 41.

78. Fenton TR et al. 2008. Meta-analysis of the quantity of calcium excretion associated with the net acid excretion of the modern diet under the acid-ash diet hypothesis. *Am J Clin Nutr* 88: 1159–1166.

79. Hunt JR et al. 2009. Dietary protein and calcium interact to influence calcium retention: a controlled feeding study. *Am J Clin Nutr* 89: 1357–1365.

80. Macdonald HM et al. 2008. Effect of potassium citrate supplementation or increased fruit and vegetable intake on bone metabolism in healthy post-menopausal women: a randomized controlled trial. *Am J Clin Nutr* 88: 465–474.

81. Estrada K et al. 2012. Genome-wide meta-analysis identifies 56 bone mineral density loci and reveals 14 loci associated with risk of fracture. *Nat Genet* 44: 491–501.

82. Dawson Hughes B et al. 1995. Calcium absorption on high and low calcium intakes in relation to vitamin D receptor genotype. *J Clin Endocrinol Metabol* 80: 3657–3661.

83. Nordin BEC. 1960. Osteomalacia, osteoporosis, and calcium deficiency. *Clin Orthop* 17: 235–258.

84. Heaney RP et al. 1978. Menopausal changes in calcium balance performance. *J Lab Clin Med* 92: 953–963.

85. Nordin BE et al. 2004. A longitudinal study of bone-related biochemical changes at the menopause. *Clin Endocrinol* 61: 123–130.

86. Prince RL et al. 1995. The effects of menopause and age on calcitropic hormones: a cross-sectional study of 655 healthy women aged 35 to 90. *J Bone Miner Res* 10: 835–842.

87. Tang BM et al. 2007. Use of calcium or calcium in combination with vitamin D supplementation to prevent fractures and bone loss in people aged 50 years and older: a meta-analysis. *Lancet* 370: 657–666.

88. Prince RL et al. 1993. The regulation of calcitriol by parathyroid hormone and absorbed dietary phosphorus in subjects with moderate chronic renal failure. *Metabolism* 42: 834–848.

89. Prince RL et al. 1988. Calcitriol deficiency with retained synthetic reserve in chronic renal failure. *Kidney Intl* 33: 722–728.

90. Need AG et al. 1993. Effects of skin thickness, age, body fat, and sunlight on serum 25-hydroxyvitamin D. *Am J Clin Nutr* 58: 882–885.

91. Thacher TD et al. 1999. A comparison of calcium, vitamin D, or both for nutritional rickets in Nigerian children. *New Engl J Med* 341: 563–568.

92. Prince RL et al. 2006. Effects of calcium supplementation on clinical fracture and bone structure: results of a 5-year, double-blind, placebo-controlled trial in elderly women. *Arch Intern Med* 166: 869–875.

93. Stein EM et al. 2013. Primary hyperparathyroidism is associated with abnormal cortical and trabecular microstructure and reduced bone stiffness in post-menopausal women. *J Bone Miner Res* 28: 1029–1040.

94. Parisien M et al. 1995. Bone structure in post-menopausal hyperparathyroid, osteoporotic, and normal women. *J Bone Miner Res* 10: 1393–1399.

95. Christensen SE et al. 2009. Skeletal consequences of familial hypocalciuric hypercalcaemia versus primary hyperparathyroidism. *Clin Endocrinol* 71: 798–807.

96. Chan FK et al. 2003. Increased bone mineral density in patients with chronic hypoparathyroidism. *J Clin Endocrinol Metabol* 88: 3155–3199.

97. Abugassa S et al. 1993. Bone mineral density in patients with chronic hypoparathyroidism. *J Clin Endocrinol Metabol* 76: 1617–1621.

98. Rubin MR et al. 2008. Dynamic and structural properties of the skeleton in hypoparathyroidism. *J Bone Miner Res* 23: 2018–2024.
99. Bilezikian JP et al. 2011. Hypoparathyroidism in the adult: epidemiology, diagnosis, pathophysiology, target organ involvement, treatment, and challenges for future research. *J Bone Miner Res* 26: 2317–2337.
100. Moe S et al. 2006. Definition, evaluation, and classification of renal osteodystrophy: a position statement from Kidney Disease: Improving Global Outcomes (KDIGO). *Kidney Int* 69: 1945–1953.
101. Parfitt AM et al. 1987. Bone histomorphometry: standardization of nomenclature, symbols, and units: report of the ASBMR Histomorphometry Nomenclature Committee. *J Bone Miner Res* 2: 595–610.
102. Asplin JR et al. 2006. Urine calcium excretion predicts bone loss in idiopathic hypercalciuria. *Kidney Intl* 70: 1463–1467.
103. Giannini S et al. 2005. Bone disease in primary hypercalciuria. *Crit Rev Clin Lab Sci* 42: 229–248.
104. Schmitt CP and Mehls O. 2004. The enigma of hyperparathyroidism in hypophosphatemic rickets. *Pediatr Nephrol* 19: 473–477.

4 Calcium Sensing Receptors: Coordinators of Mineral Metabolism and Therapeutic Targets for Metabolic Bone Disorders

Arthur D. Conigrave

CONTENTS

4.1   INTRODUCTION

The calcium sensing receptor (CaSR) was cloned for the first time from a bovine parathyroid cDNA library by Brown, Hebert, and colleagues and reported in 1993 [1]. This event paved the way for far deeper understandings of the regulatory mechanisms that underpin the control of whole body calcium and bone metabolism, particularly in the parathyroid and kidney, along with various other tissues including gut and bone [2].

It led to new understandings of the mechanisms by which calcium metabolism is perturbed during pregnancy and lactation [3,4]. It provided surprising new insights into the nutrient-dependent control of cell survival, proliferation, migration, and differentiation in tissues including bone [5], colon [6], and the central nervous system [7]. It also promoted the realization that macronutrient and micronutrient metabolisms are linked by a small subfamily of nutrient sensing receptors that detect and respond to changes in L-amino acids, Ca^{2+}, or both [8]. The CaSR opened new lines of investigation into the modulation of fetal development and growth, control of tissue mass and mineralization, and even tumorigenesis.

This chapter first considers the nature of the receptor, control of its expression, and its signaling mechanisms. These discussions are followed by considerations of the roles of the receptor in the control and modulation of calcium metabolism and new insights into its roles in the skeleton including bone cell fate and function. Finally, the status of the receptor as a target in the treatment of disorders of calcium metabolism as well as bone metabolism are discussed.

4.2   MOLECULAR CELL BIOLOGY, STRUCTURE, AND FUNCTION

4.2.1   CALCIUM SENSING RECEPTOR GENE: STRUCTURE AND TRANSCRIPTIONAL CONTROL

The CaSR gene is located on chromosome 3 in humans and chromosome 16 in mice (www.ensembl.org). Its near-neighbor genes (±0.3 Mb) are conserved in mammals but are not clearly involved in calcium metabolism or any other functional roles of the CaSR. These gene products include the SLC15A2 H^+ peptide transporter; the stefin-A cysteine protease inhibitor; a substrate receptor for the ubiquitin–E3 ligase known as WDR5B; and the α subunit of the nuclear importin KPNA1.

The CaSR gene encodes eight exons of which 1a and 1b act as alternative promoters and are not translated [9]. Exons 2 through 7 encode the full-length CaSR protein. The CaSR promoters contain binding sites for transcription factors under the control of the cytokines IL-1β and IL-6 [10,11] and the activated vitamin D receptor [12], all of which promote its expression.

The presence of cytokine-responsive elements in the CaSR promoter suggests a possible role of up-regulated CaSR expression in hypocalcemia arising in the context of systemic infections, major burns [13], and/or severe autoimmune disease in which levels of pro-inflammatory cytokines are markedly elevated. Consistent with this idea, intraperitoneal injections of IL-1β or IL-6 into rats induced hypocalcemia accompanied by enhanced expression of CaSR mRNA in parathyroid, thyroid, and kidney along with elevated serum calcitonin levels and inappropriately suppressed serum levels of PTH and calcitriol [10,11].

The presence of vitamin D response elements in the CaSR promoter supports a negative modulatory mechanism in which an elevated serum calcitriol level first promotes gastrointestinal calcium absorption to raise the serum calcium concentration, and then facilitates the detection of small increases in extracellular ionized calcium (Ca_0^{2+}) to prevent hypercalcemia via enhanced expression of CaSRs. This outcome depends on a decrease in serum PTH level, enhanced serum calcitonin level, and decreased renal Ca^{2+} reabsorption [12]. Consistent with this idea, the CaSR has a primary role in suppressing serum calcium levels that extends beyond its negative impact on PTH secretion [14–16].

4.2.2   CaSR Protein: Domain-Based Structure, Dimers, Protein Partners, and Trafficking

4.2.2.1   Domain-Based Structure

The CaSR subunit is a 1078-residue class C G protein coupled receptor (GPCR) composed of several well-defined domains that are characteristic of class C GPCRs including a Venus flytrap (VFT) domain, a cysteine (Cys)-rich domain, a heptahelical (HH) signaling domain, and an intracellular C-terminus (Figure 4.1). Immediately

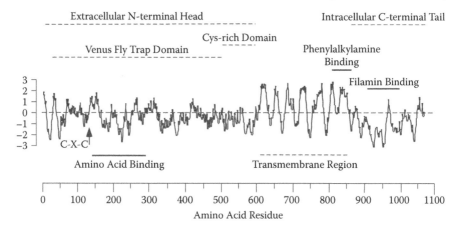

FIGURE 4.1 Annotated hydropathy plot of calcium sensing receptor. Hydropathy plot analysis (Kyte-Doolittle; window size, 13 residues; DNA Strider 1.2) was performed on the CaSR amino acid sequence (including its signal peptide, residues 1 through 19). It demonstrates a 7-transmembrane helix (heptahelical or HH) motif characteristic of G protein-coupled receptors (GPCRs) and thus defines a 612-residue N-terminal extracellular region and a 216—residue cytoplasmic C-terminus. The N-terminus conforms to a pattern established for GPCR class C, whereby residues 20 through 537 form a nutrient-binding Venus flytrap (VFT) domain and residues 538 through 612 form a domain stabilized by multiple cysteine disulfides that couples conformation changes between the VFT and HH domains. The locations of key binding sites are indicated. Ca^{2+} binding sites (not shown) have been demonstrated in both the VFT and HH domains. 'C-X-C' provides two disulfide links between the two subunts in CaSR dimers.

beyond the N-terminal signal peptide (residues 1 through 19) lies the VFT (residues 20 through 537), a bilobed domain that acts as a key site of nutrient binding. Based on models developed from the x-ray crystal structures of several metabotropic glutamate (mGlu) receptor homologs [17–19], the VFT adopts at least two primary conformations at the single subunit level. These are an inactive open conformation and an active closed conformation that is stabilized by nutrient binding.

The Cys-rich domain (residues 538 through 612) provides a structural link between the VFT and HH domains, playing an important role in signal transmission and thus activation of intracellular signaling pathways. The HH domain (residues 613 through 862) is composed of seven transmembrane helices characteristic of the GPCR superfamily and interacts with heterotrimeric G proteins including $G_{q/11}$, $G_{i/o}$ and $G_{12/13}$. An important site for Ca_o^{2+}- and calcimimetic-dependent activation of the receptor has been located in exo-loop-3 and its neighboring transmembrane domains [20].

Finally, the C-terminus (residues 863 through 1078) supports trafficking and expression, activation of phosphoinositide-specific phospholipase C (PI-PLC), and interactions that contribute to the localization of the receptor to specific intracellular compartments and the formation of signaling scaffolds [21].

4.2.2.2 Receptor Dimers: Homodimers and Heterodimers

The CaSR forms homodimers and heterodimers with other class C GPCRs in the cells of tissues engaged in the control of calcium homeostasis [21]. Homodimers are functional in CaSR-expressing HEK-293 cells and have been studied in detail. Their properties include Ca_o^{2+}-dependent activation of signaling pathways and sensitivity to positive modulators including the phenylalkylamines and NPS R568 and negative modulators including NPS 2143.

The properties of heterodimers, the conditions that favor them, and their physiological significance are less understood. Nevertheless, recent work demonstrates that the CaSR forms heterodimers with other class C GPCRs including GABA-B1 and GABA-B2 that have been demonstrated in growth plate chondrocytes and neurons [22,23], and the type-I metabotropic receptors mGlu-1 and –5, found in neurons [24]. How CaSR heterodimers differ in their sensitivities to Ca^{2+} ions, selectivities for modulators, and signaling properties are currently unknown. The roles of heterodimers in CaSR-mediated function and whether their formation and signaling properties are under tissue-specific control also remain largely unknown. Assembly of CaSR heterodimers in osteoblasts may underlie the formation of signaling complexes specific for the control of cell fate.

4.2.2.3 Protein Binding Partners

The CaSR interacts with various intracellular protein binding partners. One well-recognized partner is the actin-binding protein filamin that supports interactions between the CaSR and (1) caveolae [25], possibly via a direct interaction with caveolin-1 [26], and (2) the rho GEF Lbc, thereby activating the monomeric G protein rho to promote its transfer to the plasma membrane [27,28]. One consequence is actin stress-fiber assembly in HEK-CaSR cells [29]. Another is activated membrane phospholipid metabolism. In one example, phospholipase D acts on glycerol phospholipids to generate phosphatidate within the membrane and release various phospholipid head groups including choline [28]. In another example, choline kinase converts choline to phosphorylcholine [30]. Filamin also supports CaSR-dependent activation of the mitogen-activated protein kinase (MAPK) extracellular signal-regulated kinases (ERK)$_{1/2}$ [31], presumably by assembling a scaffold for the efficient relay of molecular signals.

Other CaSR binding partners include the ubiquitin E3 ligase, dorfin that modulates CaSR trafficking and proteasome-dependent degradation [32]; the zinc metalloproteinase AMSH (also known as STAM binding protein) that promotes bone morphogenetic protein (BMP) signaling by relieving the inhibitory actions of SMADs 6 and 7 [33]; the K$^+$ channels Kir4.1 and Kir4.2 [34] that are internalized from the luminal membrane upon CaSR activation to provide a mechanism for high Ca$_o^{2+}$-induced salt-wasting in the renal thick ascending limb of the loop of Henle [35]; the adaptor protein 14-3-3 that negatively modulates CaSR-stimulated rho kinase in HEK-293 cells [36]; the focal adhesion binding protein testin that positively modulates CaSR-stimulated rho kinase in HEK-293 cells [37]; and calmodulin that interacts with a key proximal C-terminal sequence (residues 871 to 898) in a Ca$_i^{2+}$-dependent manner [38].

4.2.2.4   CaSR Trafficking and Its Control

After translation and assembly of its seven transmembrane helices into the membrane of the endoplasmic reticulum, the rate of transfer of receptor dimers to the Golgi and plasma membrane is dependent upon delays imposed by an endoplasmic reticulum quality control apparatus that detects misfolded protein subunits and/or misassembled protein complexes and directs them to proteasomes for breakdown. The proximal C-terminus (residues 868 to 898) participates in the process of quality control as revealed by enhanced rates of transfer of the deletion mutant Δ868-1078 but not Δ898-1078 to the plasma membrane [39].

Trafficking is promoted by positive allosteric modulators including NPS R568 [40] and cinacalcet [41], and receptor-dependent signaling mechanisms such as a mechanism e.g., C-terminus interacts with chaperone binding partners [42]. Surprisingly, however, the negative modulator (calcilytic) NPS 2143 was also effective in promoting the trafficking of mutant CaSRs to the cell surface [41], raising the possibility that pharmaco-chaperone mechanisms can operate independently of receptor signaling.

Finally, rapid recruitment of labelled receptors to the plasma membranes of HEK-293 cells has been observed within seconds of receptor activation via a mechanism known as agonist-directed insertional signaling (ADIS; [43]). This mechanism may contribute to the receptor's known resistance to desensitization, which supports its role in the continual surveillance of serum calcium levels and may also enhance cooperativity in cell-types with exquisite sensitivity to small changes in Ca$_o^{2+}$ [42].

4.3   COOPERATIVITY AND RESISTANCE TO DESENSITIZATION

In support of the CaSR's primary physiological role in the surveillance of Ca$_o^{2+}$ are two important features: (1) *positive cooperativity*, whereby the receptor responds with high sensitivity to small changes in Ca_0^{2+} concentration above a threshold level around 0.5 to 1.0 mM; and (2) *resistance to desensitization*, whereby the receptor maintains signaling output in the context of continuous exposure to activating levels of agonists such as Ca_0^{2+} and extracellular magnesium (Mg_0^{2+}) and modulators such as L-amino acids.

The receptor's positive cooperativity supports its insensitivity to sub-millimolar Ca_0^{2+} concentrations. At and above threshold it also supports the receptor's exquisite sensitivity to small changes in Ca_0^{2+} of the order of 0.02 to 0.05 mM. Positive cooperativity is frequently measured in the form of Hill coefficients for the activation of signaling pathways. These are typically 3 or 4 for CaSR-mediated signaling events including inositol phosphate turnover and intracellular ionized calcium (Ca_i^{2+}) mobilization [21], suppression of cytoplasmic cAMP levels [44], and even agonist-dependent insertional signaling (ADIS) in which receptors are acutely recruited to the plasma membrane [43].

In the parathyroid, however, Ca_0^{2+}-dependent control of PTH secretion exhibits extreme positive cooperativity with Hill coefficients around 8 to 12 [45]. Cooperativity arises, in part, from interactions between Ca^{2+} binding sites within domains, e.g., between VFT domain sites 1 to 3 [46] and between domains in individual subunits, including the VFT and HH domains. Positive cooperativity also arises from interactions between subunits in receptor dimers. Thus, monomeric receptors exhibit a loss of cooperativity and reductions in maximal Ca_0^{2+}-stimulated PI-PLC activity [47]. Cooperativity also depends upon peptide determinants in the receptor's C-terminus [48].

The receptor's resistance to desensitization following activation arises, in part, from its retention in the plasma membrane or in a rapidly recycling population of sub-plasma membrane vesicles despite protein kinase C (PKC) and/or G protein receptor kinase (GRK)-dependent phosphorylation [49]. In addition, it is supported by the organization of intracellular stores of receptors in which a sizeable proportion of the total CaSR pool is available for forward trafficking to the plasma membranes under conditions of accelerated receptor uptake and delivery to lysosomes [42]. Analyses of CaSR truncations and point mutations demonstrate that the proximal C-terminal peptide (868 to 898) noted above to participate in the control of trafficking from the endoplasmic reticulum, also supports PI-PLC-dependent signaling and resistance to desensitization and cooperativity [48], possibly by coordinating interactions with the cytoskeleton and establishing signaling scaffolds.

4.4 SIGNALING PATHWAYS

The CaSR controls distinct functions within a cell and across cell populations by adjusting the relative activities of signaling pathways downstream of three main groups of heterotrimeric G proteins. This occurs in a ligand-dependent manner—a manifestation of so-called *ligand-biased signaling*. It also occurs in a cell-type specific manner dependent upon the expression of isoforms of G proteins and enzymes such as adenylyl cyclase and PKC, as well as adapter proteins that control the assembly and targeting of signaling units.

It is beyond the scope of this chapter to discuss all the pathways that the receptor has been reported to modulate, the breadth of ligand-directed signaling, and all complexities of the signaling—many of which remain unsolved—in diverse CaSR-expressing cells. Instead, attention is drawn to key G proteins and signaling pathways that are known to control cell function and fate.

4.4.1 HETEROTRIMERIC G PROTEINS

The CaSR interacts with various heterotrimeric G proteins to initiate change along a suite of intracellular signaling pathways.

4.4.1.1 $G_{i/o}$ Pertussis Toxin-Sensitive G Proteins and $G_{q/11}$

The CaSR mediates inhibition of adenylyl cyclase and thus suppression of cAMP synthesis via $G_{i/o}$ pertussis toxin-sensitive G proteins. $G_{i/o}$ contributes to the inhibitory control of PTH secretion by various agents including $PGF_{2\alpha}$ and α-adrenergic agonists [2,50]. In addition, it contributes to Ca_o^{2+}- and multivalent cation-dependent suppression of PTH secretion, presumably via CaSR-mediated signaling [51,52]. $G_{i/o}$ also contributes to the activation of the mitogen-activated protein kinase ERK ½ (ERK) in cells including CaSR-expressing HEK-293 cells and parathyroid cells [53,54]. The role of β-arrestin in adapting $G_{i/o}$ protein activation to ERK and c-Jun N-terminal kinase (JNK) activation is well established for other GPCRs [55] and probably also operates for the CaSR.

The CaSR supports the activation of PI-PLCβ, and thus inositol phosphate release and turnover, Ca_i^{2+} mobilization, and activation of conventional isoforms of PKC via $G_{q/11}$. Indeed, the demonstration that parathyroid cells exhibit Ca_o^{2+}- or Mg_o^{2+}-stimulated elevations in Ca_i^{2+} mobilization and inositol phosphate turnover allowed the development of a successful expression cloning strategy for the CaSR [56–58]. The machinery for activating this pathway relies on residues in the receptor's second and third intracellular loops [59] and on its proximal C-terminus [60,61]. $G_{q/11}$ and PI-PLC contribute to the CaSR-mediated activation of multiple downstream signaling pathways in various cell-types [62] and parathyroid-selective ablation of the α subunit of G_q on a global G_{11} α subunit null background-abolished Ca_o^{2+}-dependent negative feedback control of PTH secretion [63].

A PLC-dependent pathway also supports Ca_o^{2+}-dependent migration of pre-osteoblasts to sites of active bone resorption for remodeling [64] (see below). CaSR-mediated activation of PI-PLC provides an additional mechanism for the inhibition of cyclic AMP synthesis via Ca_i^{2+}-dependent inhibition of certain adenylyl cyclase isoforms (5, 6, and 9) as reported for CaSR-expressing HEK-293 cells [44] and for the inhibitory control of renin secretion from renal juxtaglomerular cells [65].

4.4.1.2 $G_{12/13}$

The CaSR, like various other GPCRs [66], supports the activation of guanine nucleotide exchange factors (GEFs) for the monomeric G protein rho A and downstream signaling pathways via $G_{12/13}$. This pathway links to the control of changes in cell shape and migration [67] and gene expression via the activation of rho kinase and phosphorylation of serum-response factor (SRF) [66]. In addition, $G_{12/13}$ controls (1) a key protein regulator of G protein signaling Akin that positively modulates

IMPACTS OF CALCIUM SENSING RECEPTOR ACTIVATORS ON BONE CELLS

Osteoblasts	Osteocytes
Stem cell commitment to osteoblast lineage	Suppressed sclerostin
Survival	**Osteoclastogenesis and Osteoclasts**
Chemotaxis	Suppressed RANKL expression and signaling
Proliferation	Enhanced OPG expression
Differentiation	Enhanced apoptosis
Matrix protein synthesis	Suppressed chemotaxis
Disinhibition of mineralization	Suppressed resorption

Wnt3a-frizzled signaling; (2) the release of β-catenin from E-cadherins; (3) tyrosine kinase activities; (4) protein phosphatase activities including PP2A; (5) the A-kinase anchoring protein (AKAP) and rho GEF AKAP-Lbc that provides a point of intersection between cAMP/PKA and rho A signaling; and (6) interactions with tight junction proteins [67]. The components of signaling pathways downstream of $G_{12/13}$, their organization, and full physiological implications are not understood.

Relevant to the roles of the CaSR in various cell types, and in response to distinct ligands, Ca^{2+}_o- and the calcimimetic NPS R-467-induced rho kinase-dependent formation of actin stress fibers in CaSR-expressing HEK-293 cells [29], L-amino acid-induced Ca^{2+}_i mobilization in CaSR-expressing HEK-293 cells was reported to require G_{12} and rho A [68]. A a G_{12}–rho A pathway negatively modulates RANKL expression in osteoblasts [69] and may support CaSR-mediated control [70]. In addition, $G_{12/13}$ activates adenylyl cyclase isoform-7 (AC7) [71] so that up-regulated expression of $G_{12/13}$ or AC7 may contribute to the "switching" in G protein usage as described in breast cancer [72].

$G_{12/13}$ supports various CaSR-mediated effects on cell fate. Two key effects in bone arise from positive modulation of Wnt3a–β-catenin signaling resulting osteoblast differentiation [73], negative modulation of RANKL expression [70], and thus suppression of osteoclastogenesis. With respect to Ca^{2+}_i-dependent control of acute cellular responses including chemotaxis of pre-osteoblasts (see box), $G_{12/13}$-dependent pathways may support $G_{q/11}$-dependent activation of PI-PLC via activation of PP2A, leading to dephosphorylation of CaSR residue T888 and thus sustained elevations of Ca^{2+}_i [74].

4.4.1.3   CaSR Coupling to Gs

The CaSR paradoxically stimulates adenylyl cyclase in settings such as breast cancer cells [72] and At-T20 pituitary cells that secrete ACTH and PTHrP [75]. In both cases, the CaSR was reported to couple to G_s. In the breast cancer cell example, the authors proposed receptor-dependent switching of G protein preference since normal mammary epithelial cells exhibit CaSR-dependent coupling to $G_{i/o}$ [72]. An alternative mechanism may also operate in some cell-types dependent on $G_{12/13}$ signaling to adenylyl cyclase isoform-7 [71], as noted above. Elevated Ca^{2+} also stimulates cAMP synthesis and COX2 expression in primary mouse osteoblasts [76]. Whether G_s, $G_{12/13}$-AC7, or some other mechanism is involved remains unknown.

4.4.1.4   Protein Kinases

The CaSR activates various protein kinases including conventional isoforms of PKC downstream of PI-PLC and Ca_i^{2+} mobilization, as well as mitogen-activated protein (MAP) kinases including ERK, p38, JNK [62,77], and two key protein kinase regulators of cell fate, Akt and GSK-3 [73]. The CaSR also couples to rho kinase under the control of the monomeric G protein rho A [29] and in the activation of the transcriptional modulator known as serum response factor (SRF) [78]. The roles of these protein kinases in CaSR-mediated control of cell functions were identified by the use of specific inhibitors and/or siRNAs. Studies covered the role of JNK in CaSR-mediated proliferation in rat calvarial osteoblasts [79] and p38 in PTHrP secretion from CaSR-expressing HEK-293 cells [80].

The mechanisms of activation of many CaSR-stimulated protein kinases are not well understood. As noted above, ERK lies downstream of $G_{q/11}$-stimulated PKC and also requires $G_{i/o}$, possibly via the activation of β-arrestin [53]. In addition, CaSR-mediated ERK phosphorylation depends on the transactivation of epidermal growth factor (EGF) receptors in some cell types [81,82]. Finally, cytoskeletal scaffolds support cell context-specific signaling. For example, the actin-binding protein filamin is required for CaSR-mediated activation of ERK [31].

4.4.1.5   Transcriptional Control of Gene Expression

CaSR-mediated control of gene expression is critical to its effects on cell fate and occurs downstream of the MAP kinases, ERK, p38 and JNK, as well as rho kinase, Wnt-β-catenin [73], and CREB [54]. Thus, the CaSR controls the activation of $ERK_{1/2}$-dependent factors such as c-Jun, c-Fos, Elk-1, and Egr-1 [83] as well as SRF downstream of rho kinase [78]. The identities of gene targets of CaSR-activated transcription factors are largely unknown.

4.5   RECEPTOR ACTIVATORS: Ca^{2+} IONS AND MODULATORS

Ca^{2+} ions are the primary physiological agonists of the receptor. They bind at multiple sites including at least one, and possibly as many as five, in the Venus fly trap (VFT) domain [46,84] and at least one additional site in the heptahelical (HH) domain [85,86].

Because the Ca_o^{2+} concentration in plasma and other biological fluids is typically around 1.0 mM or more, CaSRs expressed on cell surfaces are active even under normal physiological conditions and are further activated by increases in plasma Ca^{2+} concentration up to its normal maximum level around 1.3 mM. However, the threshold Ca_o^{2+} concentrations for the activation of various signaling pathways differ within a cell so that some pathways may be almost maximally activated at normal physiological Ca_o^{2+}. This situation has been described for normal osteoblasts or pre-osteoblasts [87].

In addition, CaSR-dependent signaling pathways are subject to differential modulation by natural allosteric modulators including L-amino acids [8,88] and glutathione and its analogs [89,90]. In one recent study utilizing HEK-293 cells under conditions of maximum CaSR surface expression, the Ca_o^{2+} threshold concentrations were 0.3 mM for intracellular Ca^{2+} mobilization and 1.0 mM for $ERK_{1/2}$ phosphorylation [91]. Some signaling pathways are more sensitive than others due to variations in receptor expression, e.g., arising from limiting levels of scaffold proteins in support of receptor signaling.

4.5.1 Calcimimetics

Dr. Edward Nemeth, leader of the team at NPS Pharmaceuticals that developed cinacalcet as a clinically effective positive CaSR modulator [92], first described non-Ca_o^{2+} activators as *calcimimetics* [93] and classified them as type I, agonists, which are typically inorganic or organic multivalent cations, and type-II positive modulators, which are typically uncharged organic compounds that bind at one of the receptor's allosteric sites. He also coined the term *calcilytic* to describe negative modulators of the CaSR that inhibited its response to physiological activators as well as synthetic calcimimetics [94,95].

4.5.1.1 Type I Calcimimetics (Agonists)

These agents are typically multivalent cations and are surprisingly diverse in structure. As may be expected, they include inorganic cations such as the divalent Mg^{2+} and Sr^{2+} ions and tervalent Gd^{3+} ion. Sr^{2+} is considered in more detail in Section 4.8 below. The type 1 calcimimetics also include organic multivalent cations such as the antibiotic neomycin, polyamines such as spermine, cationic proteins such as β-amyloid and even the cationic peptide polyarginine [2].

The results suggest that the CaSR is highly promiscuous with respect to cationic activators. Nevertheless, it seems feasible that the receptor is activated by endogenous organic cations in some compartments. The polyamine spermine is one example; it is obtained from the diet and also synthesized in the brain and by gut bacteria. It acts on the one hand as a modulator of colonic epithelial cell differentiation [96] and on the other as a neuromodulator [97,98].

4.5.1.2 Type II Calcimimetics (Positive Modulators)

These agents generally require threshold levels of Ca_o^{2+} for efficacy and enhance Ca_o^{2+} potency. The first selective agents of this type developed were NPS R467 and NPS R568 [93]—analogs of the phenylalkylamine fendiline. Both elicited robust Ca_i^{2+} mobilization in bovine parathyroid cells [93]. The related phenylalkylamine known as cinacalcet entered clinical practice for the treatment of secondary hyperparathyroidism in the context of chronic kidney disease [99] and poorly controlled primary hyperparathyroidism in patients unable to undergo parathyroidism or after failed parathyroidectomy or in the context of parathyroid cancer [100].

Phenylalkylamine calcimimetics bind in the receptor's HH domain [101,102]. Various other classes of CaSR-active synthetic compounds have been identified but their biological and clinical effects are not well studied [103].

In addition to these synthetic modulators, two classes of natural positive modulators have been identified: (1) L-amino acids [88] and (2) glutathione [89] and several of its analogs including S-methylglutathione [90] and γ-glutamyl-valine-glycine [104]. Both of these natural classes of modulators bind in the VFT domain [89,102].

4.5.2 L-Amino Acids as Positive Modulators

Like several other members of GPCR class-C including metabotropic glutamate receptors, GPRC6A, and $T1R_1/R_3$ heterodimers, the CaSR is activated by several endogenous L-amino acids [88,105]. Atypically, however, L-amino acids are positive modulators rather than agonists of the CaSR. Active amino acids are primarily aromatics such as L-phenylalanine, L-tryptophan, and L-histidine and small aliphatic amino acids such as L-alanine, L-threonine, and L-serine. In CaSR-expressing cells, however, more than two thirds of the 20 endogenous amino acids exhibit efficacy in Ca_i^{2+} mobilization assays dependent on the presence of a threshold level of Ca^{2+} [8,45].

Interestingly, the CaSR exhibits biased signaling whereby several pathways including PI-PLC and $ERK_{1/2}$ are either not accessible or only weakly sensitive to amino acid activators. Instead, L-amino acid modulators promote a Ca_i^{2+} mobilization pathway that in the gastrointestinal tract supports the secretion of key hormones from entero-endocrine cells including gastrin [106], cholecystokinin [107,108], GLP-1, PYY, and GIP [109].

4.5.2.1 Mediation of Dietary Protein-Derived Nutrient Signals

Dietary protein exerts various positive effects on bone growth and metabolism that are not well understood [110]. For example, dietary protein promotes intestinal calcium absorption by a jejunal macronutrient-dependent pathway that is distinct from the duodenal pathway controlled by 1,25-dihydroxyvitamin D [111]. It also negatively modulates PTH secretion so that low protein diets induce a state of secondary hyperparathyroidism [112,113] secondary to either inadequate calcium absorption, altered release of an intestinal hormone, or drops in the serum levels of L-amino acids leading to impaired Ca_o^{2+} sensitivity of CaSRs on the parathyroid [110].

Dietary protein also positively modulates serum levels of insulin-like growth factor-1 (IGF-1) and its local production by osteoblasts [114]. Interestingly, cell type-specific deletion of the CaSR gene in osteoblasts markedly reduced serum IGF-1 levels in transgenic mice [5,115]. The suggestion is that CaSRs in osteoblasts or perhaps osteocytes mediate dietary protein-dependent release of IGF-1 production directly in response to serum L-amino acids and/or secondary to enhanced intestinal calcium absorption.

4.6   BIOLOGICAL ROLES IN MINERAL
AND MACRONUTRIENT METABOLISM

4.6.1   ENDOCRINE CONTROL OF CALCIUM METABOLISM

4.6.1.1   Parathyroid Gland

The CaSR mediates the physiological feedback mechanism by which elevations in Ca_0^{2+} concentration suppress PTH secretion from the parathyroid gland [116]; see Figure 4.2. A decrease in Ca_0^{2+} (e.g,, that associated with bone mineralization and renal calcium losses during fasting) provokes an elevation of PTH secretion and serum PTH level. This, in turn, promotes Ca^{2+} retention by the kidney and calcium resorption from bone. If these effects are sufficient to restore Ca_0^{2+}, activation of the CaSR suppresses PTH secretion to lower serum PTH levels, attenuating further bone resorption and renal calcium reabsorption [117].

Although Ca_0^{2+} is the primary physiological regulator of PTH, it seems likely that its actions are supported by Mg_0^{2+}, which is a lower affinity agonist of the CaSR. Furthermore, serum levels of L-amino acids are positive modulators of CaSR and enhance the receptor's sensitivity for Ca_0^{2+} [45]. Whether increases in serum L-amino acid levels derived from dietary protein suppress PTH secretion is unclear.

The mechanism by which the CaSR mediates Ca_0^{2+}-dependent feedback regulation of PTH secretion has not been solved. PTH secretion is supported by an intrinsic mechanism that is enhanced by various hormonal, neuronal, and paracrine factors including epinephrine, glucagon, dopamine, serotonin, and histamine [2]. Many of

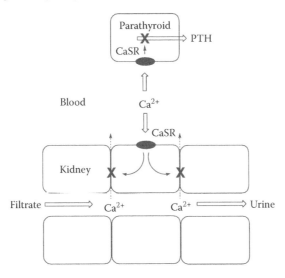

FIGURE 4.2   Primary roles of CaSRs in calcium metabolism: inhibition of PTH secretion and inhibition of renal calcium reabsorption. CaSRs expressed on parathyroid chief cells and renal cortical thick ascending limb (cTAL) cells couple in these sites to signaling pathways that respectively suppress PTH secretion via exocytosis and suppress Ca^{2+} reabsorption via a paracellular transport pathway.

these agents activate G_s-coupled GPCRs that elevate cAMP levels. Thus, exocytosis of PTH-containing secretory vesicles and PTH synthesis are stimulated by a cAMP-dependent mechanism blocked by the CaSR through various pathways including suppression of cAMP levels via $G_{i/o}$ [51,52] and/or Ca_i^{2+}-dependent inhibition of adenylyl cyclase isoforms 5 and 6 [118]—and, perhaps, Ca_i^{2+}/calmodulin-dependent activation of cyclic nucleotide phosphodiesterase.

4.6.1.2   Thyroid Gland C Cells

Thyroid parafollicular C cells secrete the peptide hormone calcitonin in response to elevated serum calcium concentrations. Calcitonin, in turn, acts to lower the serum Ca_0^{2+} concentration by suppressing bone resorption [119]. However, calcitonin does not appear to act as an essential element of the feedback mechanism for the regulation of serum calcium levels [120] that requires PTH to defend against hypocalcemia and Ca_0^{2+}-induced renal calcium excretion to combat hypercalcemia [121].

Instead, calcitonin promotes whole body calcium retention via enhancing the renal Ca^{2+} reabsorption pathway and coupled inhibition of bone resorption [111]. In bone, calcitonin acts on osteoclasts to suppress resorption via its class B GPCR coupled to the activation of G_s and adenylyl cyclase. Calcitonin modulates maternal bone metabolism during pregnancy and lactation [122] and also contributes to combating hypercalcemia [123,124].

The CaSR is a key element of the mechanism by which Ca_0^{2+} signals are detected in C cells. First, it is expressed in C cells derived from various species [125,126]. Second, it couples to Ca_i^{2+} mobilization in the form of low frequency oscillations [127,128] and triggers calcitonin release [125]. In a manner similar to islet β cells, elevations of Ca_i^{2+} in C cells depend upon the expression of voltage-operated Ca^{2+} channels including L-, N-, and T-types [129], as well as PI-PLC.

4.6.2   Regulation of Renal Calcium and Phosphate Excretion

The CaSR is expressed in various renal tubular segments including, notably, the proximal tubule, cortical thick ascending limb, and cortical collecting ducts. The receptor plays distinct roles in calcium and phosphate metabolism along with salt and water metabolism at these sites.

4.6.2.1   Modulation of Mineral Metabolism via Expression in Proximal Tubules

CaSR expression in the proximal tubules localizes to the apical membranes (those facing the luminal fluid) [130]. CaSR is thus positioned to provide sensing of Ca_0^{2+} levels in the luminal fluid following glomerular filtration and detect deviations in local Ca_0^{2+} concentrations that may arise from a mismatch of the rates of transcellular water reabsorption and paracellular Ca^{2+} reabsorption. Whether the CaSR in this location modulates the rate of water transport, as it does in the cortical collecting tubules, is unknown. Whether the CaSR modulates divalent cation transport in the proximal tubule as it does in the cortical thick ascending limb [131] is also unknown.

The CaSR has two likely functions in the proximal tubules. First, it may mediate Ca_0^{2+}-dependent suppression of expression of the gene coding for the 25-hydroxyvitamin D-1α hydroxylase (CYP27B1), reducing synthesis of 1,25-dihydroxyvitamin D_3 [130,132] as a form of feedback analogous to Ca_0^{2+}-dependent suppression of PTH secretion. Second, it negatively modulates PTH-induced suppression of phosphate reabsorption [133] acting to modestly elevate serum inorganic phosphate levels.

4.6.2.2 Regulation of Renal Calcium Reabsorption via Expression in Thick Ascending Limb Cells

CaSR expression in the cortical thick ascending limb provides a physiological mechanism by which elevated Ca_0^{2+} promotes renal calcium wasting to lower Ca_0^{2+} levels to homeostatic levels (Figure 4.2). In familial hypocalciuric hypercalcemia (FHH) associated with heterozygous inactivating mutations of the CaSR, impaired CaSR function results in unrestrained Ca^{2+} reabsorption, hypocalciuria, and hypercalcemia [116]. Similarly, selective CaSR ablation in the mouse kidney results in hypercalcemia due to defective negative control of Ca^{2+} reabsorption [14].

Ca^{2+} reabsorption in the cortical thick ascending limb is predominantly paracellular and is thus dependent on the magnitude of a lumen-positive transepithelial potential difference and the conductance of a divalent cation-selective paracellular pathway. The lumen-positive potential difference arises from (1) the transfer of positive charge from the interstitium to the lumen via Na^+/K^+-ATPase-dependent basolateral uptake of K^+ and its luminal secretion via the renal outer medullary potassium channel (ROMK) and/or (2) the transfer of negative charge from the lumen to the interstitium via luminal membrane uptake of Cl^- ions mediated by the $Na^+/K^+/2Cl^-$ co-transporter NKCC2 and basolateral efflux via the channel CLC-KB, also known as barttin [134]. Ca^{2+}- and Mg^{2+}-dependent paracellular conductance [130,135] arises from the expression of divalent cation-selective claudins (including claudins 16 and 19) in the tight junctional surfaces of the luminal plasma membranes [111, 136].

CaSR-dependent inhibitory control of renal Ca^{2+} reabsorption arises from its expression in the basolateral membranes of cortical thick ascending limb epithelial cells where it monitors Ca_0^{2+} levels. In response to elevated Ca_0^{2+}, CaSRs mediate the generation of arachidonic acid metabolites to disable luminal K^+ secretion [137] and suppress cAMP levels to inhibit basolateral Cl^- efflux [138]. In addition, recent evidence indicates that the CaSR signals via a novel microRNA-dependent pathway to promote the expression of claudin 14, a negative modulator of claudins 16 and 19, in the cortical thick ascending limb [139,140]. Interestingly, dietary calcium positively modulates claudin 14 expression at both the mRNA and protein levels [139].

4.6.2.3 Modulation of Renal Phosphate Excretion

Along with calcium, inorganic phosphate is a key component of hydroxyapatite. Phosphate is also a key regulator of growth plate maturation and bone formation and a low serum phosphate level is a common causative factor in the pathogenesis of rickets [141,142].

The activated CaSR restrains renal phosphate losses via two mechanisms. First, CaSRs expressed in the parathyroid mediate suppression of PTH secretion even at Ca_0^{2+} levels in the normal physiological range, thereby suppressing the drive for PTH-dependent phosphate losses in the proximal tubules [2]. Second, as noted above,

CaSRs expressed on the luminal membranes of proximal tubular cells negatively modulate the phosphaturic effect of PTH [130]. Thus, CaSR activation raises serum phosphate levels while lowering serum calcium levels. On the basis of the foregoing, the calcimimetic cinacalcet would be expected to lower serum calcium and raise serum phosphate. Consistent with this idea, patients with primary hyperparathyroidism treated with 40 mg oral cinacalcet twice daily for 15 days exhibited significant reductions in serum total calcium concentrations from 2.7 to 2.1 mM and a more modest but statistically significant increases in serum inorganic phosphate levels from 0.9 mM to 1.0 mM [143]. Cinacalcet has also been used successfully to elevate serum phosphate levels in hypophosphatemic rickets [144].

4.6.2.4 CaSR-Dependent Modulation of Urinary Concentration: Defense against Renal Calculus Formation

The CaSR mediates suppression of water reabsorption in the collecting ducts and thus negatively modulates renal concentrating ability [145]. One important consequence is a reduced luminal Ca_0^{2+} concentration and a reduced risk of calcium stone formation. In addition, the CaSR promotes acid excretion to enhance the solubility of calcium salts [146].

Recent work defined a mechanism by which the activated CaSR suppresses water reabsorption. Thus, CaSRs expressed on the apical membranes of cortical and medullary collecting duct cells sense elevations in luminal Ca_0^{2+} and stimulate a signaling response that: (1) suppresses intracellular cAMP levels; and (2) activates rho A [147]. Together, these effects impair vasopressin-induced insertion of aquaporin-2-containing vesicles into the apical membranes and thus lower water permeability and reabsorption. These modulatory effects provide a local mechanism for preventing precipitation of calcium phosphate and/or oxalate crystals and subsequent formation of renal calculi [148].

4.6.3 COMBATING HYPOCALCEMIA AND HYPERCALCEMIA

4.6.3.1 Hypocalcemia

Acute hypocalcemia is a serious disorder with clinical features arising from impaired Ca_0^{2+}-dependent inhibitory modulation of central and peripheral nerve excitability including the neuromuscular junctions and a conducting defect in the heart associated with prolonged QT_c intervals. Recognized consequences include neuromuscular instability, fasciculations, tetanic contractions, arrhythmias, and seizures. Key defenses against hypocalcemia are circulating parathyroid gland-derived PTH and 1,25-dihydroxyvitamin D (calcitriol), both of which are under negative feedback control mediated by CaSRs.

Serum calcitriol promotes intestinal calcium and phosphate absorption [149]) and renal calcium reabsorption [150], providing support for serum calcium levels over a 24- to 48-hour period. PTH, on the other hand, provides minute-to-minute surveillance of serum calcium levels and its levels are continuously subject to negative feedback regulation by the serum ionized Ca_0^{2+} concentration [2].

The CaSR participates in several of these homeostatic events. First, and most obviously, it mediates negative feedback control of PTH secretion by Ca_0^{2+}. When the Ca_0^{2+} level drops, PTH secretion is no longer inhibited and the serum PTH level rises sharply to drive a number of processes including (1) Ca^{2+} release from the bone matrix and possibly from a more rapidly mobilizable pool of bone calcium such as that associated with matrix microvesicles; (2) Ca^{2+} reabsorption from the renal tubules; and (3) intestinal Ca^{2+} absorption secondary to enhanced calcitriol synthesis [111]. Second, when the Ca_0^{2+} level drops, an enhanced drive for calcitriol synthesis operates primarily in the renal proximal tubules. The CaSR also appears to mediate these effects, at least in part via transcriptional down-regulation of renal CYP27B1 expression [132]. Thus, as the Ca_0^{2+} concentration drops, feedback inhibition of calcitriol synthesis is withdrawn to promote serum calcitriol levels and stimulate the drive for duodenal calcium absorption.

4.6.3.2   Hypercalcemia
The two primary defenses against hypercalcemia are (1) enhanced renal calcium excretion arising from the action of elevated Ca_0^{2+} concentration on CaSRs expressed on the basolateral membranes of renal cortical thick ascending limb cells to disable paracellular Ca^{2+} reabsorption [14] and (2) suppressed osteoclastic resorption of bone arising from enhanced calcitonin secretion via the actions of CaSRs in thyroid C cells [123,124], and possibly via direct CaSR-dependent suppression of osteoclast function. Conversely, CaSR-dependent suppression of PTH secretion plays only a limited role in the defense against hypercalcemia [14,16].

4.6.4   CaSR-Dependent Control of Calcium Metabolism during Pregnancy and Lactation

Calcium is released from bone during pregnancy and lactation through enhanced bone turnover, osteoclastic bone resorption, and lactation [151]. Recent work demonstrates that, at least during lactation, osteocytic bone resorption also occurs dependent upon up-regulated expression of genes including tartrate-resistant acid phosphatase (TRAP) and cathepsin K [152].

4.6.4.1   Placental Calcium Transport
The CaSR contributes to the control of fetal skeletal development by supporting placental calcium transport [4] within the placenta where it is expressed on both cytotrophoblasts and transporting syncytiotrophoblasts [153], and/or in fetal parathyroid cells. Interestingly, the CaSR and PTHrP appear to activate the same component of placental calcium transport [4], suggesting CaSR-dependent control of PTH/PTHrP levels and/or modulation of type I PTH receptor function. Whether the CaSR modulates expression of the epithelial Ca^{2+}-selective ion channel TRPV6, which supports placental calcium transport [154], is not yet known.

4.6.4.2   Lactation: Control of Bone Resorption and Calcium Secretion into Milk
Two hormonal signals contribute to bone resorption during lactation: suppressed serum estrogen levels and elevated serum PTHrP levels arising from the mammary glands [155]. Upon weaning, maternal bone resorption stops promptly through

a generalized apoptosis of osteoclasts that is complete within 2 or 3 days [156,157] and arises, at least in part, from suppressed RANKL expression [156]. Recovery of bone mass and mineralization are driven by enhanced osteoblastic bone formation over the succeeding weeks to months [151]. The CaSR has roles in both processes.

Calcium transport into milk during lactation is dependent upon two transcellular pathways initiated by the transfer of Ca^{2+} ions from the extracellular fluid across the basolateral membrane into the cytoplasm. Two epithelial Ca^{2+} channels, TRPV5 and TRPV6, contribute to this mechanism [158]. Upon transfer into cells, Ca^{2+} is taken up by (1) a Golgi-mediated secretory pathway in which Ca^{2+} ions are concentrated by the actions of smooth endoplasmic reticulum Ca^{2+}-ATPases (SERCAs) secretory pathway Ca^{2+}-ATPases (SPCAs), notably SPACA2 [159], into secretory vesicles containing casein micelles, or (2) a cytoplasmic pathway dependent on markedly up-regulated expression of PMCA2 in the apical membrane that pumps Ca^{2+} directly from the cytoplasm into the mammary duct [158]. Consistent with the idea that the cytoplasmic pathway is critical to lactation, PMCA2 mRNA expression peaks around 100-fold with respect to basal non-pregnant levels by day 5 of lactation [160] and lactating mice null for PMCA2 exhibited an approximate 60% reduction in calcium transport into milk despite compensatory up-regulations of SERCA2 and SPCA1 [161].

The CaSR positively modulates calcium transport into milk during lactation based on serum Ca^{2+}_0 level and, as noted above, is expressed on the basolateral membranes of mammary duct epithelial cells where it is up-regulated during lactation [158]. In support of its proposed role, low Ca^{2+}_0 levels suppressed the calcium content of mouse milk and the calcimimetic NPS R467 ameliorated the effect [3]. These activities have important consequences for the maternal and infant skeletons. First, with respect to the maternal skeleton, by stimulating calcium transfer from the blood into milk, up-regulated CaSR expression in lactating mammary epithelial cells lowers serum Ca^{2+}_0 to promote calcium mobilization and depletion from bone, requiring restoration of bone mineral content at the termination of lactation. Second, with respect to the infant skeleton, up-regulated CaSR expression in lactating mammary epithelial cells supports postnatal development.

4.6.5 CaSR-Dependent Control of Intestinal Calcium and Phosphate Absorption

The CaSR does not appear to promote small intestinal calcium and/or phosphate absorption. Based on its low level of expression and relative concentration in basal rather than apical membranes [162], the intestinal epithelial cell CaSR appears to have only a limited and perhaps negative role in the modulation of calcium absorption, analogous to its negative modulatory role in the renal thick ascending limb, particularly in the context of hypercalcemia [14]. CaSRs expressed on endocrine cells in other tissues, however, contribute to the negative control of intestinal calcium and/or phosphate absorption via suppression of calcitriol synthesis in renal proximal tubule cells [132].

4.6.6 CaSR-Dependent Control of Macronutrient Digestion and Absorption

The CaSR is expressed at high levels in entero-endocrine cells of the gastrointestinal tract and responds to elevated concentrations of Ca_0^{2+} and/or amino acids with enhanced release of gut hormones including gastrin from G cells [106,163], cholecystokinin from I cells [107,108], GIP from K cells, and GLP1 and PYY from L cells [109]. The consequences include enhanced digestion, absorption, nutrient disposition, and satiety. In addition to promoting gastric acid secretion via enterochromaffin-like (ECL) cell-dependent release of histamine, gastrin also acts outside the gut. One potentially important site with respect to metabolic bone disease is the calcitonin-secreting C cell, that expresses gastrin-sensitive type B CCK receptors [164].

Gastrin stimulates calcitonin release in support of a mechanism whereby ingested calcium and protein induce nutrient-dependent suppression of bone resorption [165]. Thus, the CaSR senses macronutrient-derived amino acid signals and modulates both macronutrient and micronutrient metabolism, providing links between dietary protein intake and calcium metabolism [45,110,166].

4.7 BIOLOGICAL ROLES IN BONE AND CARTILAGE

4.7.1 Actions in Growth Plate, Osteoblasts, and Osteoclasts

4.7.1.1 Expression and Functional Consequences in Bone Cells

The CaSR is expressed in bone cells of various lineages including mesenchymal stem cells, growth plate chondrocytes, pre-osteoblasts, osteoblasts, osteocytes, pre-osteoclasts, and osteoclasts [167]. It also modulates the functions of these cells in ways that generally promote bone formation and maintain bone mass as described in the box in Section 4.4.1.2. However, some, but not all, CaSR activators induce functional effects leading to considerable confusion. Does the CaSR mediate all the effects of Ca_0^{2+} in these cells? Why are the effects of some activators so modest? Are some divalent cation-dependent functions mediated by other candidate Ca_0^{2+}-sensing receptors, such as one of the metabotropic glutamate receptors [168,169] or the GABA(B) receptor [170], or are they mediated by heterodimers formed between the CaSR and other receptor(s) as suggested for CaSR-GABA(B1) and/or CaSR-GABA(B2) in chondrocytes [23]?

In attempting to answer these questions, the functional significance of the CaSR for skeletal growth and bone metabolism has been assessed in transgenic mice that are null for one of the CaSR's six translated exons either on a global, tissue-selective, or combined tissue-selective and developmental basis. The outcomes of these studies demonstrate that in mice and perhaps other mammals, the CaSR has critical non-redundant functions in support of pre-osteoblast and/or osteoblast differentiation and osteogenesis, as well as differentiation of growth plate chondrocytes in support of growth plate function to promote linear growth [5].

4.7.1.2 Global CaSR Exon 5-Null Mice and Double Knockout Rescues

The earliest CaSR transgenic mouse model was a global knockout in which CaSR exon 5 was disrupted by the insertion of a neomycin resistance cassette [171]. Exon 5 encodes 77 amino acids (residues 460 through 536 of the human CaSR; casrdb.mcgill. ca) that contribute to the C-terminus of the nutrient-binding VFT domain immediately prior to the Cys-rich domain. Homozygous global CaSR exon5-null mice exhibited features of severe primary hyperparathyroidism and heterozygous mice exhibited features of familial hypocalciuric hypercalcemia [171] conforming to the established patterns of human disease arising from inactivating mutations of the CaSR [172,173].

The severe bone disease in homozygous global exon 5 knockout mice was shown to arise exclusively or almost exclusively from the markedly elevated serum PTH levels by rescue of the phenotype in double null mice in which either parathyroid gland development was suppressed by deletion of Gcm2 [174] or the PreProPTH gene was disabled [175]. These findings appeared to eliminate the skeleton and, thus, growth plate chondrocytes, osteoblasts, osteocytes, and osteoclasts as key sites of CaSR expression and function. In addition, the findings were consistent with restoration of skeletal growth and normal bone metabolism following total parathyroidectomy and combined treatment with calcium supplements and active vitamin D analogs in patients with neonatal severe primary hyperparathyroidism [176].

The situation described above was "turned on its head" following the demonstration that CaSR exon 5 is subject physiologically to in-frame alternative splicing and that an exon5-minus in-frame splice variant retains residual function in endogenous cells of various lineages including keratinocytes [177,178], growth plate chondrocytes [179], and epithelial cells of the developing lung [180]. Whether residual CaSR function from the exon 5-minus splice variant arises from homodimers or requires the formation of heterodimers with other receptors is unclear.

In favor of the latter idea, exon 5-minus CaSRs expressed heterologously in HEK-293 cells were not trafficked to the plasma membranes and failed to activate phospholipase C, but when expressed endogenously in growth plate chondrocytes prepared from CaSR exon 5-null mice, they were trafficked successfully to the plasma membranes and activated phospholipase C [179]. These findings demonstrated that new transgenic mouse models were required to properly investigate the significance of the CaSR for skeletal development and growth as well as maintenance of bone mass and mineralization.

4.7.1.3 Tissue-Selective (Conditional) CaSR-Null Mice

Conditional deletions of CaSR exon 7 in a tissue and development stage-selective manner provided a radically different view of the CaSR's roles in normal endochondral bone formation and skeletal development. In these strategies, CaSR exon 7-floxed mice were cross-bred with mice expressing Cre recombinase under the control of selected promoters including the PTH promoter for parathyroid cells, the type-I collagen α1-subunit and osterix promoters for pre-osteoblasts and osteoblasts, and the type-II collagen α1-subunit for chondrocytes [5]. Since exon 7 encodes the last 35 amino acids of the N-terminal extracellular domain (residues 578 to 612), the entire HH domain, and intracellular C-terminus, its deletion eliminates signaling from the G protein-binding core of the HH domain as well as receptor interactions with cytoplasmic protein partners such as those responsible for assembling signaling scaffolds, e.g., in caveolae [25].

Tissue-selective deletion of CaSR exon 7 in the parathyroid gland induced primary hyperparathyroidism with markedly elevated serum Ca^{2+} and PTH levels arising from impaired feedback inhibition of PTH secretion together with hypercalciuria, consistent with intact CaSR function in the renal thick ascending limb [5]. On the other hand, in osteoblast-specific CaSR knockout mice specified by the type-I collagen $\alpha 1$ subunit promoter activity, parathyroid gland function and thus serum Ca^{2+}_0 and PTH levels were normal but postnatal skeletal development and linear growth were markedly impaired in association with attenuated expression of IGF-1 [5], a key local growth factor [181].

Surprisingly, tissue-selective deletion of CaSR exon 7 in chondrocytes (including growth plate chondrocytes) under the control of the type II collagen $\alpha 1$ subunit promoter was embryonic lethal. In response, the transgenic mouse model was redesigned to provide tamoxifen-dependent control of Cre recombinase expression under the col(II)$\alpha 1$-subunit promoter [5]. In late fetal and postnatal life, mice homozygous for the mutant construct were exposed to tamoxifen, resulting in selective deletion of the CaSR from chondrocytes, leading to impaired growth of the long bones. The results demonstrate that the CaSR has a positive role in the modulation of growth plate function.

4.7.1.4 Assessment of Bone Phenotypes in Humans with CaSR Mutations

Despite the foregoing observations in transgenic mice, patients with homozygous or compound heterozygous inactivating mutations of the CaSR typically present with a single disorder—neonatal severe primary hyperparathyroidism in which the key disturbances are marked elevations in the serum calcium and PTH levels [9]. In addition, these infants have high bone turnover and accelerated bone resorption leading to pathological fractures. Interestingly, the clinical problem responds to total parathyroidectomy, calcium supplements, and therapy with calcitriol [117]. Thus, it is not clear whether loss of CaSR function in humans has the same catastrophic effect on skeletal development as described above in mice.

Two possible explanations for the discrepancies between the phenotypes in conditional exon 7 knockout mice and humans bearing homozygous or compound heterozygous CaSR mutations are as follows: (1) humans with NSHPT may be protected generally from major developmental abnormalities by residual CaSR function except in the most severe cases associated with deletions or truncations of the mutant receptors [182,183]; and (2) there may be a species-related difference in function such that developmental processes that require the CaSR in mice are provided by or can be compensated by another class C GPCR in humans.

4.7.2 Cellular Basis of CaSR Functions in Cells of Osteoblast Lineage

Although these phenotypic changes demonstrate roles for the CaSR in skeletal growth and development, the cellular and molecular mechanisms that underlie them are uncertain. Furthermore, the roles of CaSRs in coordinating global nutritional responses are not well understood. The CaSR supports cell functions in the bone microenvironment via three main mechanisms:

1. Dependent upon its expression (e.g., secondary to cytokines IL-1β, IL-6, or calcitriol), alone or in the context of an expressed partner with signaling initiated by physiological levels of activators including Ca_0^{2+}, amino acids, polyamines and/or glutathione analogs;
2. In response to local increases in the concentrations of activators including Ca_0^{2+} in the resorptive pit and in the regional extracellular fluid [184] to provide signals for the chemotaxis, attachment, and subsequent differentiation of pre-osteoblasts to osteoblasts;
3. In response to general increases in the concentrations of Ca_0^{2+} and/or other nutrient activators such as following the digestion and absorption of macro- and micronutrients.

In support of the first mechanism, CaSR expression in fetal rat calvarial cells mediates proliferation, differentiation, matrix synthesis, and mineralization in the presence of physiological levels of Ca_0^{2+} (i.e., around 1.2 mM) as revealed by the inhibitory effect of the calcilytic NPS 89636 [87]. In support of the second mechanism, high Ca_0^{2+} levels (around 3 to 20 mM) suppress osteoclastogenesis [185], induce osteoclast apoptosis [186], and markedly impair osteoclast-dependent bone resorption [187]. In addition, elevated Ca_0^{2+} acts as an early signal in support of osteoblast chemotaxis to sites of active bone resorption [188]. Finally, in support of the third mechanism, the CaSR mediates positive effects of dietary calcium on trabecular bone volume, tibial length, and mineral apposition rate as well as osteoblast number and expression of genes supporting bone formation including Cbfa-1, type-I collagen, alkaline phosphatase, and osteocalcin [189]. The CaSR also couples nutrient signals to the local synthesis of insulin-like growth factor-1 (IGF-1) in bone [5] and is a candidate L-amino acid sensor for the positive effects of dietary proteins on serum IGF-1 levels [110].

4.7.3   SIGNALING MECHANISMS UNDERLYING PRO-ANABOLIC EFFECTS ON BONE

It has not been clear whether Ca_0^{2+}-sensing in bone cells is mediated by the CaSR wholly, in part, or not at all. As a result, information on the roles of signaling pathways in coupling CaSR receptor activation to biological effects including survival, chemotaxis, proliferation, and differentiation, is limited. The available information is summarized below.

4.7.3.1   Chemotaxis, Survival, and Proliferation

Studies of signaling mechanisms underlying chemotaxis have focused on MC 3T3-E1 cells in which roles have been identified for $G_{q/11}$ as revealed by the effects of inhibitors of PI-PLCβ, $G_{i/o}$ as revealed by the impact of pertussis toxin, and PLCγ downstream of PKC activity [64]. The CaSR also mediates Sr^{2+}-dependent cell survival in human fetal osteoblasts [73].

Various signaling pathways contribute to CaSR-dependent up-regulation of proliferation in pre-osteoblasts and osteoblasts. In rat calvarial osteoblasts, the JNK MAP kinase has been implicated by experiments employing SP600125 [79]. In MC3T3-E1 cells, on the other hand, phosphorylated $ERK_{1/2}$ and p38 have been implicated in CaSR-mediated up-regulation of proliferation by experiments employing inhibitors of these enzymes, PD98059 and SB203580, respectively [190].

4.7.3.2   Differentiation, Matrix Synthesis, and Suppression of Negative Modulators of Mineralization

Differentiation of osteoblasts takes the form of a tightly coupled molecular program that drives the coordinated expression of growth factors and their receptors, followed by the secretion of matrix proteins such as type-I collagen, osteocalcin, and osteopontin to provide an extracellular scaffold into which calcium- and phosphate-rich matrix microvesicles are released. Mineralization proceeds dependent on negative modulation of pyrophosphate-dependent inhibition via the actions of tissue-specific alkaline phosphatase and/or the Ank pyrophosphate transport protein [111]. CaSRs expressed on osteoblasts enhance mineralization by suppressing expression of (1) ecto-nucleotide pyrophosphatase/phosphodiesterase-1 (ENPP1), the enzyme that catalyzes the synthesis of pyrophosphate (PP_i) from nucleoside triphosphates and (2) Ank, which mediates export of PP_i from the cytoplasm into the extracellular space [115].

CaSR activation by elevated Ca_o^{2+} or Gd_o^{3+} in rat fetal calvarial cells induced differentiation as revealed by enhanced expression of Cbfa1, osteocalcin, osteopontin, alkaline phosphatase, and type-I collagen [87]. In addition, enhanced formation of mineralized nodules was noted. The signaling mechanism responsible for these effects is uncertain. However, CaSR activation was coupled to the phosphorylation of $ERK_{1/2}$, Akt, and GSK-3 [87] as observed for Sr^{2+}-induced CaSR-mediated differentiation in human fetal osteoblasts [73]. Interestingly, in this latter system, the Akt inhibitor AKT-1 suppressed nuclear translocation of β-catenin [73], consistent with the notion that Akt phosphorylation is critical to osteoblast differentiation and enhanced osteoblast-dependent matrix synthesis and mineralization. More work is required to properly describe the signaling components that support CaSR-mediated differentiation of pre-osteoblasts.

4.7.4   Roles in Osteoclastogenesis and Osteoclastic Bone Resorption

The CaSR contributes to the negative modulation of osteoclastogenesis via effects on osteoblast-dependent expression of RANKL and OPG [70,115]. In addition, it is expressed in pre-osteoclasts and osteoclasts, and negatively modulates osteoclast-dependent bone resorption [185,187]. Some reports, however, also identified pro-osteoclastogenic effects of the CaSR and appear to point to maturation-dependent positive and negative control of osteoclast function [186].

Consistent with this notion, elevated Ca_o^{2+} positively modulated osteoclast formation in co-cultures of osteoblasts and osteoclast precursors in the absence of the differentiating factors calcitriol and mCSF, but negatively modulated osteoclast formation in their presence [191]. Furthermore, RAW 264.7 osteoclasts exhibited biphasic Ca_o^{2+}

concentration-dependent control of cell migration. Thus, in the range 2 to 10 mM, Ca_o^{2+} enhanced migration; at higher concentrations from 10 to 20 mM, however, Ca_o^{2+} suppressed migration [192]. The CaSR was directly implicated in enhanced migration in the lower Ca_o^{2+} concentration range by the negative impact of CaSR-specific siRNA.

4.8   CaSR-BASED THERAPEUTICS FOR OSTEOPOROSIS

4.8.1   PHENYLALKYLAMINE CALCIMIMETICS

Despite the expression of CaSRs in cells of the osteoblast and osteoclast lineages, none of the phenylalkylamine calcimimetics including NPS R-467, NPS R-568, and cinacalcet that effectively lower serum calcium levels via positive modulatory actions on CaSRs in parathyroid and renal cortical thick ascending limb cells have been reported to act as effective modulators of osteoblast or chondrocyte survival, proliferation, or differentiation. These findings support the notion that Ca_o^{2+} sensing is mediated by a distinct receptor or by CaSR heterodimers that are resistant to the actions of these calcimimetics. If this is true, it is interesting that no such limitation on the inhibitory actions of calcilytics have been noted. Thus, the calcilytic 89636 suppressed Ca_o^{2+}-induced proliferation and differentiation of osteoblasts in primary culture [87].

4.8.2   STRONTIUM RANELATE

Strontium ranelate has been successfully introduced into clinical practice for the prevention of osteoporotic fractures [196]. It dissociates bone resorption and bone formation by promoting bone formation and suppressing bone resorption [197]. Its effects are surprisingly diverse. Thus, it promotes the commitment of mesenchymal stem cells to the osteoblast lineage and away from adipocytes [198]. It also promotes signaling pathways that promote osteoblast survival, proliferation, and differentiation, restrain osteoclastogenesis, and impair osteoclast survival and function [197].

The active component, extracellular Sr^{2+} stimulates signaling pathways in bone cells at pharmacologically relevant concentrations (around 0.01 to 0.2 mM) and several of its effects are impaired when the CaSR is knocked down [73]. In addition, Sr^{2+} exhibits biased agonism with respect to CaSR-mediated $ERK_{1/2}$ phosphorylation and calcitonin release from thyroid C cells [199]. These findings implicate the CaSR as a key target for the positive effects of Sr^{2+} in bone.

The CaSR is implicated in several actions of Sr^{2+} in osteoblasts including positive modulation of proliferation, differentiation, and survival, at least in part via effects on canonical Wnt signaling [73] and enhanced Cbfa1 (also known as Runx2) expression [70,200]. It also acts as a negative modulator of osteoclastogenesis via coordinated down-regulation of RANKL expression and up-regulation of osteoprotegerin (OPG) [70]. In osteoclasts, on the other hand, Sr^{2+} impairs RANKL signaling [201] and enhances apoptosis [202]. Whether the CaSR mediates all the effects of Sr^{2+} is currently uncertain.

4.8.3 CALCILYTICS

As noted above, calcilytics are negative modulators of the CaSR that typically bind in the receptor's HH domain [193]. Considerable effort has gone into the development of potent oral calcilytics that are rapidly absorbed, acutely inhibit parathyroid CaSRs, and thus stimulate PTH secretion [95]. If successful, an oral calcilytic with these properties would induce spikes in the serum PTH level that resemble those seen in patients receiving subcutaneous teriparatide (human PTH 1-34) and produce anabolic bone responses. Thus far, none of the calcilytics that entered clinical trials has emulated the impact of teriparatide on markers of bone formation or bone density [194]. One possible explanation is CaSR-dependent inhibition of osteoblast function in bone. Another is inadequate efficacy as revealed by peak serum PTH levels that are $\leq 25\%$ of those observed in response to subcutaneous injections of teriparatide [195].

4.9 SUMMARY

CaSR expression supports Ca_0^{2+}-dependent feedback regulation of key components of calcium homeostasis including inhibition of PTH synthesis and secretion, inhibition of renal calcium reabsorption, and activation of calcitonin secretion. Release of CaSR-dependent inhibition of PTH secretion is a key event in the defense against hypocalcemia. On the other hand, CaSR-dependent suppression of renal calcium reabsorption and activation of calcitonin act as defenses against hypercalcemia.

The CaSR also plays important roles in the skeleton by modulating the function of the growth plate and cellular activity in support of bone modeling and remodeling. Because of its key roles in calcium homeostasis and bone metabolism, the CaSR has proven an effective target, particularly in the treatment of hyperparathyroidism (cinacalcet) and osteoporosis (strontium ranelate). It remains to be seen whether potent short-acting oral calcilytics alone or in combination with other agents will be effective treatments for osteoporosis and other metabolic bone disorders.

ACKNOWLEDGMENTS

The author's research on the roles of calcium sensing receptors in the control of mineral metabolism received generous support from the NHMRC of Australia.

REFERENCES

1. Brown EM et al. 1993. Cloning and characterization of an extracellular Ca^{2+}-sensing receptor from bovine parathyroid. *Nature* 366: 575–580.
2. Brown EM and MacLeod RJ. 2001. Extracellular calcium sensing and extracellular calcium signaling. *Physiol Rev* 81: 239–297.
3. VanHouten J et al. 2004. The calcium sensing receptor regulates mammary gland parathyroid hormone-related protein production and calcium transport. *J Clin Invest* 113: 598–608.

4. Kovacs CS et al. 1998. Regulation of murine fetal-placental calcium metabolism by the calcium sensing receptor. *J Clin Invest* 101: 2812–2820.

5. Chang W et al. 2008. The extracellular calcium-sensing receptor (CaSR) is a critical modulator of skeletal development. *Sci Signal* 1: 1.

6. Rey O et al. 2012. Negative cross-talk between calcium sensing receptor and β-catenin signaling systems in colonic epithelium. *J Biol Chem* 287: 1158–1167.

7. Riccardi D and Kemp P. 2012. The calcium sensing receptor beyond extracellular calcium homeostasis: conception, development, adult physiology, and disease. *Annu Rev Physiol* 74: 271–297.

8. Conigrave AD et al. 2000. L-amino acid sensing by the extracellular Ca^{2+}-sensing receptor. *Proc Natl Acad Sci USA* 97: 4814–4819.

9. Hendy GN et al. 2000. Mutations of the calcium sensing receptor (CaSR) in familial hypocalciuric hypercalcemia, neonatal severe hyperparathyroidism, and autosomal dominant hypocalcemia. *Hum Mutat* 16: 281–296.

10. Canaff L and Hendy G. 2005. Calcium sensing receptor gene transcription is up-regulated by the proinflammatory cytokine, interleukin-1β: role of the NF-κB pathway and κB elements. *J Biol Chem* 280: 14177–14188.

11. Canaff L et al. 2008. The proinflammatory cytokine, interleukin-6, up-regulates calcium sensing receptor gene transcription via Stat1/3 and Sp1/3. *J Biol Chem* 283: 13586–13600.

12. Canaff L and Hendy GN. 2002. Human calcium sensing receptor gene: vitamin D response elements in promoters P1 and P2 confer transcriptional responsiveness to 1,25-dihydroxyvitamin D. *J Biol Chem* 277: 30337–30350.

13. Klein G. 2011. Burns: where has all the calcium (and vitamin D) gone? *Adv Nutr* 2: 457–462.

14. Kantham L et al. 2009. The calcium sensing receptor (CaSR) defends against hypercalcemia independently of its regulation of parathyroid hormone secretion. *Am J Physiol Endocrinol Metabol* 297: E915–E923.

15. Egbuna O et al. 2009. The full-length calcium sensing receptor dampens the calcemic response to 1α,25(OH)$_2$ vitamin D3 in vivo independently of parathyroid hormone. *Am J Physiol Renal Physiol* 297: F720–F728.

16. Loupy A et al. 2012. PTH-independent regulation of blood calcium concentration by the calcium sensing receptor. *J Clin Invest* 122: 3355–3367.

17. Tsuchiya D et al. 2002. Structural views of the ligand-binding cores of a metabotropic glutamate receptor complexed with an antagonist and both glutamate and Gd3+. *Proc Natl Acad Sci USA* 99: 2660–2665.

18. Kunishima N et al. 2000. Structural basis of glutamate recognition by a dimeric metabotropic glutamate receptor. *Nature* 407: 971–977.

19. Muto T et al. 2007. Structures of the extracellular regions of the group II/III metabotropic glutamate receptors. *Proc Natl Acad Sci USA* 104: 3759–3764.

20. Hu J et al. 2005. A region critical in the seven-transmembrane domain of the human Ca^{2+} receptor critical for response to Ca^{2+}. *J Biol Chem* 280: 5113–5120.

21. Khan MA and Conigrave AD. 2010. Mechanisms of multimodal sensing by extracellular Ca^{2+}-sensing receptors: a domain-based survey of requirements for binding and signalling. *Br J Pharmacol* 159: 1039–1050.

22. Chang W et al. 2007. Complex formation with the Type B γ-aminobutyric acid receptor affects the expression and signal transduction of the extracellular calcium sensing receptor: studies with HEK-293 cells and neurons. *J Biol Chem* 282: 25030–25040.

23. Cheng Z et al. 2007. Type B γ-aminobutyric acid receptors modulate the function of the extracellular Ca^{2+}-sensing receptor and cell differentiation in murine growth plate chondrocytes. *Endocrinology* 148: 4984–4992.

24. Gama L et al. 2001. Heterodimerization of calcium sensing receptors with metabotropic glutamate receptors in neurons. *J Biol Chem* 276: 39053–39059.

25. Kifor O et al. 1998. The calcium sensing receptor is localized in caveolin-rich plasma membrane domains of bovine parathyroid cells. *J Biol Chem* 273: 21708–21713.

26. Stahlhut M and Deurs Bv. 2000. Identification of filamin as a novel ligand for caveolin-1: evidence for the organization of caveolin-1-associated membrane domains by the actin cytoskeleton. *Mol Biol Cell* 11: 325–337.

27. Pi M et al. 2002. Calcium sensing receptor activation of rho involves filamin and rho-guanine nucleotide exchange factor. *Endocrinology* 143: 3830–3838

28. Huang C et al. 2004. The Ca^{2+}-sensing receptor couples to $G\alpha12/13$ to activate phospholipase D in Madin-Darby canine kidney cells *Am J Physiol Cell Physiol* 286: C22–C30.

29. Davies SL et al. 2006. Calcium sensing receptor induces rho kinase-mediated actin stress fiber assembly and altered cell morphology though not in response to aromatic amino acids. *Am J Physiol Cell Physiol* 290: 1543–1551.

30. Huang C et al. 2009. Activation of choline kinase by extracellular Ca^{2+} is Ca^{2+}-sensing receptor, $G\alpha12$ and ρ-dependent in breast cancer cells. *Cell Signal* 21: 1894–1900.

31. Hjalm G et al. 2001. Filamin-A binds to the carboxyl-terminal tail of the calcium sensing receptor, an interaction that participates in CaR-mediated activation of mitogen-activated protein kinase. *J Biol Chem* 276: 34880–34887.

32. Huang Y et al. 2006. Calcium sensing receptor ubiquitination and degradation mediated by the E3 ubiquitin ligase dorfin. *J Biol Chem* 281: 11610–11617.

33. Itoh F et al. 2001. Promoting bone morphogenetic protein signaling through negative regulation of inhibitory Smads. *EMBO J* 20: 4132–4142.

34. Huang C et al. 2007. Interaction of the Ca^{2+}-sensing receptor with the inwardly rectifying potassium channels Kir4.1 and Kir4.2 results in inhibition of channel function. *Am J Physiol Renal Physiol* 292: F1073–F1081.

35. Cha S et al. 2011. Calcium sensing receptor decreases cell surface expression of the inwardly rectifying K+ channel Kir4.1. *J Biol Chem* 286: 1828–1835.

36. Arulpragasam A et al. 2012. The adaptor protein 14-3-3 binds to the calcium sensing receptor and attenuates receptor-mediated ρ kinase signalling. *Biochem J* 441: 995–1006.

37. Magno A et al. 2011. Testin, a novel binding partner of the calcium sensing receptor, enhances receptor-mediated ρ-kinase signalling. *Biochem Biophys Res Commun* 412: 584–589.

38. Huang Y et al. 2010. Calmodulin regulates Ca^{2+}-sensing receptor-mediated Ca^{2+} signaling and its cell surface expression. *J Biol Chem* 285: 35919–35931.

39. Cavanaugh A et al. 2010. Calcium sensing receptor biosynthesis includes a co-translational conformational checkpoint and endoplasmic reticulum retention. *J Biol Chem* 285: 19854–19864.

40. Huang Y and Breitwieser G. 2007. Rescue of calcium sensing receptor mutants by allosteric modulators reveals a conformational checkpoint in receptor biogenesis. *J Biol Chem* 282: 9517–9525.

41. Leach K et al. 2012. Identification of molecular phenotypes and biased signaling induced by naturally occurring mutations of the human calcium sensing receptor. *Endocrinology* 153: 4304–4316.

42. Breitwieser G. 2012. Minireview: the intimate link between calcium sensing receptor trafficking and signaling: implications for disorders of calcium homeostasis. *Mol Endocrinol* 26: 1482–1495.

43. Grant M et al. 2011. Agonist-driven maturation and plasma membrane insertion of calcium sensing receptors dynamically control signal amplitude. *Sci Signal* 4: 78.

44. Gerbino A et al. 2005. Termination of cAMP signals by Ca^{2+} and $G(\alpha)i$ via extracellular Ca^{2+} sensors: a link to intracellular Ca^{2+} oscillations. *J Cell Biol* 171: 303–312.

45. Conigrave AD et al. 2004. L-amino acids regulate parathyroid hormone secretion. *J Biol Chem* 279: 38151–38159.

46. Huang Y et al. 2009. Multiple Ca^{2+}-binding sites in the extracellular domain of the Ca^{2+}-sensing receptor corresponding to cooperative Ca^{2+} response. *Biochemistry* 48: 388–398.

47. Ray K et al. 1999. Identification of the cysteine residues in the amino terminal extracellular domain of the human Ca^{2+} receptor critical for dimerization: implications for function of monomeric Ca^{2+} receptor. *J Biol Chem* 274: 27642–27650.

48. Gama L and Breitwieser GE. 1998. A carboxyl terminal domain controls the cooperativity for extracellular Ca^{2+} activation of the human calcium sensing receptor: a study with receptor–green fluorescent protein fusions. *J Biol Chem* 273: 29712–29718.

49. Lorenz S et al. 2007. Functional desensitization of the extracellular calcium sensing receptor is regulated via distinct mechanisms: role of G protein-coupled receptor kinases, protein kinase C and β-arrestins. *Endocrinology* 148: 2398–2404.

50. Fitzpatrick LA et al. 1986. Prostaglandin F2a and α-adrenergic agonists regulate parathyroid cell function via the inhibitory guanine nucleotide regulatory protein. *Endocrinology* 118: 2115–2119.

51. Fitzpatrick LA et al. 1986. Calcium-controlled secretion is effected through a guanine nucleotide regulatory protein in parathyroid cells. *Endocrinology* 119: 2700–2703.

52. Chen CJ et al. 1989. Divalent cations suppress 3',5'-adenosine monophosphate accumulation by stimulating a pertussis toxin sensitive guanine nucleotide-binding protein in cultured bovine parathyroid cells. *Endocrinology* 124: 233–239.

53. Kifor O et al. 2001. Regulation of MAP kinase by calcium sensing receptor in bovine parathyroid and CaR-transfected HEK-293 cells. *Am J Physiol Renal Physiol* 280: F291–F302.

54. Avlani V et al. 2013. Calcium sensing receptor-dependent activation of CREB phosphorylation in HEK-293 cells and human parathyroid cells. *Am J Physiol Endocrinol Metabol* 304, E1097–E1104.

55. Pierce K et al. 2001. New mechanisms in heptahelical receptor signaling to mitogen activated protein kinase cascades. *Oncogene* 20: 1532–1539.

56. Nemeth EF and Scarpa A. 1986. Cytosolic Ca^{2+} and the regulation of secretion in parathyroid cells. *FEBS Lett* 203: 15–19.

57. Nemeth EF and Scarpa A. 1987. Rapid mobilization of cellular Ca^{2+} in bovine parathyroid cells evoked by extracellular divalent cations: evidence for a cell surface calcium receptor. *J Biol Chem* 262: 5188–5196.

58. Brown EM et al. 1987. High extracellular Ca^{2+} and Mg^{2+} stimulate accumulation of inositol phosphates in bovine parathyroid cells. *FEBS Lett* 218: 113–118.

59. Chang W et al. 2000. Amino acids in the second and third intracellular loops of the parathyroid Ca^{2+}-sensing receptor mediate efficient coupling to phospholipase C. *J Biol Chem* 275: 19955–19963.

60. Ray K et al. 1997. The carboxyl terminus of the human calcium receptor: requirements for cell-surface expression and signal transduction. *J Biol Chem* 272: 31355–31361.

61. Chang W et al. 2001. Amino acids in the cytoplasmic C terminus of the parathyroid Ca^{2+}-sensing receptor mediate efficient cell-surface expression and phospholipase C activation. *J Biol Chem* 276: 44129–44136.

62. Brennan SC and Conigrave AD. 2009. Regulation of cellular signal transduction pathways by the extracellular calcium sensing receptor. *Curr Pharmaceut Biotechnol* 10: 270–281.

63. Wettschureck N et al. 2007. Parathyroid-specific double knockout of Gq and G11 α subunits leads to a phenotype resembling germline knockout of the extracellular Ca^{2+}-sensing receptor. *Mol Endocrinol* 21: 274–280.

64. Godwin S and Soltoff S. 2002. Calcium sensing receptor-mediated activation of phospholipase C-γ1 is downstream of phospholipase C-β and protein kinase C in MC3T3-E1 osteoblasts. *Bone* 30: 559–566.

65. Beierwaltes W. 2010. The role of calcium in the regulation of renin secretion. *Am J Physiol Renal Physiol* 298: F1–F11.

66. Siehler S. 2009. Regulation of ρ GEF proteins by G12/13-coupled receptors. *Br J Pharmacol* 158: 41–49.

67. Kelly P et al. 2007. Biologic functions of the G12 subfamily of heterotrimeric G proteins: growth, migration, and metastasis. *Biochemistry* 46: 6677–6687.

68. Rey O et al. 2005. Amino acid-stimulated Ca^{2+} oscillations produced by the Ca^{2+}-sensing receptor are mediated by a phospholipase C/inositol 1,4,5-trisphosphate-independent pathway that requires G12, rho, filamin-A, and the actin cytoskeleton. *J Biol Chem* 280: 22875–22882.

69. Wang J and Stern P. 2010. Osteoclastogenic activity and RANKL expression are inhibited in osteoblastic cells expressing constitutively active Gα(12) or constitutively active rho A. *J Cell Biochem* 111: 1531–1536.

70. Brennan T et al. 2009. Osteoblasts play key roles in the mechanisms of action of strontium ranelate. *Br J Pharmacol* 157: 1291–1300.

71. Jiang L et al. 2008. Regulation of cAMP responses by the G12/13 pathway converges on adenylyl cyclase VII. *J Biol Chem.* 283: 23429–23439.

72. Mamillapalli R et al. 2008. Switching of G protein usage by the calcium sensing receptor reverses its effect on parathyroid hormone-related protein secretion in normal versus malignant breast cells. *J Biol Chem* 283: 24435–24447.

73. Rybchyn MS et al. 2011. An Akt-dependent increase in canonical Wnt signaling and a decrease in sclerostin protein levels are involved in strontium ranelate-induced osteogenic effects in human osteoblasts. *J Biol Chem* 286: 23771–23779.

74. McCormick WD et al. 2010. Increased receptor stimulation elicits differential calcium sensing receptor T888 dephosphorylation. *J Biol Chem* 285: 14170–14177.

75. Mamillapalli R and Wysolmerski J. 2010. The calcium sensing receptor couples to Galpha(s) and regulates PTHrP and ACTH secretion in pituitary cells. *J Endocrinol* 204: 287–297.

76. Choudhary S et al. 2004. Extracellular calcium induces COX-2 in osteoblasts via a PKA pathway. *Biochem Biophys Res Commun* 322: 395–402.

77. Magno A et al. 2011. The calcium sensing receptor: a molecular perspective. *Endocr Rev* 32: 330.

78. Pi M and Quarles L. 2005. Osteoblast calcium sensing receptor has characteristics of ANF/7TM receptors. *J Cell Biochem* 95: 1081–1092.

79. Chattopadhyay N et al. 2004. Mitogenic action of calcium sensing receptor on rat calvarial osteoblasts. *Endocrinology* 145: 3451–3462.

80. MacLeod RJ et al. 2003. PTHrP stimulated by the calcium sensing receptor requires MAP kinase activation. *Am J Physiol Endocrinol Metab* 284: E435–E442.

81. MacLeod RJ et al. 2004. Extracellular calcium sensing receptor transactivates the epidermal growth factor receptor by a triple membrane-spanning signaling mechanism. *Biochem Biophys Res Commun* 320: 455–460.

82. Yano S et al. 2004. Calcium sensing receptor activation stimulates parathyroid hormone-related protein secretion in prostate cancer cells: role of epidermal growth factor receptor transactivation. *Bone* 35: 664–672.

83. Thiel G et al. 2012. Transcriptional response to calcium sensing receptor stimulation. *Endocrinology* 153: 4716–4728.
84. Huang Y et al. 2007. Identification and dissection of Ca^{2+}-binding sites in the extracellular domain of Ca^{2+}-sensing receptor. *J Biol Chem* 282: 19000–19010.
85. Ray K and Northup J. 2002. Evidence for distinct cation and calcimimetic compound (NPS 568) recognition domains in the transmembrane regions of the human Ca^{2+} receptor. *J Biol Chem* 277: 18908–18913.
86. Mun H et al. 2005. A double mutation in the extracellular Ca^{2+}-sensing receptor's Venus fly trap domain that selectively disables L-amino acid sensing. *J Biol Chem* 280: 29067–29072.
87. Dvorak MM et al. 2004. Physiological changes in extracellular calcium concentration directly control osteoblast function in the absence of calciotropic hormones. *Proc Natl Acad Sci USA* 101: 5140–5145.
88. Conigrave AD and Hampson DR. 2010. Broad-spectrum amino acid-sensing class C G-protein coupled receptors: molecular mechanisms, physiological significance and options for drug development. *Pharmacol Therap* 127: 252–260.
89. Wang M et al. 2006. Activation of family C G-protein-coupled receptors by the tripeptide glutathione. *J Biol Chem* 281: 8864–8870.
90. Broadhead G et al. 2011. Allosteric modulation of the calcium sensing receptor by γ-glutamyl peptides: inhibition of PTH secretion, suppression of intracellular cAMP levels and a common mechanism of action with L-amino acids. *J Biol Chem* 286: 8786–8797.
91. Davey A et al. 2012. Positive and negative allosteric modulators promote biased signaling at the calcium sensing receptor. *Endocrinology* 153: 1232–1241.
92. Nemeth E et al. 2004. Pharmacodynamics of the type II calcimimetic compound cinacalcet HCl. *J Pharmacol Exp Ther* 308: 627–635.
93. Nemeth EF et al. 1998. Calcimimetics with potent and selective activity on the parathyroid calcium receptor. *Proc Natl Acad Sci USA* 95: 4040–4045.
94. Nemeth EF et al. 2001. Calcilytic compounds: potent and selective Ca^{2+} receptor antagonists that stimulate secretion of parathyroid hormone. *J Pharmacol Exp Therap* 299: 323–331.
95. Nemeth EF. 2002. The search for calcium receptor antagonists (calcilytics). *J Mol Endocrinol* 29: 15–21.
96. Larqué E et al. 2007. Biological significance of dietary polyamines. *Nutrition* 23: 87–95.
97. Anderson DJ et al. 1975. The actions of spermidine and spermine on the central nervous system. *Neuropharmacology* 14: 571–577.
98. Kroigaard M et al. 1992. Polyamines in nerve terminals and secretory granules isolated from neurohyophyses. *Acta Physiol Scand* 146: 233–239.
99. Drüeke T and Ritz E. 2009. Treatment of secondary hyperparathyroidism in CKD patients with cinacalcet and/or vitamin D derivatives. *Clin J Am Soc Nephrol* 4: 234–241.
100. Wüthrich R et al. 2007. The role of calcimimetics in the treatment of hyperparathyroidism. *Eur J Clin Invest* 37: 915–922.
101. Hauache OM et al. 2000. Effects of a calcimimetic compound and naturally activating mutations on the human Ca^{2+} receptor and on Ca^{2+} receptor/metabotropic glutamate chimeric receptors. *Endocrinology* 141: 4156–4163.
102. Mun H et al. 2004. The Venus fly trap domain of the extracellular Ca^{2+}-sensing receptor is required for L-amino acid sensing. *J Biol Chem* 279: 51739–51744.
103. Kiefer L et al. 2011. Novel calcium sensing receptor ligands: a patent survey. *Expert Opin Ther Pat* 21: 681–698.
104. Ohsu T et al. 2010. Involvement of the calcium sensing receptor in human taste perception. *J Biol Chem* 285: 1016–1022.

105. Conigrave AD and Hampson DR. 2006. Broad-spectrum amino acid sensing by class 3 G protein-coupled receptors. *Trends Endocrinol Metabol* 17: 398–407.
106. Feng J et al. 2010. Calcium sensing receptor is a physiologic multimodal chemosensor regulating gastric G cell growth and gastrin secretion. *Proc Natl Acad Sci USA* 107: 17791–17796.
107. Wang Y et al. 2011. Amino acids stimulate cholecystokinin release through the Ca^{2+}-sensing receptor. *Am J Physiol Gastrointest Liver Physiol* 300: G528–G537.
108. Liou A et al. 2011. The extracellular calcium sensing receptor is required for cholecystokinin secretion in response to L-phenylalanine in acutely isolated intestinal I cells. *Am J Physiol Gastrointest Liver Physiol* 300: G538–G546.
109. Mace O et al. 2012. The regulation of K and L cell activity by GLUT2 and the calcium sensing receptor CaSR in rat small intestine. *J Physiol* 590: 2917–2936.
110. Conigrave AD et al. 2008. Dietary protein and bone health: toles of amino acid–sensing receptors in the control of calcium metabolism and bone homeostasis. *Annu Rev Nutr* 28: 131–155.
111. Conigrave AD. 2012. Regulation of calcium and phosphate metabolism. In *Diseases of the Parathyroid Glands*, Licata AA and EV Lerma, Eds. Springer-Verlag: Heidelberg, pp. 13–53.
112. Kerstetter JE et al. 1997. Increased circulating concentrations of parathyroid hormone in healthy, young women consuming a protein-restricted diet. *Am J Clin Nutr* 66: 1188–1196.
113. Kerstetter JE et al. 2000. A threshold for low-protein-diet-induced elevations in parathyroid hormone. *Am J Clin Nutr* 72: 168–173.
114. Ammann P et al. 2000. Protein undernutrition-induced bone loss is associated with decreased IGF-I levels and estrogen deficiency. *J Bone Miner Res* 15: 683–690.
115. Dvorak-Ewell M et al. 2011. Osteoblast extracellular Ca^{2+}-sensing receptor regulates bone development, mineralization, and turnover. *J Bone Miner Res* 26: 2935–2947.
116. Brown EM et al. 1995. Calcium-ion-sensing cell-surface receptors. *New Engl J Med* 333: 234–240.
117. Brown EM. 2007. Clinical lessons from the calcium sensing receptor. *Nature Clin Pract Endocrinol Metabol* 3: 122–133.
118. Taussig R and Gilman AG. 1995. Mammalian membrane-bound adenylyl cyclases. *J Biol Chem* 270: 1–4.
119. Inzerillo A et al. 2002. Calcitonin: the other thyroid hormone. *Thyroid* 791–798.
120. Hirsch P and Baruch H. 2003. Is calcitonin an important physiological substance? *Endocr Rev* 21: 201–208.
121. Brown E, 2013. Role of the calcium-sensing receptor in extracellular calcium homeostasis. In *Calcium-Sensing Receptors in Health and Disease*, Best Practice & Research Clinical Endocrinology and Metabolism Series.
122. Woodrow J et al. 2006. Calcitonin plays a critical role in regulating skeletal mineral metabolism during lactation. *Endocrinology* 147: 4010–4021.
123. Davey RA et al. 2008. Calcitonin receptor plays a physiological role to protect against hypercalcemia in mice. *J Bone Miner Res* 23: 1182–1193.
124. Turner A et al. 2011. The role of the calcitonin receptor in protecting against induced hypercalcemia is mediated via its actions in osteoclasts to inhibit bone resorption. *Bone* 48: 354–361.
125. Freichel M et al. 1996. Expression of a calcium sensing receptor in a human medullary thyroid carcinoma cell line and its contribution to calcitonin secretion. *Endocrinology* 137: 3842–3848.
126. Garrett JE et al. 1995. Calcitonin-secreting cells of the thyroid gland express an extracellular calcium sensing receptor gene. *Endocrinology* 136: 5202–5211.

127. Fajtova VT et al. 1991. Cytosolic calcium responses of single rMTC 44-2 cells to stimulation with external calcium and potassium. *Am J Physiol* 261: E151–158.
128. McGehee DS et al. 1997. Mechanism of extracellular Ca^{2+} receptor-stimulated hormone release from sheep thyroid parafollicular cells. *J Physiol* 502: 31–44.
129. Raue F and Scherubl H. 1995. Extracellular calcium sensitivity and voltage-dependent calcium channels in C cells. *Endocr Rev* 16: 752–764.
130. Riccardi D and Brown E. 2010. Physiology and pathophysiology of the calcium sensing receptor in the kidney. *Am J Physiol Renal Physiol* 298: F485–F499.
131. Ba J and Friedman PA. 2004. Calcium sensing receptor regulation of renal mineral ion transport. *Cell Calcium* 35: 229–237.
132. Bajwa A et al. 2008. Specific regulation of CYP27B1 and VDR in proximal versus distal renal cells. *Arch Biochem Biophys* 477: 33–42.
133. Ba J et al. 2003. Calcium sensing receptor regulation of PTH-inhibitable proximal tubule phosphate transport. *Am J Physiol* 285: F1233–F1243.
134. Estévez R et al. 2001. Barttin is a Cl⁻ channel β subunit crucial for renal Cl⁻ reabsorption and inner ear K⁺ secretion. *Nature* 414: 558–561.
135. Gamba G and Friedman PA. 2009. Thick ascending limb: the Na+: K+: 2Cl– cotransporter, NKCC2 and the calcium sensing receptor. *Pflugers Arch* 458: 61–76.
136. Günzel D and Yu A. 2009. Function and regulation of claudins in the thick ascending limb of Henle. *Pflugers Arch* 458: 77–88.
137. Wang W et al. 1997. Phospholipase A2 is involved in mediating the effect of extracellular Ca^{2+} on apical K+ channels in rat TAL. *Am J Physiol* 273: F421–429.
138. Ferreira MCJ et al. 1998. Co-expression of a Ca^{2+}-inhibitable adenylyl cyclase and of a Ca^{2+}-sensing receptor in the cortical thick ascending limb cell of the rat kidney: inhibition of hormone-dependent cAMP accumulation by extracellular Ca^{2+}. *J Biol Chem* 15192–15202.
139. Gong Y et al. 2012. Claudin-14 regulates renal Ca^{2+} transport in response to CaSR signalling via a novel microRNA pathway. *EMBO J* 31: 1999–2012.
140. Hou J. 2012. New light on the role of claudins in the kidney. *Organogenesis* 8: 1–9.
141. Sabbagh Y et al. 2005. Hypophosphatemia leads to rickets by impairing caspase-mediated apoptosis of hypertrophic chondrocytes. *Proc Natl Acad Sci USA* 102: 9637–9642.
142. Tiosano D and Hochberg Z. 2009. Hypophosphatemia: the common denominator of all rickets. *J Bone Miner Metabol* 27: 392–401.
143. Shoback DM et al. 2003. The calcimimetic cinacalcet normalizes serum calcium in subjects with primary hyperparathyroidism. *J Clin Endocrinol Metabol* 88: 5644–5649.
144. Alon U et al. 2008. Calcimimetics as adjuvant treatment for familial hypophosphatemic rickets. *Clin J Am Soc Nephrol* 3: 658–664.
145. Hebert SC et al. 1997. Role of the Ca^{2+}-sensing receptor in divalent mineral ion homeostasis. *J Exp Biol* 200: 295–302.
146. Renkema K et al. 2009. The calcium sensing receptor promotes urinary acidification to prevent nephrolithiasis. *J Am Soc Nephrol* 20: 1705–1713.
147. Procino G et al. 2012. Calcium sensing receptor and aquaporin 2 interplay in hypercalciuria-associated renal concentrating defect in humans: an in vivo and in vitro study. *PLoS* 7: e33145.
148. Renkema K et al. 2011. Role of the calcium sensing receptor in reducing the risk for calcium stones. *Clin J Am Soc Nephrol* 6: 2076–2082.
149. Bouillon R et al. 2008. Vitamin D and human health: lessons from vitamin D receptor-null mice. *Endocr Rev* 29: 726–776.
150. Li Y et al. 2001. Effects of vitamin D receptor inactivation on the expression of calbindins and calcium metabolism. *Am J Physiol Endocrinol Metabol* 281: E558–E564.

151. Wysolmerski J. 2010. Interactions between breast, bone, and brain regulate mineral and skeletal metabolism during lactation. *Ann NY Acad Sci* 192: 161–169.

152. Qing H et al. 2012. Demonstration of osteocytic perilacunar/canalicular remodeling in mice during lactation. *J Bone Miner Res* 27: 1018–1029.

153. Bradbury RA et al. 2002. Localization of the extracellular Ca^{2+}-sensing receptor in the human placenta. *Placenta* 23: 192–200.

154. Suzuki Y et al. 2008. Calcium channel TRPV6 is involved in murine maternal–fetal calcium transport. *J Bone Miner Res* 23: 1249–1256.

155. Ardeshirpour L et al. 2010. Increased PTHrP and decreased estrogens alter bone turnover but do not reproduce the full effects of lactation on the skeleton. *Endocrinology* 151: 5591–5601.

156. Ardeshirpour L et al. 2007. Weaning triggers a decrease in receptor activator of nuclear factor-κB ligand expression, widespread osteoclast apoptosis, and rapid recovery of bone mass after lactation in mice. *Endocrinology* 148: 3875–3876.

157. Miller S and Bowman B. 2007. Rapid inactivation and apoptosis of osteoclasts in the maternal skeleton during the bone remodeling reversal at the end of lactation. *Anat Rec* 290: 65–73.

158. VanHouten J and Wysolmerski J. 2007. Transcellular calcium transport in mammary epithelial cells. *J Mammary Gland Biol Neoplasia* 12: 223–235.

159. Faddy H et al. 2008. Localization of plasma membrane and secretory calcium pumps in the mammary gland. *Biochem Biophys Res Commun* 369: 977–981.

160. VanHouten J et al. 2007. The calcium sensing receptor regulates plasma membrane calcium adenosine triphosphatase isoform 2 activity in mammary epithelial cells: a mechanism for calcium-regulated calcium transport into milk. *Endocrinology* 148: 5943–5954.

161. Reinhardt T et al. 2004. Null mutation in the gene encoding plasma membrane Ca^{2+}-ATPase isoform 2 impairs calcium transport into milk. *J Biol Chem* 279: 42369–42373.

162. Chattopadhyay N et al. 1998. Identification and localization of extracellular Ca^{2+}-sensing receptor in rat intestine. *Am J Physiol* 274: G122–G130.

163. Buchan A et al. 2001. Mechanism of action of the calcium sensing receptor in human antral gastrin cells. *Gastroenterology* 120: 1128–1139.

164. Blaker M et al. 2002. Expression of the cholecystokinin 2-receptor in normal human thyroid gland and medullary thyroid carcinoma. *Eur J Endocrinol* 146: 89–96.

165. Bevilacqua M et al. 2006. Dissimilar PTH, gastrin, and calcitonin responses to oral calcium and peptones in hypocalciuric hypercalcemia, primary hyperparathyroidism, and normal subjects: a useful tool for differential diagnosis. *J Bone Miner Res* 21: 406–412.

166. Conigrave AD et al. 2002. L-Amino acid sensing by the calcium sensing receptor: a general mechanism for coupling protein and calcium metabolism? *Eur J Clin Nutr* 56: 1072–1080.

167. Marie P. 2010. The calcium sensing receptor in bone cells: a potential therapeutic target in osteoporosis. *Bone* 46: 571–576.

168. Kubo Y et al. 1998. Structural basis for a Ca^{2+} sensing function of the metabotropic glutamate receptors. *Science* 279: 1722–1725.

169. Jiang Y et al. 2010. Elucidation of a novel extracellular calcium-binding site on metabotropic glutamate receptor 1α (mGluR1α) that controls receptor activation. *J Biol Chem* 285: 33463–33474.

170. Galvez T et al. 2000. Ca^{2+} requirement for high-affinity γ-aminobutyric acid (GABA) binding at GABA(B) receptors: involvement of serine 269 of the GABA(B)R1 subunit. *Mol Pharmacol* 57: 419–426.

171. Ho C et al. 1995. A mouse model of human familial hypocalciuric hypercalcemia and neonatal severe hyperparathyroidism. *Nat Genet* 11: 389–394.

172. Pollak MR et al. 1994. Familial hypocalciuric hypercalcemia and neonatal severe hyperparathyroidism: effects of mutant gene dosage on phenotype. *J Clin Invest* 93: 1108–1112.

173. Pollak MR et al. 1993. Mutations in the human Ca^{2+}-sensing receptor gene cause familial hypocalciuric hypercalcemia and neonatal severe hyperparathyroidism. *Cell* 75: 1297–1303.

174. Tu Q et al. 2003. Rescue of the skeletal phenotype in CaSR-deficient mice by transfer onto the Gcm2-null background. *J Clin Invest* 111: 1029–1037.

175. Kos CH et al. 2003. The calcium sensing receptor is required for normal calcium homeostasis independent of parathyroid hormone. *J Clin Invest* 117: 1021–1028.

176. Hendy G et al. 2009. Calcium sensing receptor and associated diseases. *Progr Mol Biol Transl Sci* 89: 31–95.

177. Oda Y et al. 1998. The calcium sensing receptor and its alternatively spliced form in keratinocyte differentiation. *J Biol Chem* 273: 23344–23352.

178. Oda Y et al. 2000. The calcium sensing receptor and its alternatively spliced form in murine epidermal differentiation. *J Biol Chem* 275: 1183–1190.

179. Rodriguez L et al. 2005. Expression and functional assessment of an alternatively spliced extracellular Ca^{2+}-sensing receptor in growth plate chondrocytes. *Endocrinology* 146: 5294–5303.

180. Finney B et al. 2011. An exon 5-less splice variant of the extracellular calcium sensing receptor rescues absence of the full-length receptor in the developing mouse lung. *Exp Lung Res* 37: 269–273.

181. Brennan-Speranza T et al. 2011. Selective osteoblast overexpression of IGF-I in mice prevents low protein-induced deterioration of bone strength and material level properties. *Bone* 49: 1073–1079.

182. Ward BK et al. 2004. Functional deletion of the calcium sensing receptor in a case of neonatal severe hyperparathyroidism. *J Clin Endocrinol Metabol* 89: 3721–3730.

183. Al-Khalaf F et al. 2011. Neonatal severe hyperparathyroidism: further clinical and molecular delineation. *Eur J Pediatr* 170: 625–631.

184. Berger CEM et al. 2001. Scanning electrochemical microscopy at the surface of bone-resorbing osteoclasts: evidence for steady-state disposal and intracellular functional compartmentalization of calcium. *J Bone Miner Res* 16: 2092–2102.

185. Kanatani M et al. 1999. High extracellular calcium inhibits osteoclast-like cell formation by directly acting on the calcium sensing receptor existing in osteoclast precursor cells. *Biochem Biophys Res Commun* 261: 144–148.

186. Mentaverri R et al. 2006. The calcium sensing receptor is directly involved in both osteoclast differentiation and apoptosis. *FASEB J* 20: 2562–2564.

187. Kameda T et al. 1998. Calcium sensing receptor in mature osteoclasts, which are bone resorbing cells. *Biochem Biophys Res Commun* 245: 419–422.

188. Yamaguchi T et al. 1998. Mouse osteoblastic cell line (MC3T3-E1) expresses extracellular calcium (Ca_{o}^{2+})-sensing receptor and its agonists stimulate chemotaxis and proliferation of MC3T3-E1 cells. *J Bone Miner Res* 13: 1530–1538.

189. Shu L et al. 2011. The calcium sensing receptor mediates bone turnover induced by dietary calcium and parathyroid hormone in neonates. *J Bone Miner Res* [Epub ahead of print].

190. Yamaguchi T et al. 2000. Activation of p42/44 and p38 mitogen-activated protein kinases by extracellular calcium sensing receptor agonists induces mitogenic responses in the mouse osteoblastic MC3T3-E1 cell line. *Biochem Biophys Res Commun* 279: 363–368.

191. Shin M et al. 2003. High extracellular Ca^{2+} alone stimulates osteoclast formation but inhibits in the presence of other osteoclastogenic factors. *Exp Mol Med* 35: 167–174.

192. Boudot C et al. 2010. Implication of the calcium sensing receptor and the phospho-inositide 3-kinase/Akt pathway in the extracellular calcium-mediated migration of RAW 264.7 osteoclast precursor cells. *Bone* 46: 1416–1423.

193. Miedlich SU et al. 2004. Homology modeling of the transmembrane domain of the human calcium sensing receptor and localization of an allosteric binding site. *J Biol Chem* 279: 7254–7263.

194. Nemeth EF and Shoback D. 2013. Calcimimetic and calcilytic drugs. In *Calcium Sensing Receptors in Health and Disease*, Conigrave AD and EM Brown, Eds.

195. Kimura S et al. 2011. JTT-305: an orally active calcium sensing receptor antagonist, stimulates transient parathyroid hormone release and bone formation in ovariectomized rats. *Eur J Pharmacol* 668: 331–336.

196. Ringe J. 2010. Strontium ranelate: an effective solution for diverse fracture risks. *Osteoporosis Intl* 21: S431–S436.

197. Saidak Z and Marie PJ. 2012. Strontium signaing: molecular mechanisms and therapeutic implications. *Pharmacol Therap* 136: 216–226.

198. Fournier C et al. 2012. Reduction by strontium of the bone marrow adiposity in mice and repression of the adipogenic commitment of multipotent C3H10T1/2 cells. *Bone* 50: 499–509.

199. Thomsen A et al. 2012. Strontium is a biased agonist of the calcium-sensing receptor in rat medullary thyroid carcinoma 6-23 cells. *J Pharmacol Exp Ther* 343: 638–649.

200. Bonnelye E et al. 2008. Dual effect of strontium ranelate: stimulation of osteoblast differentiation and inhibition of osteoclast formation and resorption in vitro. *Bone* 42: 129–138.

201. Caudrillier A et al. 2010. Strontium ranelate decreases receptor activator of nuclear factor-κB ligand-induced osteoclastic differentiation in vitro: involvement of the calcium sensing receptor. *Mol Pharmacol* 78: 569–576.

202. Hurtel-Lemaire A et al. 2009. The calcium sensing receptor is involved in strontium ranelate-induced osteoclast apoptosis: new insights into the associated signaling pathways. *J Biol Chem* 284: 575–584.

5 Parathyroid Hormone: Its Role in Calcium and Phosphate Homeostasis

David Goltzman

CONTENTS

5.1   SYNTHESIS AND SECRETION

Parathyroid hormone (PTH) is the major secretory product of the chief cells of the parathyroid glands and is transcribed from a gene located on chromosome 11 [1]. The major translation product is an 84-amino acid straight chain polypeptide [PTH (1–84)] extended at the amino (NH2)-terminus by a leader (signal) or pre-sequence that facilitates its entry into the secretory apparatus of the cell, and by a short pro-hormone sequence, both of which are cleaved before exit from the parathyroid cell. The entire precursor of PTH (1–84) is called preproPTH. The 84 amino acid moiety is both the major glandular form and the major bioactive secreted and circulating form, although perhaps some short-lived NH2-terminal fragments circulate under special circumstances [2].

Extracellular fluid (ECF) ionized calcium [Ca^{++}] appears to be the predominant regulator of PTH production (Figure 5.1). Thus, Ca^{++} binding to and activation of a 7-transmembrane spanning G protein coupled receptor (GPCR) results in the dimerization of the calcium sensing receptor (CaSR). Via the guanine nucleotide-binding (G) proteins $Ga'_{q/11}$ or $Ga'_{i/0}$, Ca^{++} also activates several signalling pathways including phospholipase A2 (PLA_2), phospholipase D (PLD), phospholipase C (PLC), protein kinase (PKC), phosphoinositide-3-kinase (PI3K), and mitogen-activated protein kinases (MAPKs) such as extracellular signal related kinases 1/2 (ERK-1/2).

The critical pathways transducing the biological effects of CaSR are yet to be identified [3]. CaSR signaling inhibits PTH secretion. This inhibition occurs in a curvilinear fashion, characterized by a steep inverse sigmoidal curve. Half-maximal inhibition of PTH secretion (the set point) may occur at a Ca^{++} concentration of about 1 mM. In human parathyroid tissue in vitro, maximal Ca^{++}-induced inhibition of PTH secretion with continued non-suppressible PTH secretion generally occurs at Ca^{++} concentrations about 2 mM or higher. Maximal secretion of PTH generally occurs at Ca^{++} concentrations around 0.5 mM or lower. However, the actual Ca^{++} concentrations regulating these parameters of secretion vary based on both physiologic and pathologic circumstances [4]. The rate at which Ca^{++} falls may also determine the magnitude of the secretory response, with a rapid fall in ECF Ca^{++} stimulating a more robust secretory response.

Increased Ca^{++} concentrations have also been linked to increased degradation of bioactive PTH within parathyroid cells and release of bio-inactive carboxyl (COOH)-terminal fragments [5–7]. Bio-inactive PTH fragments that may be generated also in the liver are cleared by the kidney [8].

Increased Ca^{++} may also inhibit PTH gene transcription and stability, although this regulatory mechanism is considerably slower than others [9–11], and reduced Ca^{++} concentrations have also been shown to increase parathyroid cell proliferation [12]. Thus, sustained hypocalcemia can eventually lead to an increase in the total secretory capacity of the parathyroid gland. In contrast, although sustained hypercalcemia can reduce parathyroid gland size, hypercalcemia appears less effective in diminishing the numbers of the major PTH-synthesizing cells—the chief parathyroid cells—after a prolonged stimulus to hyperplasia has occurred.

The active form of vitamin D, 1,25 dihydroxyvitamin D [$1,25(OH)_2D$] has been reported to inhibit both PTH gene transcription [13] and parathyroid cell proliferation

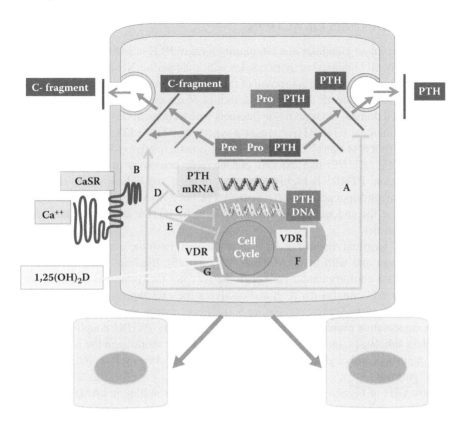

FIGURE 5.1 Regulation of parathyroid cell activity by calcium and vitamin D. (A) Calcium (Ca++), acting via the calcium-sensing receptor (CaSR), can inhibit secretion of intact PTH. (B) Ca++ can also increase intracellular proteolysis of PTH to inactive C(COOH) fragments, (C) inhibit PTH gene transcription, and (D) inhibit PTH mRNA translation, thereby reducing production of the biosynthetic precursor PrePrePTH. (E) Ca++ can also inhibit parathyroid cell cycle progression and reduce parathyroid cell proliferation. (F) The active form of vitamin D, 1,25(OH)₂D can inhibit PTHrP gene transcription via the vitamin D receptor (VDR). (G) The 1,25(OH)₂D can also inhibit cell cycle progression and reduce parathyroid cell proliferation. ↑ = increased; ⊤ = inhibited.

in part by its regulation of the myc gene complex [12,14]. PTH gene transcription by both Ca++ and 1,25(OH)₂D may involve the GCMB parathyroid transcription factor (GCM2) [15]. CaSR gene transcription may also be up-regulated by 1,25(OH)₂D. Consequently Ca++ and 1,25(OH)₂D appear to act in concert to regulate parathyroid cell growth and function.

Additional modulators of PTH secretion including cations such as lithium [16], transforming growth factor α (TGFa) [17], prostaglandins [18], and inorganic phosphate (Pi) [19] have been reported. Recent evidence indicates a regulatory role for the phosphaturic factor known as fibroblast growth factor 23 (FGF23) that appears to decrease PTH mRNA expression and PTH secretion [20].

5.2 MECHANISMS OF ACTION

Although the major glandular and circulating form of PTH is an 84-amino acid peptide, virtually all biological activity resides within its amino(NH_2)-terminal domain such that a synthetic peptide composed of the NH_2-terminal 34 residues [PTH (1-34)] appears to recapitulate all the biologic activities of the entire molecule [21,22]. The NH_2-terminal domain in target tissue interacts with a classical GPCR of the B family (class II) termed the PTH/PTHrP receptor type 1, or PTHR1 [23,24].

This receptor also transduces signalling of a genetic relative of PTH termed PTH-related protein (PTHrP) that exhibits considerable homology to PTH in its NH_2-terminal region. PTHR1 is highly expressed in bone and kidney where the major physiologic ligand appears to be circulating PTH, but is also expressed in many other tissues, where the endogenous ligand is likely to be PTHrP acting in a paracrine/autocrine manner.

The NH_2-terminal domain of PTH interacts with both the extracellular domain of the receptor and with juxtamembrane regions [25]. Binding of the receptor by PTH induces a conformational change in the receptor that promotes coupling with heterotrimeric G proteins (α, β, γ) and catalyzes the exchange of GDP for GTP on the α subunits of the G proteins (Figure 5.2). This exchange triggers conformational and/or dissociation events between the α and $\beta\gamma$ subunits. PTHR1 couples to several G protein subclasses, including Gs, Gq/11, and G12/13, resulting in the activation of many pathways, although the best studied are the adenylate cyclase and phospholipase C pathways.

Thus, $G\alpha s$ of Gs activates adenylate cyclase (AC), resulting in cAMP synthesis; cAMP then activates protein kinase A (PKA). $G\alpha q$ of Gq activates phospholipase C(PLC), which cleaves phosphatidylinositol (4,5)-bisphosphate (PIP_2) into diacylglycerol (DAG) and inositol (1,4,5)-trisphosphate (IP_3). IP_3 then diffuses through the cytoplasm and activates IP_3-gated Ca^{++} channels in the membranes of the endoplasmic reticulum, causing the release of stored Ca^{++} into the cytoplasm. The increase of cytosolic Ca^{++} promotes PKC translocation to the plasma membrane and then activation by DAG [26]. $G\alpha 12/13$ activates phospholipase D [27,28].

PTH binding to PTHR1 is also followed by phosphorylation of serines on the COOH-terminal intracellular tail of PTHR1, by G protein-coupled receptor kinases (GRKs), a process that initiates desensitization–internalization of the receptor [29]. Thus, binding of β-arrestins to these phosphorylated sites uncouples receptors from heterotrimeric G proteins and terminates PTH-mediated G protein-signaling. The PTH–receptor complex is then internalized into clathrin-coated pits to which β-arrestin binds and then into early endocytic vesicles. At least some of the internalized receptor can undergo rapid recycling to the cell surface.

β-arrestins may also serve as multifunctional scaffolding proteins linking PTHR1 to signaling molecules independent of the classic G protein-coupled second messenger-dependent pathways [30]. Thus β-arrestins also serve as adaptors that assemble intracellular complexes between internalized PTHR1 and signaling proteins to activate MAPK pathways, among others. Alternatively AC and Gs may be internalized with the PTH/PTHR1/β-arrestin complex. Within early endosomes,

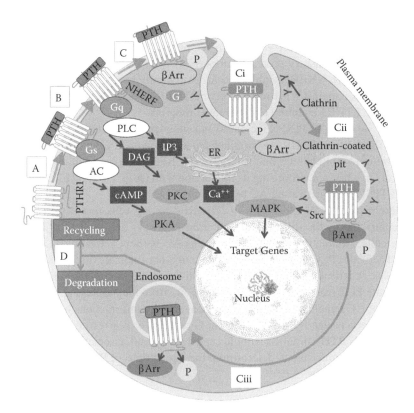

FIGURE 5.2 Mechanism of PTH action via PTHR1. (A) After PTH binding to the PTHR1 GPCR, GS activates AC, leading to cAMP synthesis that in turn activates PKA and ultimately increased transcriptional activity. (B) In cells expressing the NHERF cytoplasmic adaptor protein, NHERF binds to PTHR1, inhibits β-arrestin binding to PTHR1, and facilitates PTHR1 coupling to Gq proteins without compromising the ability of PTHR1 to stimulate Gs and AC. PTHR1 signaling to PLC is increased and leads to increased DAG and IP3 production. IP3 then causes the release of stored Ca^{++} from the ER into the cytoplasm that promotes PKC translocation to the plasma membrane and then activation by DAG. Activated PLC can ultimately increase transcriptional activity. (C) PTH activation of PTHR1 may also increase the phosphorylation of PTHR1 which may then interact with β-arrestin, causing termination of receptor-mediated cAMP and DAG/IP3 signaling through steric inhibition of G protein binding. The phosphorylation ligand–receptor complex (Ci) can be internalized via clathrin-coated vesicles and into clathrin-coated pits (Cii). Arrestins can serve as scaffolds for internalized PTHR1 to initiate G protein–independent MAPK signaling and transcriptional activity (Ciii). The PTHR1 complex in endosomes may be alternatively degraded or recycled (D). AC = adenylate cyclase; βArr = β-arrestin; ER = endoplasmic reticulum; G = heterotrimeric G protein; Gs = G protein α subunit that activates adenylate cyclase; Gq = G protein α subunit that activates phospholipase C; DAG = diacylglycerol; GPCR = heterotrimeric GTP-binding protein (G protein)-coupled receptor; IP3 = inositol (1,4,5) trisphosphate; MAPK = Src-mediated MAP kinase; NHERF = Na/H exchanger regulatory protein factor; P = phosphorylation; PKA = protein kinase A; PKC = protein kinase C; PLC = phospholipase C; PTH = parathyroid hormone; PTHR1 = PTH/PTHrP receptor type 1.

functional interactions between PTHR1, Gs, and AC may then allow sustained cAMP production within cells.

PTHR1 may also interact with other cytoplasmic adaptor proteins such as the Na/H exchanger regulatory protein factors (NHERFs) that bind to the intracellular tail of PTHR1 [31]. NHERF1 inhibits β-arrestin binding to PTHR1. NHERF1 may therefore protect against PTH resistance or PTHR down-regulation. NHERFs also modulate the PTHR1 coupling to different G proteins.

PTHR1 signaling to PLC is increased in cells expressing NHERF1. Association with NHERF1 allows PTHR1 to stimulate Gq and thereby PLC without compromising its ability to stimulate Gs and AC [32]. NHERF2 promotes coupling of PTHR1 to Gq and Gi, while compromising its interaction with Gs [33]. NHERF2 can thereby switch PTHR1 from activating AC to activating PLC.

Different patterns of expression of NHERFs among cells that express PTHR1 likely contribute to the diversity of signaling pathways activated by PTH. Thus, in some cells, stimulation of PTHR1 activates AC without activating PLC [34]. In others, it activates PLC and not AC [33], while in others, notably osteoblasts and kidney tubules, it activates both [34]. Even within the same proximal tubule cell, PTH may activate PLC from the apical surface and AC from the basolateral surface [35].

Different PTH analogues stabilize different active conformations of PTHR1 that may then interact selectively with different G proteins or β-arrestins. Therefore, the intensity of the PTH stimulus, stimulus trafficking, and association with scaffold proteins may all contribute to determining the interactions of PTHR1 with intracellular signalling proteins.

5.3 CONTRIBUTIONS TO PLASMA CALCIUM AND PHOSPHATE HOMEOSTASIS

PTH plays a central role in regulating ECF Ca^{++} and Pi homoeostasis and in modulating bone turnover. Thus, when a reduction in ECF Ca^{++} (potentially caused by an increase in ECF Pi) stimulates release of PTH from the parathyroid glands, this hormone can then act to enhance Ca^{++} reabsorption in the kidney, while at the same time inhibiting Pi reabsorption and producing phosphaturia.

In the kidney, PTH (and hypocalcemia) can also stimulate the conversion of the inactive metabolite of vitamin D known as 25-hydroxyvitamin D [25OHD] to the active moiety 1,25-dihydroxyvitamin D [$1,25(OH)_2D$] that can then travel through the bloodstream to increase intestinal absorption of Ca^{++} and to a lesser extent Pi. PTH can also increase bone turnover, leading to enhanced bone resorption and liberation of both Ca^{++} and Pi from the skeleton. The PTH-mediated renal effects to maintain Ca^{++} homeostasis appear more rapid than the skeletal effects.

The net effect of the increased stimulation of PTH release in response to hypocalcemia, therefore is to increase reabsorption of renal Ca^{++} (direct effect), increase absorption of Ca^{++} from the gut (indirect effect), mobilize Ca^{++} from bone (direct effect), and therefore to restore the ECF Ca^{++} to normal and thereby inhibit further production of PTH and $1,25(OH)_2D$.

In the kidney, Ca^{++} reabsorption primarily takes place in the distal tubules and connecting ducts [36]. Calcium ions cross the apical membrane from the tubular lumen via TRPV5, a highly selective Ca^{++}channel, and are then transported across the basolateral membrane into the blood system by the sodium/calcium exchanger 1 (NCX1) and the plasma membrane ATPase. PTH regulates the expression of Ca^{++} transport proteins and their activity. Thus PTH regulates expression of TRPV5 and NCX1 [37]. The PTH regulation of, at least TRPV5, appears to occur through PKC [38]. TRPV5 is also regulated through the PKC signaling pathway by CaSR [39].

Pi reabsorption across the apical membranes of renal proximal tubules mainly occurs through two sodium-dependent phosphate co-transporters, NaPi-IIa and NaPi-IIc, that are exclusively expressed in the brush border membranes (BBMs) of the proximal tubules [40]. PTH increases Pi excretion in the proximal tubules mainly by reducing these sodium-coupled co-transporters. Thus, PTH binding to PTHR1 at either apical or basolateral membranes results in the down-regulation of BBM NaPi-IIa and NaPi-IIc in which the transporter is removed from the BBM via clathrin-coated pits [41,42]. PTH activation of apical PTHR1 leads to PLC-PKC stimulation mediated by NHERF, whereas activation of basolateral PTHR1 utilizes the AC/PKA pathway [43]. Following endocytosis, NaPi-II is eventually transported to the lysosome for degradation [44].

PTH stimulates the conversion of 25OHD to 1,25(OH)2D in kidney by transcriptional activation of the 25-hydroxyvitamin D 1[α] hydroxylase [1α(OH)ase or CYP27B1], apparently by the AC/PKA pathway [45]. Thus, in kidney, $Ca++$ reabsorption in the distal tubules seems to be regulated mainly through the PKC pathway. The renal 1(OH)ase seems to be stimulated mainly by PKA, and both PKA and PKC pathways are activated by PTH in the proximal tubules for regulation of Pi reuptake.

The effects of PTH in bone appear complex. Bone undergoes constant remodeling in response to endocrine, autocrine/paracrine, and intracrine signals and is maintained through a balance between bone formation and resorption. PTH binds to PTHR1 on cells of the osteoblastic lineage [46] including progenitor cells, osteoblasts, and osteocytes and can stimulate a variety of factors ultimately leading to increased proliferation of mesenchymal stem cells, the commitment of these cells into the osteoblast lineage, and then enhanced differentiation and activity of osteoblastic cells resulting in new bone matrix production and its mineralization.

The anabolic effects of PTH in bone seem to be mediated at least in part via the stimulation of the Wnt signaling system [46], a critical system in osteoblast activation. Thus, for example, PTH has been demonstrated to inhibit production of sclerostin, an inhibitor of the Wnt system produced by osteocytes [47], leading to activation of the canonical Wnt signalling pathway.

However osteoblastic cells also produce the TNF-related cytokine, receptor activator of nuclear factor κ-B (RANK) ligand (RANKL), a critical stimulator of osteoclast production and action, as well as the soluble RANKL decoy receptor, osteoprotegerin (OPG) [48]. While stimulating osteoblastic cells, PTH also enhances production of RANKL and inhibits production of OPG leading to increased osteoclastic bone resorption [49]. Bone resorption leads to the release of Ca^{++} and Pi as a result of the degradation of hydroxyapatite, a major mineral component of bone matrix.

Consequently PTH can stimulate bone turnover, leading to either a net increase in bone formation or a net increase in bone resorption. In animal studies, continuous infusion of exogenous PTH primarily produced a bone catabolic effect with hypercalcemia whereas intermittent administration of exogenous PTH to animals or to humans produced a net bone anabolic effect. In fetal and neonatal animals, endogenous PTH appears to play predominantly an anabolic role especially in trabecular bone [50]. As the animals mature and maternal sources of calcium are limited, endogenous PTH acts mainly to resorb bone (primarily cortical bone) [51,52]. Thus PTH appears to also exert a compartmental effect, primarily forming trabecular bone and resorbing cortical bone. Even in mature animals, however, the anabolic effect of endogenous PTH is critical, for example, for optimal fracture healing [53].

PTH seems to primarily utilize the PKA pathway in exerting both its catabolic and anabolic effects [54–56], however PKC activation by PTH and intracellular Ca^{++} signaling pathways may play an important role in bone as well [57].

5.4 BONE DISEASE ASSOCIATED WITH INCREASED PTH ACTION

5.4.1 PRIMARY HYPERPARATHYROIDISM (PHPT)

5.4.1.1 Sporadic PHPT

At least 85 to 90% of cases of sporadic PHPT are associated with a single parathyroid adenoma that overproduces PTH. About 10 to 15% of cases may be associated with multi-gland hyperplasia or multiple adenomas, in which case the possibility of a familial syndrome should be considered. Parathyroid carcinoma as a cause of sporadic PHPT is a relatively rare event occurring in about 1% of cases. Parathyroid tumors constitute the most common forms of endocrine neoplasia with an incidence of 1 in 1000 in the general population. These are more common in females than males (ratio of 3:1) and the prevalence of parathyroid tumors is about 1 to 2% in postmenopausal women.

Genes definitively implicated in sporadic benign PHPT account for less than 50% of sporadic parathyroid adenomas [58]. Somatic mutations in MEN1, a gene also implicated in familial multiple endocrine neoplasia type I that encodes the menin protein, have been reported in approximately 15 to 25% of parathyroid adenomas. Most demonstrated loss of the second allele in keeping with the role of MEN1 as a tumor suppressor gene [59]. Somatic (and germ line) mutations in CDC73 (HRPT2), a tumor suppressor gene associated with the hyperparathyroidism–jaw tumor syndrome, were reported in a high proportion (15 to 100%) of parathyroid carcinomas but have been reported in only about 4% of parathyroid adenomas [60].

A pericentromeric inversion of chromosome 11p localizing the cyclin D1 (CCND1) gene under the control of tissue-specific enhancer elements of the PTH gene promoter and somatic and germ line cyclin-dependent kinase 1B (CDKN1B) mutations are all reported to occur in about 5% of sporadic parathyroid adenomas [61]. In addition, abnormalities of β-catenin (CTNNB1) are involved in fewer than 2% of sporadic parathyroid adenomas [62]. Therefore, mutations in MEN1 appear the most common event in parathyroid tumorigenesis with parathyroid adenomas overall displaying relatively few somatic variants, in keeping with their benign nature.

Other important parathyroid regulatory pathways that may play a role in the pathogenesis of hyperparathyroidism are related to the principal regulators of parathyroid cell proliferation and PTH secretion, i.e., Ca^{++}, $1,25(OH)_2D$, and, Pi. Rarely, sporadic hyperparathyroidism with hypocalciuria may occur, caused by blocking antibodies to the calcium-sensing receptor that inhibits its function. This syndrome is known as autoimmune hypocalciuric hypercalcemia [63].

In sporadic PHPT, increased PTH secretion leads to a net increase in skeletal resorption with release of Ca^{++} and Pi from bone. PTH-induced increases in production of $1,25(OH)_2D$ lead to increased Ca^{++} and Pi absorption from the small intestine. PTH also enhances renal Ca^{++} reabsorption and inhibits Pi reabsorption, resulting in increased urine Pi excretion and hypophosphatemia. The net result is an increase in ECF Ca^{++} that does not, however, completely suppress circulating PTH levels. Consequently, the presence of easily detectable or elevated PTH in association with hypercalcemia is diagnostic for sporadic PHPT.

About 80% of cases of the most common form of PHPT, i.e., benign sporadic PHPT present as mild or asymptomatic hyperparathyroidism in which hypercalcemia is generally less than 0.25 mM (1 mg/dL) above the upper limit of normal and may be normal intermittently [64]. However, significant increases in serum calcium may occur even after 13 years of follow-up. Rarely, primary sporadic PHPT may present with severe acute hypercalcemia (parathyroid crisis).

Excess PTH production can produce significant bone loss. Classically this is manifested by discrete lesions including subperiosteal bone resorption of the distal phalanges, osteitis fibrosa cystica characterized by bone cysts and "brown tumors" (collections of osteoclasts intermixed with poorly mineralized woven bone), and ultimately fractures. However, these manifestations are rarely seen today and the more common skeletal manifestation of excess circulating PTH now appears to be resorption of cortical bone, reflecting the "catabolic bone activity" of PTH, with relative preservation of trabecular bone, reflecting its "anabolic activity" [65]. This reduction in the severity of bone disease is possibly a result of a reduced prevalence of associated vitamin D deficiency.

The less marked hypercalcemia generally observed possibly occurs as a consequence of less severe bone disease, less calcium mobilization from bone, and therefore a lower filtered load of renal calcium. Consequently, the incidence of hypercalciuria, kidney stones, and particularly nephrocalcinosis declined as well. Nevertheless, hypercalciuria still occurs in 35 to 40% of patients with sporadic benign PHPT and kidney stones occur in 15 to 20% [66]. About 25% of patients with even mild (asymptomatic) sporadic PHPT have been reported to develop renal manifestations within 10 years, including renal concentrating defects or kidney stones.

Abnormalities other than skeletal and renal disease have been associated with benign sporadic PHPT. These include gastrointestinal manifestations such as peptic ulcers and acute pancreatitis. The incidence of peptic ulcer disease in sporadic PHPT is currently estimated to be about the same as in the general population but the presence of multiple peptic ulcers may suggest the presence of multiple endocrine neoplasia type I (MENI). Acute pancreatitis may be a manifestation of hypercalcemia per se but is estimated to occur in only 1.5% of those with sporadic PHPT.

Neuromuscular abnormalities manifested by weakness and fatigue and accompanied by EMG changes may occur although the pathophysiology is uncertain. The relationship of hypertension and other cardiovascular manifestations and neuropsychiatric symptoms to hyperparathyroidism remains unclear.

To establish the diagnosis of PHPT, documentation of at least two elevated corrected (or ionized) serum calcium levels with concomitant elevated (or at least normal) serum PTH levels is required. Although second-generation two-site immunoradiometric (IRMA) and ELISA assays that measure intact PTH are usually acceptable, third-generation assays that have less capacity to interact with large NH_2 terminally truncated fragments are preferable (especially in renal failure). If mild PHPT is documented, in addition to measuring the level of urine calcium, bone densitometry, calculation of estimated glomerular filtration rate (GFR), and a renal ultrasound or renal CT scan for evidence of nephrolithiasis may help determine the extent of the disease.

For severe PHPT, appropriate skeletal x-rays would be indicated to provide a baseline of disease extent before parathyroidectomy. Imaging is not recommended to establish or confirm the diagnosis of PHPT, but has become routine for preoperative localization of the abnormal parathyroid tissue, generally by nuclear imaging (MIBI scans) or ultrasound [64]. Computed tomography, magnetic resonance imaging, positron emission tomography scanning, arteriography, and selective venous sampling for PTH are usually reserved for patients who have not been cured by previous explorations or for whom other localization techniques are not informative or are discordant.

Although estrogen therapy has been advocated for the treatment of PHPT in postmenopausal women, potential adverse effects of estrogen therapy including breast cancer and cardiovascular complications make this option unattractive. Although selective estrogen receptor modulators may be alternatives, few long-term studies have been done to assess them.

Bisphosphonates [64] may increase bone mineral density (BMD) at the lumbar spine and hip regions but generally do not reduce hypercalcemia substantially. Calcimimetic agents (that mimic or potentiate the action of calcium at the CaSR) [64] can reduce hypercalcemia effectively and have been approved for use in parathyroid carcinomas but generally do not significantly improve skeletal abnormalities. Calcimimetic agents may also be useful to treat severe hypercalcemia in patients with PHPT who are unable to undergo parathyroidectomy.

Surgical removal of a parathyroid adenoma currently remains the treatment of choice (1) if the ECF calcium exceeds 0.25 mM (1 mg/dL) above normal, (2) if there is evidence of bone disease (BMD T-score <−2.5 at the lumbar spine, total hip, femoral neck, 33% radius (1/3 site), and/or previous fracture fragility), (3) if calculated creatinine clearance is reduced to <60 ml/min or the patient is younger than age 50 [67]. Surgery is also indicated in patients for whom medical surveillance is not desired or is not possible [67]. In addition, although hypercalciuria is only one of several risk factors affecting the development of kidney stones, some physicians still regard 24-hour urinary calcium excretion exceeding 10 mmol (400 mg) as an indication for surgery.

The type of surgical procedure (non-invasive or standard) and the use of operative adjuncts (e.g., rapid PTH assay) is institution-specific and should be based on the expertise and resource availabilities of the surgeon and institution. Severe chronic hypercalcemia is more commonly associated with parathyroid carcinoma, and complete resection of the primary lesion is urgent in this case.

5.4.1.2   Familial PHPT

Multiple endocrine neoplasia type I (MENI)—MENI is a familial disorder with an autosomal dominant pattern of inheritance characterized by tumors of the parathyroid glands, the anterior pituitary, and the pancreatic islets [68]. Patients exhibit mutations in the MENI gene that encodes the menin nuclear protein [69]. Tumors in at least two of these sites in a proband and in at least one of these sites in a first-degree relative confirm the clinical phenotype. The most common and the earliest endocrinopathy is PHPT (80 to 100% of cases) [70].

In contrast to sporadic PHPT, however, MENI occurs in both sexes equally and patients are younger at the time of diagnosis. Furthermore, in contrast to the frequent occurrence of a single adenoma in sporadic disease, multi-gland involvement in an asymmetric fashion is the norm in MENI. Entero-pancreatic tumors are usually multiple and gastrinomas are the most common. These produce the Zollinger-Ellison syndrome, and occur in the duodenum and pancreatic islets. Gastrinomas can produce considerable morbidity due to the potential for ulcers and the possibility of metastatic disease. Insulinomas, glucagonomas, VIPomas and other islet tumors can occur as well. A variety of functioning anterior pituitary tumors can occur although prolactinomas are most frequent and anterior pituitary tumors may also be non-functioning. Finally, foregut carcinoids and other endocrine tumors have been described with lesser frequency and skin tumors such as facial angiofibromas and truncal collagenomas may occur and appear specific for MENI.

Patients with hyperparathyroidism due to MENI have multi-glandular disease. Surgical resection of fewer than three glands leads to high rates of recurrence. Consequently, either subtotal parathyroidectomy with 3 ½ gland removal or total parathyroidectomy is recommended. The latter may be accompanied by auto-transplantation of resected parathyroid gland fragments.

Multiple endocrine neoplasia type IIA (MENIIA)—MENIIA is an autosomal dominant familial syndrome characterized by medullary thyroid carcinoma (MTC), bilateral pheochromocytomas, and hyperparathyroidism [70,71]. It results from activating mutations in the RET proto-oncogene which is a receptor tyrosine kinase [72]. Two variants of this disorder are MENIIB which includes mucosal and intestinal neuromas and a marfanoid habitus but no hyperparathyroidism and familial medullary thyroid carcinoma.

The dominant feature of the MENIIA syndrome is MTC, a calcitonin-secreting neoplasm of thyroid C cells. Genetic testing for mutations in the RET oncogene is of value in considering prophylactic thyroidectomy to prevent MTC. Another major feature is pheochromocytomas that have high malignant potential. Hyperparathyroidism is milder and less frequent (5 to 20%) in MENIIA than in MENI but is also associated with multi-gland involvement in which gland enlargement may be asymmetric. The treatment of the hyperparathyroidism is as for MENI.

Hyperparathyroidism–jaw tumor (HPT-J) syndrome—HPT-J syndrome is an autosomal dominant familial disorder characterized by early onset of single or multiple cystic parathyroid adenomas that may develop asynchronously, and ossifying fibromas of the mandible and maxilla. These jaw tumors lack osteoclasts and therefore differ from brown tumors. Affected individuals also present increased risk (15 to 20%) of developing parathyroid carcinoma. Surgical removal of the affected parathyroid tissue is clearly indicated.

A variety of renal tumors have been described in some kindred and pancreatic, testicular and thyroid tumors have been described in others. Mutations in the HRPT2 tumor suppressor gene that encodes a protein called parafibromin have been implicated in this syndrome [73], in sporadic parathyroid cancer, and in a minority of families with isolated hyperparathyroidism. HRPT2 DNA testing in relatives can identify individuals at risk for parathyroid carcinoma, enabling preventative or curative parathyroidectomy.

Familial hypocalciuric hypercalcemia (FHH) and neonatal severe primary hyperparathyroidism (NSHPT)—FHH [74] is an autosomal dominant trait characterized by moderate hypercalcemia and relative hypocalciuria, i.e., urine calcium that is low in relationship to the prevailing hypercalcemia. The molecular basis is usually an inactivating mutation in the CaSR gene [75]. As a consequence, in heterozygotes, diminished ability of the CaSR in the cortical thick ascending limb of the kidney to detect ECF Ca^{++} occurs leading to enhanced renal tubular reabsorption of Ca^{++} and magnesium, to hypercalcemia, and often to hypermagnesemia.

The calcium-to-creatinine clearance ratio is usually low, i.e., below 0.01 in patients with FHH and above this level in sporadic PHPT. This increased ECF Ca^{++} is also inadequately sensed by the altered CaSR in the parathyroid gland so that mild hyperplasia may occur and normal or elevated levels of PTH are secreted despite the hypercalcemia. Patients are generally asymptomatic. Testing serum and urine calcium in three relatives appears to have a lower false negative rate in diagnosing FHH than CaSR gene testing in a proband. However, CaSR gene testing may be of value when hypocalciuric hypercalcemia occurs in an isolated patient without access to additional family members or familial isolated hyperparathyroidism (FIH) occurs in the absence of classical features of FHH.

Because renal lesions and therefore hypercalcemia persist after parathyroidectomy and patients are generally asymptomatic, it is important to identify these patients to ensure that they are not subjected to parathyroidectomy. Individuals who are homozygous for the mutated CaSR or are compound heterozygotes and therefore have little functional CaSR may develop NSHPT [76].

This disorder generally presents within a week of birth and is characterized by severe life-threatening hypercalcemia, hypermagnesemia, increased circulating PTH concentrations, massive hyperplasia of the parathyroid glands, and relative hypocalciuria. Skeletal abnormalities including demineralization, widening of the metaphyses, osteitis fibrosa, and fractures may occur. Inasmuch as the course of NSHPT can be self-limited, aggressive medical management is first indicated in all cases of NSHPT. Prompt surgical intervention including total parathyroidectomy with immediate or delayed parathyroid auto-transplantation should be performed in patients who deteriorate.

Familial isolated hyperparathyroidism (FIH)—Familial hyperparathyroidism can occur in the MENI syndrome in which menin is mutated; in the MENII syndrome in which RET is mutated; in FHH and NSHPT in which CaSR is mutated; and in the

HPT-J syndrome in which HRPT2 is mutated. FIH refers to familial hyperparathyroidism in the absence of the specific features of the other documented syndromes including the known genetic mutations and suggests that other genes relevant to parathyroid neoplasia await identification.

5.4.1.3   Tertiary Hyperparathyroidism

Tertiary hyperparathyroidism appears to represent the autonomous function of parathyroid tissue that develops in the face of long-standing secondary hyperparathyroidism [77]. This may occur with monoclonal expansion of nodular areas of the parathyroid gland. These in turn may be associated with decreased VDR and decreased CaSR expression that may lead to an increased set point for PTH secretion.

The most common circumstance in which this occurs is chronic renal failure where $1,25(OH)_2D$ deficiency hypocalcemia and hyperphosphatemia produce chronic stimulation of the parathyroid glands. However, hypercalcemic hyperparathyroidism has also been described in some cases of X-linked hypophosphatemic rickets and other hypophosphatemic osteomalacias. Long-term treatment with supplemental phosphate is believed to induce intermittent slight decreases in ECF Ca^{++} and stimulation of PTH secretion. In symptomatic patients, surgical treatment— subtotal removal of the parathyroid mass or total parathyroidectomy with autografting of parathyroid tissue—is indicated.

5.4.1.4   Drug-Associated PHPT

PHPT has been reported in 4.3 to 6.3% of patients treated for many years with lithium, a well-established psychiatric medication [78]. Lithium appears to antagonize CaSR, thereby reducing the suppression of PTH by serum calcium. Serum calcium levels are elevated, although usually only slightly above the normal range. Intact PTH levels are typically mildly elevated or inappropriately normal in relationship to the increase in serum calcium along with a decrease in urinary calcium excretion with resultant hypocalciuria and generally normal serum phosphate levels.

An increase in $1,25(OH)_2D$ levels is thought to result from the normal physiologic actions of PTH on vitamin D metabolism as opposed to a direct effect of lithium on vitamin D metabolism. There appears to be an increase in multi-glandular disease associated with lithium therapy in keeping with its apparent action via CaSR. Surgical treatment may be required if other causes of hypercalcemia have been excluded, if lithium cannot be discontinued, or the patient cannot be transitioned to another psychiatric medication and significant hypercalcemia [exceeding 0.25 mM (1 mg/dL) above the reference range] persists.

5.4.1.5   Ectopic HPT

Inasmuch as PTH per se is expressed virtually exclusively in the parathyroid gland, the secretion of PTH by non-parathyroid tumors constitutes true ectopic hyperparathyroidism. However, true ectopic hyperparathyroidism as a cause of malignancy-associated hypercalcemia (MAH) is rare. A number of such cases of MAH with true PTH production have been well documented by immunological and molecular biological techniques. The tumors involved include ovarian, lung, thyroid, thymus, and gastric malignancies [79].

5.5   BONE DISEASE ASSOCIATED WITH INCREASED PTHR1 ACTION

5.5.1   JANSEN'S METAPHYSEAL CHONDRODYSPLASIA (JMC)

JMC is a rare autosomal dominant disorder, due to gain-of-function mutations in PTHR1 causing agonist-independent cAMP accumulation. It is characterized by short-limbed dwarfism and by persistent hypercalcemia, hypophosphatemia, and hypercalciuria. Activation of PTHR1 leads to excessive action of the receptor in the cartilaginous growth plate independent of PTHrP, the natural ligand for PTHR1 in the growth plate, and consequently to increased chondrocyte proliferation and delayed chondrocyte differentiation causing dysplastic growth plates, short-limbed dwarfism, and bowing of long bones [80]. Hypercalcemia and phosphaturia appear to arise from PTH-independent excess action of PTHR1 in bone and kidney, with the resultant hypercalcemia causing suppression of circulating PTH.

5.5.2   CHRONIC KIDNEY DISEASE (CKD)

PTH is an integral part of the CKD–mineral and bone disorder (MBD) syndrome, a systemic disorder characterized by abnormal calcium, phosphorus, PTH, and vitamin D metabolism. Renal osteodystrophy is the term traditionally used to describe the abnormalities in bone pathology that develop in CKD, but it is just one of several components of the mineral and bone disorders that occur as complications of CKD. Thus, in addition to affecting the skeletal system, CKD-MBD is related to the appearance of cardiovascular and soft tissue calcifications [81] that are associated with cardiovascular pathology [82–84].

As the GFR declines, one of the earliest alterations in mineral regulating hormones is an increase in the phosphaturic hormone called fibroblast growth factor (FGF) 23. This hormone can inhibit CYP27B1 production and reduce the production of 1,25 $(OH_2)D$. The lower circulating levels of $1,25(OH)_2D$ can reduce calcium absorption and circulating Ca^{++} levels. Reduced Ca^{++} and $1,25(OH)_2D$ then can enhance PTH secretion and parathyroid cell proliferation, leading to secondary hyperparathyroidism. PTH levels generally begin to increase as GFR declines to less than 60 mL/min/1.73 m^2.

As CKD worsens and renal mass declines, Pi retention occurs, accentuating the reductions of $1,25(OH)_2D$ production and circulating Ca^{++} and further increasing secondary hyperparathyroidism. Secondary hyperparathyroidism can lead to increased bone turnover with a high turnover state and net bone resorption. In advanced CKD, this can lead to bone pain and fractures; and the liberated skeletal Ca^{++} and Pi may enhance extra-skeletal calcification, including vascular calcification that may predispose to myocardial infarction.

In the past, the presence of aluminum in dialysis fluid and the use of aluminum-based phosphate binders resulted in aluminum toxicity characterized by increased mineralization lag time in bone, leading to osteomalacia and also to inhibition of PTH synthesis and release, leading to decreased circulating PTH. This syndrome was associated with increased bone pain and fractures. With the switch to calcium-based phosphate binders, the excess use of these binders coupled with excess use of active vitamin D compounds to replace low circulating $1,25(OH)_2D$ levels has been reported to cause hypercalcemia, suppress circulating PTH levels and also lead to reduced bone turnover and a state of adynamic bone disease [85]. This low turnover state in bone can also lead to bone pain, fractures, increased vascular calcification, and myocardial infarction.

Therefore, the most common forms of renal osteodystrophy are attributable largely to variations in the circulating levels of PTH. For this reason, these levels have been used as surrogate indicators of bone turnover. Circulating PTH levels are best determined with assays that specifically measure bioactive PTH rather than inert fragments that may accumulate due to reduced clearance in CKD. These are used together with measurements of serum calcium, phosphorus, and alkaline phosphatase levels (total or bone-specific) to evaluate, diagnose, and guide the treatment of renal osteodystrophy.

Although the specificity of PTH as an indicator of bone turnover has been questioned and several other circulating biochemical markers of bone formation and resorption have been investigated, their clinical applicability remains to be established. If inconsistencies in biochemical markers (e.g., high PTH and low alkaline phosphatase), unexplained bone pain, or unexplained fractures are present, a bone biopsy would be indicated. In children with CKD, additional tests are needed to assess linear growth rate. In addition to bone histology and serum biomarkers, imaging has become an important component of evaluating renal bone disease and remains the main tool in assessing extra-skeletal calcification in CKD patients.

5.5.3 RICKETS AND OSTEOMALACIA

Rickets is a disorder of the developing growth plate associated with altered mineralization and changes in chondrocyte proliferation and hypertrophy [86,87]. Decreased mineralization of bone, i.e., osteomalacia, generally accompanies rickets and after closure of the epiphyses, only the alterations of osteomalacia are seen. Often the *rickets* term is used to describe both rickets and osteomalacia in children prior to closure of the growth plate. Rickets and osteomalacia can be defined as calciopenic or phosphopenic, but whether decreased systemic or local mineralization ever occurs in the absence of phosphopenia remains unclear.

5.5.3.1 Calciopenic Rickets and Osteomalacia

Calciopenic rickets results from a deficiency of or resistance to the action of vitamin D or from insufficient calcium absorption from the intestine from lack of dietary calcium. It may present as early as 6 to 24 months of age although hypocalcemia may be evident in younger infants and is characterized clinically by hypotonia, growth retardation, muscle weakness, craniotabes, and delayed fontanelle closure, hypocalcemic seizures in early infancy, dental caries and tooth abcesses in older children and adults, and radiographic features of rickets. Typical laboratory findings include hypocalcemia, elevated serum PTH, hypophosphatemia, and reduced urine calcium excretion.

Secondary hyperparathyroidism is a prominent feature and contributes to the pathophysiologies in all forms of calciopenic rickets. Initially, in response to hypocalcemia, increased PTH secretion appears to temporarily restore normocalcemia in the course of the development of rickets and osteomalacia by stimulating $1,25(OH)_2D$ production and mobilizing Ca^{++} from bone. PTH appears to be the major factor causing phosphaturia and hypophosphatemia and therefore making an essential contribution to the mineralization defect. Ultimately, however, vitamin D and calcium deficiencies worsen and secondary hyperparathyroidism is unable to maintain normocalcemia [87].

Radiological evidence indicates widened epiphyseal growth plates and frayed and cupped metaphyses. Clinical evidence includes short stature, widened wrists, and beaded (rachitic rosary) ribs secondary to enlarged costochondral junctions. Osteomalacia is characterized radiologically by bowing of long bones, especially the femur, after walking begins (usually by age 2 to 3), and by pseudo-fractures (Looser's zones) in long bones.

Vitamin D deficiency, 25OHD deficiency, $1,25(OH)_2D$ deficiency, and $1,25(OH)_2D$ resistance may all contribute to the decreased capacity of the active form of vitamin D to enhance intestinal calcium absorption.

Vitamin D deficiency—Although $1,25(OH)_2D$ is the active form of vitamin D, the best measure of vitamin D sufficiency is provided by circulating levels of the inactive 25OHD metabolite that best integrates vitamin D sources from both cutaneous synthesis and intestinal absorption and has a longer circulating half-life than $1,25(OH)_2D$. Levels of 25OHD below 30 nmol/L (12 ng/mL) generally indicate vitamin D deficiency. Levels exceeding 50 nmol/L (20 ng/mL) or in some cases 75 nmol/L (30 ng/mL) reflect vitamin D sufficiency. Although frank vitamin D deficiency is rare in industrialized countries, vitamin D insufficiency as determined from 25OHD levels is relatively common, especially in winter months [88,89] and is still common in developing countries.

Deficiency of vitamin D per se may be nutritional or associated with malabsorption states, both of which limit intestinal absorption or may arise from habitation in higher latitudes, extensive use of sunscreens or customs of dress, or darkly pigmented skin, all which can decrease cutaneous synthesis of vitamin D. In addition, adiposity may reduce circulating 25OHD levels. Infants whose mothers had poor vitamin D status during pregnancy and those exclusively breast-fed for prolonged periods with little skin exposure to UVB are also at increased risk of vitamin D deficiency [90].

Deficiency of 25OHD—Because 25-hydroxylation of vitamin D may be performed by multiple hepatic enzymes, insufficient hepatic production of 25OHD is seldom a problem, even with diffuse liver disease. However 25OHD deficiency appears more common in primary biliary cirrhosis inasmuch as bile salts are needed for the entero-hepatic circulation of vitamin D metabolites. Chronic administration of anticonvulsant drugs has been associated with accelerating the disappearance of 25OHD from the circulation and the appearance of inactive polar metabolites of vitamin D in the bile and urine [92]. However, anticonvulsant drugs may display a variety of mechanisms for producing metabolic bone disease including high turnover bone loss seemingly independent of effects on bone mineralization [93].

Both vitamin D deficiency and 25OHD deficiency respond well to treatment with vitamin D but the dose must be monitored to ensure adequate resolution of the biochemical and radiologic changes and to prevent overtreatment that can lead to hypercalciuria and nephrocalcinosis.

Deficiency of 1,25(OH)$_2$D (pseudodeficiency rickets or vitamin D-dependent rickets type I)—CKD-MBD is the most common clinical entity characterized by 1,25(OH)$_2$D deficiency. However, loss of 1α(OH)ase (CYP27B1) enzyme function can also occur in a rare autosomal recessive disorder termed vitamin D-dependent rickets type 1 (VDDR-I). Mutations in the CYP27B1 gene are the molecular bases of VDDR-I [94]. Individuals who are compound heterozygous or homozygous for loss-of-function mutations in CYP27B1 have little or no capacity to convert 25OHD to 1,25(OH)$_2$D and develop congenital rickets and osteomalacia. Patients appear normal at birth but manifest signs between the ages of 2 to 24 months. They have low or undetectable serum levels of 1,25(OH)$_2$D despite normal or increased serum 25OHD. Treatment with calcitriol is generally successful but monitoring of the response is required to prevent hypercalciuria and nephrocalcinosis.

Resistance to 1,25(OH)$_2$D (vitamin D-dependent rickets type II)—Vitamin D-dependent rickets type II (VDDR- II) is a rare autosomal recessive disorder characterized by rickets, alopecia, and resistance to vitamin D therapy [95]. The resistance to 1,25(OH)$_2$D is caused by heterogeneous loss-of-function mutations in the vitamin D receptor (VDR), a member of the nuclear family of receptors. Serum concentrations of 1,25(OH)$_2$D are highly elevated in affected individuals due to the failure of the VDR to inhibit CYP27B1 and stimulate CYP24A1 that encodes the vitamin D 24-hydroxylase enzyme [24(OH)ase]. Alopecia is considered one of the indicators of severe hormone resistance in patients with VDDR-type II [96]. Treatment with intravenous calcium infusion and oral phosphate generally results in a significant gain in height and healing of rickets but not the alopecia.

Calcium deficiency—Studies in Africa and Bangladesh identified rickets in children, typically 3 to 5 years old at first presentation, in whom circulating 25OHD concentrations are higher than those characteristic of primary vitamin D deficiency. Calcium deficiency per se has been implicated. Calcium deficiency appears to be the major cause of rickets in Africa and some parts of tropical Asia, but is recognized increasingly in other parts of the world. Chronic calcium deficiency may be due to very low intakes and also due to poor absorption as a result, for example, of competing dietary factors, enteropathy, and intestinal bacterial or parasitic infestations. Genetic susceptibility may also occur [97]. Vitamin D supplementation alone therefore may not prevent or treat rickets in populations with limited calcium intakes.

5.5.3.2 Phosphopenic Rickets

Phosphopenic rickets may be classified as FGF23-related or associated with renal tubular dysfunction.

FGF23-related—FGF23 is a potent osteocyte-derived phosphaturic hormone [98] that reduces transcription of SLC34A1 and SLC34A3 that encode the renal Pi transporters, NaPi-IIa and NaPi-IIc, respectively. It is also a powerful inhibitor of the renal 1α(OH)ase enzyme, CYP27B1, and therefore of 1,25(OH)$_2$D production, and a stimulator of the transcription of renal CYP24A1 that encodes the 24(OH)ase enzyme, causing increased clearance of plasma $1,25(OH)_2D$.

Although both FGF23 and PTH can induce renal phosphate wasting, the contrasting effects on circulating $1,25(OH)_2D$ of elevated FGF23 (inhibition) and of elevated PTH (stimulation) result in more profound hypophosphatemia in association with elevated FGF23 because of reduced intestinal absorption of phosphate due to suppressed $1,25(OH)_2D$. Rickets and osteomalacia associated with increased FGF23 are therefore accompanied by hypophosphatemia, a low tubular maximum for phosphorus reabsorption per glomerular filtration rate (TMP/GFR) resulting in phosphaturia, inappropriately normal or low circulating $1,25(OH)_2D$, and normal or elevated circulating PTH. Despite the increased FGF23 levels reported to inhibit PTH release, the increased PTH is believed to arise from low $1,25(OH)_2D$ with resultant decreased intestinal Ca^{++} absorption. Studies in a mouse model of X-linked hypophosphatemic rickets (XLH) have shown that animals die of hypocalcemia in the absence of parathyroid function [99].

Consequently although treatment with phosphate replacement, especially in the absence of concomitant calcitriol, may aggravate the secondary hyperparathyroidism and lead to tertiary hyperparathyroidism, secondary hyperparathyroidism appears to be a required compensatory mechanism in FGF23-related rickets and osteomalacia to maintain normal Ca^{++} in the presence of reduced $1,25(OH)_2D$.

Increased FGF23 production—Increased FGF23 production occurs in XLH, the most common inherited form of rickets (prevalence of 1 in 20,000). In addition to the usual rachitic manifestations, children may also develop frontal bossing, oxycephaly, and craniosynostosis; adults may develop enthesophytes. The elevated FGF23 levels appear due to a mutation in the PHEX gene (phosphate-regulating gene with homologies to endopeptidases on the X chromosome) [101]. However, the exact mechanism whereby PHEX leads to increased FGF23 levels is presently unknown.

Increased FGF23 production can occur in autosomal recessive hypophosphatemic rickets (ARHR) due to homozygous inactivating mutations of the gene encoding dentin matrix protein 1 (DMP1). Again, the mechanism whereby DMP1 mutations increase FGF23 is unknown. A form of ARHR associated with homozygous loss-of-function mutations in ectonucleotide pyrophosphatase/phophodiesterase 1 (ENPP1) and a predisposition to vascular calcifications has also been described [104] but the mechanism whereby increased FGF23 occurs is uncertain.

Fibrous dysplasia (FD) lesions may have postzygotic somatic activating mutations in GNAS-1, which encodes the α subunit of stimulatory G protein (Gsα) and appears to stimulate the release of FGF23 [105]. FD lesions may be monostotic or polyostotic and mineralization defects may involve bones with FD lesions and bones without such lesions. Patients may also exhibit hypophosphatemia.

A closely related condition known as McCune-Albright syndrome (MAS) is caused by activating mutations in GNAS, which encodes the AC-stimulating Gsα G protein and is characterized by polyostotic fibrous dysplasia, cutaneous hyperpigmented patches, and hyperfunctioning endocrine disorders (e.g., precocious puberty). Some patients with MAS develop a hypophosphatemic phenotype similar to ARHR patients, and may have increased circulating FGF23 levels that roughly correlate with the number of skeletal fibrous dysplastic lesions [106]. Consequently Gsα appears to be a stimulator of FGF23 release from bone.

Increased FGF23 production may also occur in tumor-induced osteomalacia (TIO), often in adults. Tumors are generally of mesenchymal origin (e.g., hemangiopericy-tomas), usually benign, and small and difficult to localize, but can recur. Prostate cancer has also been reported to produce this syndrome [107]. Neurofibromatosis has been associated with hypophosphatemic osteomalacia [108].

Decreased FGF23 degradation—Missense mutations causing reduced FGF23 degradation by furin-like enzymes, leading to increased circulating bioactive FGF23 have been reported in autosomal dominant hypophosphatemic rickets (ADHR) [109]. This disorder can present in children, adolescents, or adults, displays incomplete penetrance, delayed onset at times (pregnancy may be a precipitating factor), and is occasionally reversible (e.g., in children at puberty).

Increased co-receptor or receptor activity—Hypophosphatemic rickets has also been described due to increased production of klotho, the co-receptor that trans-duces FGF23 signaling. Markedly elevated circulating FGF23 levels and hyperpara-thyroidism due to parathyroid hyperplasia have been described in this syndrome, which may be caused by a translocation of the klotho gene. How klotho regulates FGF23 levels is unknown.

Linear sebaceous or epidermal nevus syndrome (ENS) may be caused by a mosaicism of activating FGF receptor (FGFR) 3 mutations in the human epidermis [110]. Osteoglophonic dysplasia (OD) is a disorder characterized by craniosynosto-sis, prominent supraorbital ridge, and depressed nasal bridge, as well as rhizomelic dwarfism and non-ossifying bone lesions. It is caused by activating mutations in FGFR1 [111]. In both cases, increased FGF23 and rickets were reported, but how the increased FGFR activity increases FGF23 is presently unknown.

Renal tubular dysfunction, isolated renal Pi loss—Hereditary hypophospha-temic rickets with hypercalciuria (HHRH) is a disorder due to a mutation within the gene encoding the type IIc sodium–phosphate co-transporter [112,113] and is associ-ated with hypophosphatemia, hyperphosphaturia, normal serum calcium and 25OHD concentrations, elevated 1,25(OH)$_2$D, and hypercalciuria. Secondary hyperparathy-roidism does not appear to be a prominent feature, at least in untreated patients.

Renal tubular dysfunction, complex renal tubular defects—Fanconi's syn-drome, a generalized transport defect in the proximal tubules leading to renal losses of a variety of organic compounds including phosphate [114] and distal renal tubu-lar acidosis (RTA), may also be associated with hypophosphatemia and rickets. Secondary hyperparathyroidism may occur in cases where chronic hypocalcemia is also present.

5.6   BONE DISEASE ASSOCIATED WITH DECREASED PTH ACTION

5.6.1   Primary Hypoparathyroidism

Reduction or absence of circulating PTH results in a loss of renal effects includ-ing 1,25(OH)$_2$D production, calcium reabsorption, increased phosphate clearance; loss of the intestinal absorption of calcium facilitated by 1,25(OH)$_2$D; and a loss of bone effects including a reduction of bone resorption. The resulting biochemical abnormalities include low or undetectable circulating serum PTH, hypocalcemia, hyperphosphatemia, and low circulating $1,25(OH)_2D$ levels. Hypocalcemia must be confirmed by measurement of ionized calcium or by correction for serum albumin by the following formulas:

Corrected calcium (mg/dL) = measured total serum calcium (mg/dL) +
$\qquad$ [4.0 – serum albumin (g/dL) × 0.8]
Corrected calcium (mM) $\quad$ = measured total Ca (mM) +
$\qquad$ [40 – serum albumin (g/L)] × 0.02

Despite an increase in fractional excretion of calcium, intestinal calcium absorption and bone resorption are both suppressed, resulting in a reduced renal filtered load of calcium and consequent hypocalciuria; nephrogenous cyclic AMP excretion is low and fractional excretion of phosphate in the urine is reduced.

Animal models of PTH deficiency showed increases in both trabecular and cortical bone volume [115,116]. Human studies largely recapitulated the findings in animals. However, virtually all studies in humans have involved children or adults on long-term vitamin D and calcium therapy, and frequently on thiazide diuretics, all of which may alter skeletal activity. Nevertheless, the studies also show a profound reduction in the bone turnover rate in hypoparathyroidism, accompanied by an increase in bone mass in both trabecular and cortical compartments [117].

5.6.1.1 Clinical Manifestations

The signs and symptoms of hypoparathyroidism include evidence of latent or overt neuromuscular hyperexcitability due to hypocalcemia. The effect may be aggravated by hyperkalemia or hypomagnesemia, but the severity of symptoms shows wide variation. Thus, "idiopathic hypoparathyroidism" has been traditionally used to describe isolated cases of glandular hypofunction when a cause is not obvious and there is no family history. However, hypoparathyroidism may also occur in a variety of inherited and acquired disorders that may color the presentation of the hypoparathyroidism.

The most common manifestations of hypocalcemia include circumoral numbness, paresthesias of the distal extremities, or muscle cramping that may progress to carpopedal spasm or tetany. Laryngospasm or bronchospasm and seizures may also occur. Other less specific manifestations include fatigue, irritability, and personality disturbance.

Severe hypocalcemia may be associated with a prolonged Q-Tc interval on electrocardiography, which reverses with treatment. More extensive cardiomyopathic changes are occasionally seen, particularly in adults. These include chest pain, elevated enzymes (CPK), left ventricular impairment, and T-wave inversion suggestive of a myocardial infarction. Patients with chronic hypocalcemia may have calcification of the basal ganglia or more widespread intracranial calcification, detected by skull x-ray or computerized tomography.

Also seen are extrapyramidal neurological symptoms (more often with intracranial calcification), subcapsular cataracts, band keratopathy, and abnormal dentition. Increased neuromuscular irritability may be demonstrated by eliciting a Chvostek or

Trousseau sign. The Chvostek sign is a prolonged reflex contraction of the facial muscle in response to a digital tap on the cheek just anterior to the ear. As with other hyper-reflexias, up to 20% of normal individuals may demonstrate slight positive reactions. The Trousseau sign is carpopedal spasm induced by inflation of a blood pressure cuff covering the upper arm to 20 mm Hg above systolic blood pressure for 3 minutes. A positive response reflects the heightened irritability of nerves undergoing pressure ischemia.

5.6.1.2   Causes of Hypoparathyroidism

The most common acquired cause of hypoparathyroidism in adults is postoperative hypoparathyroidism [118] due to inadvertent or unavoidable removal of or damage to the parathyroid glands and/or their blood supply. Surgery on the thyroid or parathyroid glands or adjacent neck structures or neck dissection surgery for malignancy may lead to transient or chronic hypoparathyroidism (when the hypoparathyroidism persists for more than 6 months).

Autoimmune disease may be a significant cause of hypoparathyroidism. Antibodies directed against parathyroid tissue have been detected in over 30% of patients with isolated hypoparathyroid disease and over 40% of patients having hypoparathyroidism combined with other endocrine deficiencies. Activating antibodies against the parathyroid CaSR have been reported either as isolated events producing acquired autoimmune hypoparathyroidism also called autosomal dominant hypocalcemia [119,120] or in type 1 autoimmune polyglandular syndrome (APS-1) [121].

APS-1, also known as autoimmune polyendocrinopathy–candidiasis–ectodermal dystrophy (APECED) usually presents in infancy with candidiasis followed by hypoparathyroidism in the first decade and adreno-cortical failure in the third decade. Additional features may include pernicious anemia, chronic active hepatitis, alopecia, keratitis, gonadal failure, autoimmune thyroid disease, pancreatic insufficiency, and diabetes mellitus [122,123] although the phenotype is highly variable.

The responsible gene, called the autoimmune regulator (AIRE), maps to chromosome 21q22 and encodes a protein regulator that plays an important role in induction of T cell tolerance [123]. APS-1/APECED may be sporadic or inherited as an autosomal-recessive disorder and has been associated with more than 40 mutations of the AIRE gene (http://bioinf.uta.fi/AIREbase/).

Radiation therapy to the neck may also be followed by loss of parathyroid gland function and parathyroid insufficiency. Hypoparathyroidism is occasionally seen in inherited metabolic disorders, e.g., those leading to excess storage of iron such as hemachromatosis [124], thalassemia [125], and other inherited anemias or to excess storage of copper (Wilson's disease) [126]. In most instances, similar dysfunctions appear in other endocrine glands and the parathyroid disease is mild. Granulomatous [127] or neoplastic invasion [128] can occasionally destroy parathyroid structure and function but other manifestations of these underlying disorders are usually evident.

In addition to genetic causes of parathyroid tissue destruction, genetic defects, have been described in PTH biosynthesis, PTH secretion, and parathyroid gland development and may be associated with or without other congenital anomalies such as dysmorphic facies, immunodeficiency, lymphedema, nephropathy, nerve deafness, and cardiac malformation. Genetic causes of hypoparathyroidism [119,129–132] are listed in Table 5.1.

TABLE 5.1

Hypoparathyroidism Forms Having Genetic Bases

Hypoparathyroid Condition	Gene/Chromosome Locus
Isolated	

Isolated

Autosomal Dominant

PTH dominant-negative gene mutation (impaired PTH translocation into secretory apparatus) [129]	*PTH*/11p15
CaSR activating mutation	*CaSR*/3q21.1 (119)
GCMB (glial cells missing, B gene) mutation (parathyroid developmental defect)	*GCMB*/6p24.2 (130)

Autosomal Recessive

PTH gene homozygous mutation (reduced production of preproPTH) [131]	*PTH*/11p15
GCMB mutation [132]	*GCMB*/6p24.2

X-linked

Parathyroid developmental defect [133]	*SOX3*/Xq26-27

Congenital Multi-System Syndromes

DiGeorge and velocardiofacial (mutated T-box transcription factor in embryonic tissues [134], loss of other contiguous genes	*TBX1*/22q11
Barakat hypoparathyroidism, deafness, renal dysplasia (HDR syndrome), haplo insufficiency of transcription for parathyroid, renal, and auditory development [135]	*GTA3*/10p13-14
Kenny-Caffey and Sanjad-Sakati (hypoparathyroidism–retardation–dysmorphism syndrome), mutated protein required for microtubule assembly [136]	*TBCE*/1q42-43

Metabolic Diseases

Mitochondrial neuromyopathies such as mitochondrial encephalopathy, lactic acidosis, and stroke-like episodes (MELAS) syndrome, Kearns-Sayre syndrome, Pearson's syndrome, tRNA-Leu mutations	Mitochondrial genome
Long-chain hydroxyacyl-CoA dehydrogenase (LCHAD) deficiency	Unknown
Heavy metal storage disorders such as Wilson's disease, mutations in copper-transporting P-type ATPase gene (ATP7B)	*ATP7B*/2p13-p16
Hemochromatosis	*HFE*/6p21.3

Autoimmune Disease

Autoimmune polyendocrine syndrome type I (APS-1 or APECED)	*AIRE*/21q22.3

Therapy of symptomatic hypocalcemia (carpal or pedal spasm, seizures, bronchospasm, or laryngospasm) can be a medical emergency requiring acute administration of intravenous calcium. If the serum calcium is above 1.9 mM (7.5 mg/dL) and the patient is asymptomatic, therapy consists of vitamin D or analogues and calcium. Occasionally, thiazide diuretics are added to reduce renal calcium excretion, which may be elevated in association with vitamin D treatment, in order to facilitate normalization of the serum calcium. Studies are ongoing to evaluate use of PTH and analogues for the treatment of hypoparathyroidism [137].

5.7 BONE DISEASE ASSOCIATED WITH DECREASED PTHR1 ACTION: PARATHYROID RESISTANCE SYNDROMES

5.7.1 PSEUDOHYPOPARATHYROIDISM

Several clinical disorders characterized by end-organ resistance to PTH have been described and are collectively termed pseudohypoparathyroidism (PHP). They are generally associated with hypocalcemia, hyperphosphatemia, and increased circulating PTH. CKD, vitamin D deficiency, and magnesium deficiency must, of course, first be excluded. Exogenous PTH administration fails to increase nephrogenous cAMP and phosphate excretion, indicating target tissue unresponsiveness to the hormone [138]. The biochemical characteristics of these disorders are compared in Table 5.2.

5.7.1.1 Pseudohypoparathyroidism Type 1a (PHP-1a)

Patients with PHP-1a display about a 50% reduction in Gsα activity, which is caused by maternally inherited heterozygous GNAS mutations. Gsα is derived in the proximal renal tubules only from the maternal GNAS allele, in view of the fact that the paternal copy is imprinted and therefore silenced [139]. Consequently these maternal GNAS mutations lead to virtually complete absence of this signaling protein in the proximal but not the distal renal tubules. This therefore leads to renal PTH resistance with reduced phosphaturia, reduced $1,25(OH)_2D$ production, hypocalcemia, and hyperphosphatemia.

The importance of cAMP in mediating the effects of PTH is evident from these disturbances. In addition to these biochemical findings, as a result of deficiency of Gsα alleles in relevant tissues during development, patients affected by PHP-1a can

TABLE 5.2
Biochemical Characteristics of Pseudohypoparathyroidism

	PHP1a	PHP1b	Type 1c	PHP2	PPHP
↑PTH	Yes	Yes	Yes	Yes	No
↓Ca/↑P/↓$1,25(OH)_2D$	Yes	Yes	Yes	Yes	No
Response to IV PTH					
↑U cAMP	No	No	No	Yes	Yes
↑U PO_4	No	No	No	No	Yes
AHO	Yes	Variable	Yes	No	Yes
Hormonal resistance	Multiple	PTH	Multiple	PTH	None

↑ = Increased; ↓ = decreased.

present with clinical features referred to as Albright hereditary osteodystrophy (AHO) [140]. The features include changes in body habitus such as short stature and obesity, craniofacial abnormalities including round face, strabismus, frontal bossing and mental retardation, brachydactyly, including brachymetacarpia, brachymetatarsia, brachyphalangia, and other connective tissue features such as ectopic calcification.

Reduction in Gsα may reduce AC coupling of other GPCRs such as the thyroid-stimulating hormone (TSH) receptor and the growth hormone–releasing hormone (GHRH) receptor. Hypothyroidism may therefore also develop in these patients because of resistance to TSH; hypogonadism can occur as a result of gonadotropin resistance; and GHRH resistance may contribute to short stature, which responds favorably to recombinant human growth hormone treatment [141].

5.7.1.2 Pseudopseudohypoparathyroidism (Pseudo-PHP)

Patients who inherit a paternal GNAS mutation do not display hormonal resistance because although the genetic imprinting of the paternal allele silences this allele, the Gsα protein in the proximal renal tubule is derived only from the maternal allele which is functional. However, in other tissues the paternal allele is required and Gsα protein is consequently reduced as a result of the paternal mutation. These patients therefore have phenotypic features of AHO. This syndrome is known as pseudo-PHP.

5.7.1.3 Pseudohypoparathyroidism Type 1b (PHP-1b)

Individuals with PHP-1b exhibit abnormal GNAS methylation on the maternal allele and consequent Gsα deficiency in the renal proximal tubules leading to PTH resistance. This may be autosomal dominant in inheritance or may occur sporadically. Typically, these patients do not present with the skeletal abnormalities of AHO, but recent reports identified some cases with mild AHO, indicating overlap between PHP-1a and PHP-1b [140].

5.7.1.4 Pseudohypoparathyroidism Type 1c (PHP-1c)

Patients with PHP-1c exhibit mutations that reside in the last exon encoding Gsα and the reduced Gsα is not detectable in the assay usually used to detect Gsα deficiency. Nevertheless, although the assay does not demonstrate a reduction in Gsα activity, these patients exhibit renal resistance to both PTH and AHO as do patients with PHP-1a.

5.7.1.5 Pseudohypoparathyroidism Type 2 (PHP-2)

In individuals affected by PHP-2, PTH resistance is characterized by a normal increase in urinary cAMP in response to exogenous PTH and a reduced phosphaturic response [142]. The defect was therefore postulated to exist downstream of cAMP production, i.e., in PKA, one of its substrates or targets, or in a component of the PTH-PKC signaling pathway. However, a clear genetic or familial basis has not been documented. It has been proposed that PHP-2 may be an acquired defect.

5.7.2 Blomstrand Chondrodysplasia and Related PTH Receptor Defects

Blomstrand chondrodysplasia is a lethal autosomal recessive disorder caused by homozygous or compound heterozygous loss-of-function mutations in PTHR1 [143–145]. It is characterized by abnormal endochondral bone formation with accelerated differentiation and premature mineralization of the cartilaginous growth plates consistent with the action of PTHrP via PTHR1, and results in short-limbed dwarfism. In addition, it is associated with craniofacial malformations, hydrops, hypoplastic lungs, and aortic coarctation. Secondary hyperplasia of the parathyroid glands occurs, presumably as a result of hypocalcemia.

A milder form of recessively inherited skeletal dysplasia known as Eiken syndrome has also been linked to mutations of PTHR1, suggesting that a wider range of skeletal phenotypes may be attributed to this gene [146].

A PTHR1 mutation was identified in two out of six patients with enchondromatosis (Ollier's disease), a familial disorder with evidence of autosomal dominance characterized by multiple benign cartilage tumors and a predisposition to malignant osteosarcomas [147]. A follow-up study failed to reveal any PTHR1 mutations, and it is likely that the condition is genetically heterogeneous [148].

In all of these syndromes, decreased PTHR1 function probably reflects resistance to the action of PTHrP rather than to the action of PTH.

5.7.3 Hypomagnesemia

Hypomagnesemia leads to decreased PTH release and to some degree of peripheral resistance, but the precise molecular mechanisms underlying these defects are unknown [149]. Laboratory testing of patients with hypocalcemia should therefore include measurement of serum magnesium, particularly in newborns.

5.8 PTH IN OSTEOPOROSIS

Although a picture of reduced bone mineral density (BMD) simulating primary osteoporosis has been observed in mild PHPT and in other disorders associated with increased circulating concentrations of PTH such as vitamin D deficiency, the role of PTH in the pathophysiology of post-menopausal osteoporosis and in male osteoporosis remains uncertain.

Secondary increases in PTH have been reported in patients using anti-resorptive therapy for osteoporosis as a result of hypocalcemia induced by decreased Ca^{++} efflux from bone due to reduced bone turnover. Whether these contribute to the increases in BMD observed with these agents remains uncertain [150]. It seems reasonable to assume, however, that the resorptive effects of increased PTH in these cases are mitigated by the anti-resorptive agents and that the secondary increases in endogenous PTH may indeed be beneficial and reflect largely its anabolic activity.

Exogenous recombinant PTH (1-34), known as teriparatide, and intact recombinant PTH (1-84) have both been effective anabolic therapies for post-menopausal, male, and glucocorticoid-induced osteoporosis when administered intermittently (daily) by the subcutaneous route. Their use has generally been restricted to less than 2 years, partly because initial studies in Fischer rats revealed an increase incidence of osteosarcoma [151].

To date, despite widespread use in humans, the incidence of osteosarcomas is no greater in users of these agents than in non-users [152]. Based on bone marker evidence, the increase in bone formation is the primary response after PTH administration to osteoporotic humans followed by an increase in bone resorptive activity reflecting PTH-induced osteoclastic stimulation. Consequently, a therapeutic anabolic window exists before resorption matches formation and BMD increases cease [153]. Thus, a plateauing of the net anabolic effect appears to occur after 18 to 24 months.

In animals, co-treatment of PTH with anti-resorptive agents (bisphosphonates or RANKL inhibitors) enhances its anabolic activity [154], whereas pre-treatment appears to blunt, but not eliminate, the anabolic effects [155]. Thus, the anti-resorptives appear to prolong the anabolic window. In humans, both co-treatment [156] and pre-treatment [157] with oral daily alendronate has been reported to blunt its activity while a single intravenous dose of zoledronic acid [158] has been reported to enhance its activity.

In all cases, however, discontinuation of PTH after a course of therapy for osteoporosis results in loss of accrued bone due to unopposed bone resorption. Consequently, anti-resorptive therapy is required after PTH use to maintain the bone gains [159]. Administered PTH reduces spine fractures to a much greater degree than fractures in non-vertebral bones, perhaps because the compartmental effect of PTH with cortical bone is less positively affected than trabecular bone [160].

Different PTH formulations are being developed to circumvent the use of daily subcutaneous injections, including transdermal [161], oral, and inhaled [162] forms. Whether these will be successful in clinical use remains to be determined. Attempts have also been made to enhance intermittent release of endogenous PTH by the use of CaSR antagonists (calcilytics). To date, however, the release of PTH with the calcilytic employed was too sustained to produce an anabolic effect [163]. As the armamentarium for osteoporosis increases, the role and timing of PTH anabolic therapy may have to be re-assessed.

REFERENCES

1. Naylor, S.L., Sakaguchi, A.Y., Szoka, P. et al. 1983. Human parathyroid hormone gene (PTH) is on short arm of chromosome 11. *Somatic Cell Genet* 9: 609–616.
2. Goltzman, D., Henderson, B., and Loveridge, N. 1980. Cytochemical bioassay of parathyroid hormone: characteristics of the assay and analysis of circulating hormonal forms. *J Clin Invest* 65: 1309–1317.
3. Brown, E.M. 2004. Calcium sensing by endocrine cells. *Endocrine Pathology* 15: 187–220.
4. Brown, E.M. 1983. Four-parameter model of the sigmoidal relationship between parathyroid hormone release and extracellular calcium concentration in normal and abnormal parathyroid tissue. *J Clin Endocrinol Metabol* 56: 572–581.
5. Mayer, G.P., Keaton, J.A., Hurst, J.G. et al. 1979. Effects of plasma calcium concentration on the relative proportion of hormone and carboxyl fragments in parathyroid venous blood. *Endocrinology* 104: 1778.
6. Hanley, D.A. and Ayer, L.M. 1986. Calcium-dependent release of carboxyl-terminal fragments of parathyroid hormone by hyperplastic human parathyroid tissue in vitro. *J Clin Endocrinol Metabol* 63: 1075
7. D'Amour, P., Palardy, J., Bahsali, G., et al. 1992. The modulation of circulating parathyroid hormone immunoheterogeneity in man by ionized calcium concentration. *J Clin Endocrinol Metabol* 74: 525.

8. Segre, G.V., D'Amour, P., Hultman, A. et al. 1981. Effects of hepatectomy, nephrectomy, and nephrectomy/uremia on the metabolism of parathyroid hormone in the rat. *J Clin Invest* 67: 439.

9. Yamamoto, M., Igarishi, T., Muramatsu, M. et al. 1989. Hypocalcemia increases and hypercalcemia decreases the steady state level of parathyroid hormone messenger RNA in the rat. *J Clin Invest* 83: 1053.

10. Naveh-Many, T. and Silver, J. 1990. Regulation of parathyroid hormone gene expression by hypocalcemia, hypercalcemia, and vitamin D in the rat. *J Clin Invest* 86: 1313.

11. Kilav, R., Silver, J., and Naveh-Many, T. 1987. A conserved cis-acting element in the parathyroid hormone 3′-untranslated region is sufficient for regulation of RNA stability by calcium and phosphate. *J Biol Chem* 276: 8727–8733.

12. Kremer, R., Bolivar, I., Goltzman, D. et al. 1989. Influence of calcium and 1,25-dihydroxycholecalciferol on proliferation and proto-oncogene expression in primary cultures of bovine parathyroid cells. *Endocrinology* 125: 935.

13. Russell, J., Lettieri, D., and Sherwood, L.M. 1986. Suppression by 1,25(OH)2D3 of transcription of the pre-proparathyroid hormone gene. *Endocrinology* 119: 2864–2866.

14. Salehi-Tabar, R., Nguyen-Yamamoto, L., Tavera-Mendoza, L.E. et al. 2012. Vitamin D receptor as a master regulator of the c-MYC/MXD1 network. *Proc Natl Acad Sci USA* 109: 18827–18832.

15. Kawahara, M., Iwasaki, Y., Sakaguchi, K. et al. 2010. Involvement of GCMB in the transcriptional regulation of the human parathyroid hormone gene in a parathyroid-derived cell line PT-r: effects of calcium and 1,25(OH)$_2$D3. *Bone* 47: 534–541.

16. Wallace, J. and Scarpa, A. 1983. Similarities of Li+ and low Ca^{2+} in the modulation of secretion by parathyroid cells in vitro. *J Biol Chem* 258: 6288–6292.

17. Dusso, A., Cozzolino, M., Lu, Y. et al. 2004. 1,25-Dihydroxyvitamin D down-regulation of TGF-α/EGFR expression and growth signaling: a mechanism for the antiproliferative actions of the sterol in parathyroid hyperplasia of renal failure. *J Steroid Biochem Mol Biol* 89–90: 507–511.

18. Xu, M., Choudhary, S., Goltzman D. et al. 2005. Do cycloxygenase-2 knockout mice have primary hyperparathyroidism? *Endocrinology* 146: 1843.

19. Nakajima, K., Umino, K., Azuma, Y. et al. 2009. Stimulating parathyroid cell proliferation and PTH release with phosphate in organ cultures obtained from patients with primary and secondary hyperparathyroidism for a prolonged period. *J Bone Miner Metabol* 27: 224–235.

20. Silver, J. and Naveh-Many, T. 2012. FGF23 and the parathyroid. *Adv Exp Med Biol* 728: 92–99.

21. Tregear, G.W., Van Rietschoten, J., Greene, E. et al. 1973. Bovine parathyroid hormone: minimum chain length of synthetic peptide required for biological activity. *Endocrinology* 93: 1349–1353.

22. Goltzman, D., Peytremann, A., Callahan, E. et al. 1975. Analysis of requirements for parathyroid hormone action in renal membranes with the use of inhibiting analogues. *J Biol Chem* 250: 3199–3203.

23. Jüppner, H., Abou-Samra, A.B., Freeman, M. et al. 1991. A G protein-linked receptor for parathyroid hormone and parathyroid hormone-related peptide. *Science* 254: 1024.

24. Abou-Samra, A.B., Jüppner, H., Force, T. et al. 1992. Expression cloning of a common receptor for parathyroid hormone and parathyroid hormone-related peptide from rat osteoblast-like cells: a single receptor stimulates intracellular accumulation of both cAMP and inositol trisphosphates and increases intracellular free calcium. *Proc Natl Acad Sci USA* 89: 2732–2733.

25. Vilardaga, J.P., Romero, G., Friedman, P.A. et al. 2011. Molecular basis of parathyroid hormone receptor signaling and trafficking: a family B GPCR paradigm. *Cell Mol Life Sci* 68: 1–13.

26. Datta, N.S. and Abou-Samra, A.B. 2009. PTH and PTHrP signaling in osteoblasts. *Cell Signal* 21: 1245–1254.

27. Singh, A.T., Gilchrist, A., Voyno-Yasenetskaya, T. et al. 2005. Gα12/Gα13 subunits of heterotrimeric G proteins mediate parathyroid hormone activation of phospholipase D in UMR-106 osteoblastic cells. *Endocrinology* 146: 2171–2175.

28. Radeff, J.M., Nagy, Z., and Stern, P.H. 2004. Rho and rho kinase are involved in parathyroid hormone-stimulated protein kinase C α translocation and IL-6 promoter activity in osteoblastic cells. *J Bone Miner Res* 19: 1882–1891.

29. Ferrari, S.L., Behar, V., Chorev, M. et al. 1999. Endocytosis of ligand-human parathyroid hormone receptor 1 complexes is protein kinase C-dependent and involves β-arrestin 2: real-time monitoring by fluorescence microscopy. *J Biol Chem* 274: 29968–29975.

30. Bohinc, B.N. and Gesty-Palmer, D. 2011. β-arrestin-biased agonism at the parathyroid hormone receptor uncouples bone formation from bone resorption. *Endocr Metabol Immune Disord Drug Targets* 11: 112–119.

31. Sneddon, W.B., Syme, C.A., Bisello, A. et al. 2003. Activation-independent parathyroid hormone receptor internalization is regulated by NHERF1 (EBP50). *J Biol Chem* 278: 43787–43796.

32. Wang, B., Ardura, J.A., Romero, G. et al. 2010. Na/H exchanger regulatory factors control parathyroid hormone receptor signaling by facilitating differential activation of Gα protein subunits. *J Biol Chem* 285: 26976–26986.

33. Mahon, M.J., Donowitz, M., Yun, C.C. et al. 2002. Na+/H+ exchanger regulatory factor 2 directs parathyroid hormone 1 receptor signalling. *Nature* 417: 858–886.

34. Maeda, S., Wu, S., Jüppner, H. et al. 1996.Cell-specific signal transduction of parathyroid hormone (PTH)-related protein through stably expressed recombinant PTH/PTHrP receptors in vascular smooth muscle cells. *Endocrinology* 137: 3154–3162.

35. Murer, H., Hernando, N., Forster, I. et al. 2003. Regulation of Na/Pi transporter in the proximal tubule. *Annu Rev Physiol* 65: 531–542.

36. Lambers, T.T., Bindels, R.J., and Hoenderop, J.G. 2006. Coordinated control of renal Ca^{2+} handling. *Kidney Intl* 69: 650–654.

37. van Abel, M., Hoenderop, J.G., van der Kemp, A.W. et al. 2005. Coordinated control of renal Ca^{2+} transport proteins by parathyroid hormone. *Kidney Intl* 68: 1708–1721.

38. Cha, S.K., Wu, T., and Huang, C.L. 2008. Protein kinase C inhibits caveolae-mediated endocytosis of TRPV5. *Am J Physiol Renal Physiol* 294: F1212–F1221.

39. Topala, C.N., Schoeber, J.P., Searchfield, L.E. et al. 2009. Activation of the Ca^{2+}-sensing receptor stimulates the activity of the epithelial Ca^{2+} channelTRPV5. *Cell Calcium* 45: 331–339.

40. Custer, M., Lotscher, M., Biber, J. et al. 1994. Expression of Na-P(i) co-transport in rat kidney: localization by RT-PCR and immunohistochemistry. *Am J Physiol* 266: F767–F774.

41. Bacic, D., Lehir, M., Biber, J. et al. 2006. The renal Na+/phosphate co-transporter NaPi-IIa is internalized via the receptor-mediated endocytic route in response to parathyroid hormone. *Kidney Intl* 69: 495–503.

42. Segawa, H., Yamanaka, S., Onitsuka, A. et al. 2007. Parathyroid hormone-dependent endocytosis of renal type IIc Na-Pi co-transporter. *Am J Physiol Renal Physiol* 292: F395–F403.

43. Traebert, M., Volkl, H., Biber, J. et al. 2000. Luminal and contraluminal action of 1-34 and 3-34 PTH peptides on renal type IIa Na-P(i) co-transporter. *Am J Physiol Renal Physiol* 278: F792–F798.

44. Brenza, H.L., Kimmel-Jehan, C., Jehan, F. et al. 1998. Parathyroid hormone activation of the 25-hydroxyvitamin D3-1alpha-hydroxylase gene promoter. *Proc Natl Acad Sci USA* 95: 1387–1391.

45. Rouleau, M.F., Mitchell, J., and Goltzman, D.1990. Characterization of the major parathyroid hormone target cell in the endosteal metaphysis of rat long bones. *J Bone Miner Res* 5: 1043–1053.
46. Kramer, I., Keller, H., Leupin, O. et al. 2010. Does osteocytic SOST suppression mediate PTH bone anabolism? *Trends Endocrinol Metabol* 21: 237–244.
47. Rhee, Y., Allen, M.R., Condon, K. et al. 2011. PTH receptor signaling in osteocytes governs periosteal bone formation and intracortical remodeling. *J Bone Miner Res* 26: 1035–1046.
48. Boyle, W.J., Simonet, W.S., and Lacey, D.L. 2003. Osteoclast differentiation and activation. *Nature* 423: 337–442.
49. Silva, B.C., Costa, A.G., Cusano, N.E. et al. 2011. Catabolic and anabolic actions of parathyroid hormone on the skeleton. *Endocrinol Invest* 34: 801–810.
50. Miao, D., He, B., Karaplis, A.C., and Goltzman, D. 2002. Parathyroid hormone is essential for normal fetal bone formation. *J Clin Invest* 109: 1173–1182.
51. Miao, D., He, B., Lanske, B. et al. 2004. Skeletal abnormalities in Pth-null mice are influenced by dietary calcium. *Endocrinology* 145: 2046–2053.
52. Yan, J., Sun, W., Zhang, J. et al. 2012. Bone marrow ablation demonstrates that excess endogenous parathyroid hormone plays distinct roles in trabecular and cortical bone. *Am J Pathol* 181: 234–244.
53. Ren, Y., Liu, B., Feng, Y. et al. 2011. Endogenous PTH deficiency impairs fracture healing and impedes the fracture-healing efficacy of exogenous PTH(1-34). *PLoS 1* 6: e23060.
54. Li, X., Liu, H., Qin, L. et al. 2007. Determination of dual effects of parathyroid hormone on skeletal gene expression *in vivo* by microarray and network analysis. *J Biol Chem* 282: 33086–33097.
55. Yang, D., Singh, R., Divieti, P. et al. 2007. Contributions of parathyroid hormone (PTH)/ PTH-related peptide receptor signaling pathways to the anabolic effect of PTH on bone. *Bone* 40: 1453–1461.
56. Li, X., Liu, H., Qin, L. et al. 2007. Determination of dual effects of parathyroid hormone on skeletal gene expression in vivo by microarray and network analysis. *J Biol Chem* 282: 33086–33097.
57. Guo, J., Liu, M., Yang, D. et al. 2010. Phospholipase C signaling via the parathyroid hormone (PTH)/PTH-related peptide receptor is essential for normal bone responses to PTH. *Endocrinology* 151: 3502–3513.
58. Newey, P.J., Nesbit, M.A., Rimmer, A.J. et al. 2012. Whole-exome sequencing studies of nonhereditary (sporadic) parathyroid adenomas. *J Clin Endocrinol Metabol* 97: E1995–E2005.
59. Heppner, C.,Kester, M.B., Agarwal, S.K. et al. 1997. Somatic mutation of the MEN1 gene in parathyroid tumours. *Nat Genet* 16: 375–378.
60. Shattuck, T.M., Välimäki, S., Obara, T. et al. 2003. Somatic and germ-line mutations of the HRPT2 gene in sporadic parathyroid carcinoma. *New Engl J Med* 349: 1722–1729.
61. Costa-Guda, J., Marinoni, I., Molatore, S. et al. 2011. Somatic mutation and germ line sequence abnormalities in CDKN1B encoding p27Kip1 in sporadic parathyroid adenomas. *J Clin Endocrinol Metabol* 96: E701–E706.
62. Haglund, F., Andreasson, A., Nilsson, I.L. et al. 2010. Lack of S37A CTNNB1/β-catenin mutations in a Swedish cohort of 98 parathyroid adenomas. *Clin Endocrinol* 73: 552–553.
63. Kifor, O., Moore, F.D., Delaney, M. et al. 2003. A syndrome of hypocalciuric hypercalcemia caused by antibodies directed against the calcium-sensing receptor. *J Clin Endocrinol Metabol* 88: 60–72.

64. Eastell, R., Arnold, A., Brandi, M.L. et al. 2009. Diagnosis of asymptomatic primary hyperparathyroidism: proceedings of third international workshop. *J Clin Endocrinol Metabol* 94: 340–350.

65. Silverberg, S.J., Shane, E., De La Cruz, L. et al. 1989. Skeletal disease in primary hyperparathyroidism. *J Bone Miner Res* 4: 283.

66. Silverberg, S.J., Shane, E., Jacobs, T.P. et al. 1990. Nephrolithiasis and bone involvement in primary hyperparathyroidism. *Am J Med* 89: 327.

67. Bilezikian, J.P., Khan, A.A, and Potts, J.T. Jr. 2009. Guidelines for the management of asymptomatic primary hyperparathyroidism: summary statement from third international workshop. *J Clin Endocrinol Metabol* 94: 335–339.

68. Wermer, P. 1954. Genetic aspects of adenomatosis of endocrine glands. *Am J Med* 16: 363.

69. Chandrasekharappa, S.C., Guru, S.C., Manickam, P. et al. 1997. Positional cloning of the gene for multiple endocrine neoplasia type 1. *Science* 276: 404.

70. Marx, S.J. and Stratakis, C.A. 2005. Multiple endocrine neoplasia: introduction. *J Intern Med* 257: 2–5.

71. Sipple, J.H. 1961. The association of pheochromocytoma with carcinoma of the thyroid gland. *Am J Med* 31: 163.

72. Mulligan, L.M., Kwok, J.B., Healey, C.S. et al. 1993. Germ line mutations of the RET proto-oncogene in multiple endocrine neoplasia type 2A. *Nature* 363: 458.

73. Carpten, J.D., Robbins, C.M., Villablanca, A. et al. 2002. HRPT2 encoding parafibromin is mutated in hyperparathyroidism–jaw tumor syndrome. *Nat Genet* 32: 676.

74. Marx, S.J., Attie, M.F., Levine, M.A. et al. 1981. The hypocalciuric or benign variant of familial hypercalcemia: clinical and biochemical features in fifteen kindreds. *Medicine* 60: 397.

75. Pollak, M.R., Brown, E.M., Chou, Y.H. et al. 1993. Mutations in the human Ca^{2+}-sensing receptor gene cause familial hypocalciuric hypercalcemia and neonatal severe hyperparathyroidism. *Cell* 75: 1297.

76. Marx, S.J., Attie, M.F., Spiegel, A.M. et al. 1982. An association between neonatal severe primary hyperparathyroidism and familial hypocalciuric hypercalcemia in three kindreds. *New Engl J Med* 306: 257.

77. Fraser, W.D. 2009. Hyperparathyroidism. *Lancet* 374: 145–158.

78. Broome, J.T. and Solorzano, C.C. 2011. Lithium use and primary hyperparathyroidism. *Endocr Pract* 17: 31–35.

79. Nakajima, K., Tamai, M., Okaniwa, S. et al. 2013. Humoral hypercalcemia associated with gastric carcinoma secreting parathyroid hormone: a case report and review of the literature. *Endocr J* 2013 Jan 9. [Epub ahead of print] PMID 23303131.

80. Schipani, E., Jensen, G.S., Pincus, J. et al. 1997. Constitutive activation of the cyclic adenosine 3′,5′-monophosphate signaling pathway by parathyroid hormone (PTH)/PTH-related peptide receptors mutated at the two loci for Jansen's metaphyseal chondrodysplasia. *Mol Endocrinol* 11: 851–858.

81. Moe, S., Drüeke, T., Cunningham, J. et al. 2006. Kidney Disease: Improving Global Outcomes (KDIGO). Definition, evaluation, and classification of renal osteodystrophy: position statement. *Kidney Intl* 69: 1945–1953.

82. Mizobuchi, M., Towler, D., and Slatopolsky, E. 2009. Vascular calcification: the killer of patients with chronic kidney disease. *J Am Soc Nephrol* 20: 1453–1464.

83. Young, E.W., Albert, J.M., Satayathum, S. et al. 2005. Predictors and consequences of altered mineral metabolism: the Dialysis Outcomes and Practice Patterns Study. *Kidney Intl* 67: 1179–1187.

84. Wald, R., Tentori, F., Tighiouart, H. et al. 2007. Impact of the Kidney Disease Outcomes Quality Initiative (K/DOQI) Clinical Practice Guidelines for Bone Metabolism and Disease in a large dialysis network. *Am J Kidney Dis* 49: 257–266.

85. Martin, K.J. and González, E.A.2012. Long-term management of CKD-mineral and bone disorder. *Am J Kidney Dis* 60: 308–315.
86. Shore, R.M. and Chesney, R.W. 2013. Rickets: Part I. *Pediatr Radiol* 43: 140–151.
87. Shore, R.M. and Chesney, R.W. 2013. Rickets: Part II. *Pediatr Radiol* 43: 152–172.
88. Greene-Finestone, L.S., Berger, C., de Groh, M. et al. 2011. CaMos Research Group: 25-hydroxyvitamin D in Canadian adults: biological, environmental, and behavioral correlates. *Osteoporosis Intl* 22: 1389–1399.
89. Berger, C., Greene-Finestone, L.S., Langsetmo, L. et al. 2012. Temporal trends and determinants of longitudinal change in 25-hydroxyvitamin D and parathyroid hormone levels. *J Bone Miner Res* 27: 1381–1389.
90. Prentice, A. 2012. Nutritional rickets around the world. *J Steroid Biochem Mol Biol.* doi: pii: S0960-0760(12)00251-8. 10.1016/j.jsbmb.2012.11.018.
91. Hahn T.J. and Halstead, L.R.1979. Anticonvulsant drug-induced osteomalacia: alterations in mineral metabolism and response to vitamin D3 administration. *Calcif Tiss Intl* 27: 13–18.
92. Drezner, M.K. 2004. Treatment of anticonvulsant drug-induced bone disease. *Epilepsy Behav* 5: S41–S47.
93. Glorieux, F.H., Edouard, T., and St, Arnaud, R. 2011. Pseudo-vitamin D deficiency. In *Vitamin D,* 3rd ed., Feldman, D., Ed. Elsevier: London, pp. 1187–1195.
94. Liberman, U.A. and Marx, S.J. 2003. Vitamin D-dependent rickets. In *Primer on the Metabolic Bone Diseases and Disorders of Mineral Metabolism,* 5th ed., Favus, M.J., Ed. American Society for Bone and Mineral Research: Washington, pp. 407–413.
95. Malloy, P.J. and Feldman, D. 2010. Genetic disorders and defects in vitamin D action. *Endocrinol Metabol Clin North Am* 39: 333–346.
96. Marx, S.J., Bliziotes, M.M., and Nanes, M. 1986. Analysis of the relation between alopecia and resistance to 1, 25-dihydroxyvitamin D. *Clin Endocrinol* 25: 373–381.
97. Thacher, R.D., Fischer, P.R., Strand, M.A. et al. 2006. Nutritional rickets around the world: causes and future directions. *Ann Trop Paediatr* 26: 1–16.
98. Kuro, M. 2012. Klotho in health and disease. *Curr Opin Nephrol Hypertens* 21: 362–368.
99. Bai, X., Miao, D., Goltzman, D. et al. 2007. Early lethality in Hyp mice with targeted deletion of Pth gene. *Endocrinology* 148: 4974–4983.
100. Carpenter, T.O. 2012. The expanding family of hypophosphatemic syndromes. *J Bone Miner Metabol.* Jan;30(1): 1-9. doi: 10.1007/s00774-011-0340-2 [Epub Dec. 14, 2011].
101. Francis, F. 1995. A gene (PEX) with homologies to endopeptidases is mutated in patients with X-linked hypophosphatemic rickets: the HYP Consortium. *Nat Genet* 11: 130–136.
102. Lorenz-Depiereux, B., Bastepe, M., Benet-Pagès, A. et al. 2006. DMP1 mutations in autosomal recessive hypophosphatemia implicate a bone matrix protein in the regulation of phosphate homeostasis. *Nat Genet* 38: 1248–1250.
103. Feng, J.Q., Ward, L.M., Liu, S. et al. 2006. Loss of DMP1 causes rickets and osteomalacia and identifies a role for osteocytes in mineral metabolism. *Nat Genet* 38: 1310–1315.
104. Lorenz-Depiereux, B., Schnabel, D., Tiosano, D. et al. 2010. Loss-of-function ENPP1 mutations cause both generalized arterial calcification of infancy and autosomal-recessive hypophosphatemic rickets. *Am J Hum Genet* 86: 267–272.
105. Bhattacharyya, N., Wiench, M., Dumitrescu, C. et al. 2012. Mechanism of FGF23 processing in fibrous dysplasia. *J Bone Miner Res* 27: 1132–1141.
106. Collins, M.T., Singer, F.R., and Eugster, E. 2012. *Orphanet J Rare Dis* 7: S4.
107. Weidner, N. and Santa Cruz, D. 1987. Phosphaturic mesenchymal tumors: a polymorphous group causing osteomalacia or rickets. *Cancer* 59: 144–154.
108. Konishi, K., Nakamura, M., Yamakawa, H. et al. 1991. Hypophosphatemic osteomalacia in von Recklinghausen neurofibromatosis. *Am J Med Sci* 301: 322–328.
109. White, K.E. 2000. Autosomal dominant hypophosphatemic rickets is associated with mutations in FGF23. *Nat Genet* 26: 345–348.

110. Sethi, S.K., Hari, P., and Bagga, A. 2010. Elevated FGF-23 and parathormone in linear nevus sebaceous syndrome with resistant rickets. *Pediatr Nephrol* 25: 1577–1578.

111. White, K.E., Cabral, J.M., Davis, S.I. et al. 2005. Mutations that cause osteoglophonic dysplasia define novel roles for FGFR1 in bone elongation. *Am J Hum Genet* 76: 361–367.

112. Bergwitz, C., Roslin, N.M., Tieder, M. et al. 2006. SLC34A3 mutations in patients with hereditary hypophosphatemic rickets with hypercalciuria predict a key role for the sodium–phosphate co-transporter NaPi-IIc in maintaining phosphate homeostasis. *Am J Hum Genet* 78: 179–192.

113. Lorenz-Depiereux, B., Benet-Pages, A., Eckstein, G. et al. 2006. Hereditary hypophosphatemia rickets with hypercalciuria is caused by mutations in the sodium–phosphate co-transporter gene SLC34A3. *Am J Hum Genet* 78: 193–201.

114. Izzedine, H., Launay-Vacher, V., Isnard-Bagnis, C. et al. 2003. Drug-induced Fanconi's syndrome. *Am J Kidney Dis* 41: 292–309.

115. Miao, D., He, B., Lanske, B. et al. 2004. Skeletal abnormalities in Pth-null mice are influenced by dietary calcium. *Endocrinology* 145: 2046–2053.

116. Miao, D., Li, J., Xue, Y. et al. 2004. Parathyroid hormone-related peptide is required for increased trabecular bone volume in parathyroid hormone-null mice. *Endocrinology* 145: 3554–3562.

117. Cohen, A., Dempster, D.W., Muller, R. et al. 2010. Assessment of trabecular and cortical architecture and mechanical competence of bone by high-resolution peripheral computed tomography: comparison with transiliac bone biopsy. *Osteoporosis Intl* 21: 263–273.

118. Marx, S.J. 2000. Hyperparathyroid and hypoparathyroid disorders. *New Engl J Med* 343: 1863–1875.

119. Pollak, M.R., Brown, E.M., Estep, H.L. et al. 1994. Autosomal dominant hypocalcemia caused by a calcium-sensing receptor gene mutation. *Nat Genet* 8: 303–307.

120. Mayer, A., Ploix, C., Orgiazzi, J. et al. 2004. Calcium-sensing receptor autoantibodies are relevant markers of acquired hypoparathyroidism. *J Clin Endocrinol Metabol* 89: 4484–4488.

121. Gavalas, N.G., Kemp, E.H., Krohn, K.J.E. et al. 2007. The calcium-sensing receptor is a target of autoantibodies in patients with autoimmune polyendocrine syndrome type 1. *J Clin Endocrinol Metabol* 92: 2107–2114.

122. Ahonen, P., Myllarniemi, S., Sipila, I. et al. 1990. Clinical variation of autoimmune polyendocrinopathy–candidiadis–ectodermal dystrophy (APECED) in a series of 68 patients. *New Engl J Med* 322: 1829–1836.

123. Eisenbarth, G.S. and Gottlieb, P.A. 2004. Autoimmune polyendocrine syndromes. *New Engl J Med* 350: 2068–2079.

124. de Sèze, S., Solnica, J., Mitrovic, D. et al. 1972. Joint and bone disorders and hypoparathyroidism in hemochromatosis. *Semin Arthritis Rheum* 2: 71–94.

125. Toumba, M., Sergis, A., Kanaris, C. et al. 2007. Endocrine complications in patients with thalassemia major. *Pediatr Endocrinol Rev* 5: 642–648.

126. Carpenter, T.O., Carnes, D.L. Jr., and Anast, C.S. 1983. Hypoparathyroidism in Wilson's disease. *New Engl J Med* 309: 873–877.

127. Badell, A., Servitje, O., Graells, J. et al 1998. Hypoparathyroidism and sarcoidosis. *Br J Dermatol* 138: 915–917.

128. Goddard, C.J. 1990. Symptomatic hypocalcaemia associated with metastatic invasion of the parathyroid glands. *Br J Hosp Med* 43: 72.

129. Datta, R., Waheed, A., Shah, G.N. et al. 2007. Signal sequence mutation in autosomal dominant form of hypoparathyroidism induces apoptosis that is corrected by a chemical chaperone. *Proc Natl Acad Sci USA* 104: 19989–19994.

130. Ding, C., Buckingham, B., and Levine, M.A. 2001. Familial isolated hypoparathyroidism caused by a mutation in the gene for the transcription factor GCMB. *J Clin Endocrinol* 108: 1215–1220.
131. Sunthornthepvarakul, T., Churesigaew, S., and Ngowngarmratana, S. 1999. A novel mutation of the signal peptide of the pre-pro-parathyroid hormone gene associated with autosomal recessive familial isolated hypoparathyroidism. *J Clin Endocrinol Metabol* 84: 3792–3796.
132. Bowl, M.R., Mirczuk, S.M, Grigorieva, I.V. et al. 2010. Identification and characterization of novel parathyroid-specific transcription factor glial cells missing homolog B (GCMB) mutations in eight families with autosomal recessive hypoparathyroidism. *Hum Mol Genet* 19: 2028–2038.
133. Bowl, M.R., Nesbit, M.A., Harding, B. et al. 2005. An interstitial deletion-insertion involving chromosome 2p25.3 and Xq27.1 near SOX3 causes X-linked recessive hypoparathyroidism. *J Clin Invest* 115: 2822–2831.
134. Kobrynski, L.J. and Sullivan, K.E. 2007. Velocardiofacial syndrome, DiGeorge syndrome: the chromosome 22q11.2 deletion syndromes. *Lancet* 370: 1443–1452.
135. Ali, A., Christie, P.T., Grigorieva, I.V. et al. 2007. Functional characterization of GATA3 mutations causing the hypoparathyroid–deafness–renal (HDR) dysplasia syndrome: insight into mechanisms of DNA binding by the GATA3 transcription factor. *Hum Mol Genet* 16: 265–275.
136. Parvari, R., Diaz, G.A., and Hershkovitz, E. 2007. Parathyroid development and the role of tubulin chaperone E. *Horm Res* 358: 12–21.
137. Winer, K.K., Zhang, B., Shrader, J.A. et al. 2012. Synthetic human parathyroid hormone 1-34 replacement therapy: a randomized crossover trial comparing pump versus injections in the treatment of chronic hypoparathyroidism. *J Clin Endocrinol Metabol* 97: 391–399.
138. Chase, R.L., Melson, G.L., and Aurbach, G.D. 1969. Pseudohypoparathyroidism: defective excretion of 3′,5′-AMP in response to parathyroid hormone. *J Clin Invest* 48: 1832–1844.
139. Weinstein, L.S., Shu-Hua, Y., Warner, D.R. et al. 2001. Endocrine manifestations of stimulatory G protein α subunit mutations and the role of genomic imprinting. *Endocr Rev* 22: 675–705.
140. Mantovani, G., de Sanctis, L., Barbieri, A.M. et al. 2010. Pseudohypoparathyroidism and GNAS epigenetic defects: clinical evaluation of Albright hereditary osteodystrophy and molecular analysis in 40 patients. *J Clin Endocrinol Metabol* 95: 651–658.
141. Mantovani, G., Ferrante, E., Giavoli, C. et al. 2010. Recombinant human GH replacement therapy in children with pseudohypoparathyroidism type 1a: first study on the effect on growth. *J Clin Endocrinol Metabol* 95: 5011–5017.
142. Drezner, M., Neelon, F.A., and Lebovitz, H.E. 1973. Pseudohypoparathyroidism type II: a possible defect in the reception of the cyclic AMP signal. *New Engl J Med* 289: 1056.
143. Jobert, A.S., Zhang, P., Couvineau, A. et al. 1998. Absence of functional receptors for parathyroid hormone and parathyroid hormone-related peptide in Blomstrand chondrodysplasia. *J Clin Invest* 102: 4069–4071.
144. Zhang, P., Jobert, A.S., Couvineau, A. et al. 1998. A homozygous inactivating mutation in the parathyroid hormone/parathyroid hormone-related peptide receptor causing Blomstrand's chondrodysplasia. *J Clin Endocrinol Metabol* 83: 3373–3376.
145. Karaplis, A.C., He, B., Nguyen, M.T. et al. 1998. Inactivating mutation in the human parathyroid hormone receptor type I gene in Blomstrand's chondrodysplasia. *Endocrinology* 139: 5255–5258.
146. Duchatelet, S., Ostergaard, E., Cortes, D. et al. 2005. Recessive mutations in PTHR1 cause contrasting skeletal dysplasias in Eiken and Blomstrand syndromes. *Hum Mol Genet* 14: 1–5.

147. Couvineau, A., Wouters, V., Bertrand, G. et al. 2008. PTHR1 mutations associated with Ollier disease result in receptor loss of function. *Hum Mol Genet* 17: 2766–2775.

148. Silve, C. and Jüppner, H. 2006. Ollier disease. *Orphanet J Rare Dis* 1: 37.

149. Tong, G.M., and Rude, R.K. 2005. Magnesium deficiency in critical illness. *J Intensive Care Med* 20: 3–17.

150. Coin, A., Veronese, N., Bolzetta, F. et al. 2012. Relationship between increased endogenous parathormone levels and bone density in postmenopausal women treated with bisphosphonates. *Panminerva Med* 54: 277–282.

151. Tashjian, A.H. Jr, and Goltzman, D. 2008. On the interpretation of rat carcinogenicity studies for human PTH (1-34) and human PTH (1-84). *J Bone Miner Res* 23: 803–811.

152. Subbiah, V., Madsen, V.S., Raymond, A.K. et al. 2010. Of mice and men: divergent risks of teriparatide-induced osteosarcoma. *Osteoporosis Intl* 21: 1041–1045.

153. Girotra, M., Rubin, M.R., and Bilezikian, J.P. 2006. The use of parathyroid hormone in the treatment of osteoporosis. *Rev Endocr Metabol Disord* 7: 113–121.

154. Samadfam, R, Xia, Q., and Goltzman, D. 2007. Co-treatment of PTH with osteoprotegerin or alendronate increases its anabolic effect on the skeleton of oophorectomized mice. *J Bone Miner Res* 22: 55–63.

155. Samadfam, R., Xia, Q., and Goltzman, D. 2007. Pretreatment with anticatabolic agents blunts but does not eliminate the skeletal anabolic response to parathyroid hormone in oophorectomized mice. *Endocrinology* 148: 2778–2787.

156. Finkelstein, J.S., Wyland, J.J., Lee, H., and Neer, R.M. 2010. Effects of teriparatide, alendronate, or both in women with postmenopausal osteoporosis. *J Clin Endocrinol Metab* 95: 1838–1845.

157. Black, D.M., Greenspan, S.L., Ensrud, K.E. et al. 2003. The effects of parathyroid hormone and alendronate alone or in combination in postmenopausal osteoporosis. *New Engl J Med* 349: 1207–1215.

158. Cosman, F., Eriksen, E.F., Recknor, C. et al. 2011. Effects of intravenous zoledronic acid plus subcutaneous teriparatide [rhPTH(1–34)] in postmenopausal osteoporosis. *J Bone Miner Res* 26: 503–511.

159. Black, D.M., Bilezikian, J.P., Ensrud, K.E. et al. 2005. One year of alendronate after one year of parathyroid hormone (1–84) for osteoporosis. *New Engl J Med* 353: 555–565.

160. Neer, R.M., Arnaud, C.D., Zanchetta, J.R. et al. 2001. Effect of parathyroid hormone (1–34) on fractures and bone mineral density in postmenopausal women with osteoporosis. *New Engl J Med* 344: 1434–1441.

161. Cosman, F., Lane, N.E., Bolognese, M.A. et al. 2010. Effect of transdermal teriparatide administration on bone mineral density in postmenopausal women. *J Clin Endocrinol Metabol* 95: 151–158.

162. Shoyele, S.A., Sivadas, N., and Cryan, S.A. 2011. The effects of excipients and particle engineering on the biophysical stability and aerosol performance of parathyroid hormone (1–34) prepared as a dry powder for inhalation. *AAPS Pharm Sci Tech* 12: 304–311.

163. Fitzpatrick, L.A., Dabrowski, C.E., Cicconetti, G. et al. 2011. The effects of ronacaleret, a calcium-sensing receptor antagonist, on bone mineral density and biochemical markers of bone turnover in postmenopausal women with low bone mineral density. *J Clin Endocrinol Metab* 96: 2441–2449.

6 Phosphate Homeostasis and Metabolic Bone Disease

Farzana Perwad and Anthony A. Portale

CONTENTS

6.1 INTRODUCTION

Inorganic phosphate (Pi) is fundamental to cellular metabolism and, in vertebrates, to skeletal mineralization. To accomplish these functions, transport systems evolved to permit the efficient transfer of negatively charged Pi ions across hydrophobic membranes. Ingested Pi is absorbed by the small intestine, deposited in bone, and filtered by the kidney where it is reabsorbed and excreted in amounts determined by the specific organism. The kidney is a major determinant of Pi homeostasis due to its ability to increase or decrease its Pi reabsorptive capacity to accommodate Pi need. Recent significant advances have been made in our understanding of the molecular mechanisms involved in renal tubular Pi reabsorption and its hormonal regulation and modulation by dietary Pi intake. This chapter describes the mechanisms regulating Pi homeostasis and the cellular and molecular aspects of renal Pi transport and their regulation.

6.2 PHOSPHATE HOMEOSTASIS

6.2.1 DISTRIBUTION AND CHEMISTRY

Phosphorus and Pi account for about 0.6% of body weight at birth and about 1% of body weight or 600 to 700 gm in adults (1). Approximately 85% of body Pi is in the skeleton and teeth, approximately 15% in soft tissue, and the remainder (~0.3%) in extracellular fluid. Pi is an important constituent of bone mineral and the balance of Pi must be positive to meet the needs of skeletal growth and consolidation in growing individuals; in adults, Pi balance is zero. Pi deficiency results in hypophosphatemia, which causes rickets in children and osteomalacia in adults.

Pi exists in plasma in an organic form consisting principally of phospholipids and phosphate esters and in an inorganic form (2). Of the total plasma Pi concentration of approximately 4.52 mmol/L (14 mg/dL), about 1.29 mmol/L (4 mg/dL) is inorganic. Of this, about 10 to 15% is protein-bound and the remainder filtered by the renal glomeruli exists principally as undissociated or "free" Pi ions or as Pi complexed with sodium, calcium, or magnesium.

At physiological pH, only HPO_4^{2-} and $H_2PO_4^-$ are present at significant concentrations in plasma. The ratio of the divalent to monovalent forms can be determined by the Henderson-Hasselbach equation. The dissociation constant (pKa) for Pi is 6.8. Thus, at a pH of 7.4, the ratio of divalent (HPO_4^{2-}) to monovalent ($H_2PO_4^-$) Pi anions is essentially 4 to 1 and the composite valence of Pi in serum (or intravenous solution) is 1.8. At this pH, 1 mmol Pi is equal to 1.8 meq. In clinical settings, only the inorganic orthophosphate form of Pi is routinely measured.

The *phosphorus concentration* and *phosphate concentration* terms are often used interchangeably and for clinical purposes the choice matters little. Phosphorus in the form of the phosphate ion circulates in blood, is filtered by the renal glomeruli, and is transported across plasma membranes. However, the content of phosphate in plasma, urine, tissue, or foodstuffs is measured and expressed as the amount of elemental phosphorus contained in a specimen, hence, the use of the incorrect *phosphorus concentration* term.

6.2.2 EXTRACELLULAR PHOSPHATE HOMEOSTASIS

In an adult in zero Pi balance, net intestinal Pi absorption (dietary Pi minus fecal Pi) is approximately 60 to 65% of dietary intake. To satisfy the demands of rapid growth of bone and soft tissue, intestinal Pi absorption in infants is higher than in adults and can exceed 90% of dietary intake (3,4). Metabolic balance studies in normal adult humans reveal that over the customary range of dietary Pi, net absorption is a linear function of intake (5), with no indication of saturation. Thus, inadequate Pi absorption results primarily from decreased Pi availability rather than from changes in the intrinsic capacity of intestinal Pi transport.

A small amount of Pi is secreted into the intestinal lumen in digestive fluids. Absorbed Pi enters the extracellular Pi pool, which is in equilibrium with the bone and soft tissue Pi pools. Pi is filtered at the glomeruli and reabsorbed to a large extent by the renal tubules. In subjects in zero Pi balance, the amount of Pi excreted by the kidney is equal to the net amount absorbed by the intestine, but in growing children it is less than the net amount absorbed due to deposition of Pi in bone. Thus, renal tubular reabsorption of Pi plays a central role in the regulation of Pi homeostasis. An overall schema of Pi metabolism is depicted in Figure 6.1.

Plasma Pi concentration and Pi homeostasis are maintained by a complex interaction of hormones produced by bone, kidney, and parathyroid gland as described below. In response to an increase in the extracellular Pi concentration, urine Pi excretion increases promptly due to an increase in filtered load at the glomeruli (Figure 6.2). This acute response reflects both an increase in the filtered load of Pi and an adaptive decrease in proximal tubule Pi reabsorption.

Hyperphosphatemia suppresses renal synthesis of 1,25-dihydroxyvitamin D (1,25D) and the opposite occurs with hypophosphatemia (6–11). A decrease in serum 1,25D decreases intestinal absorption of Pi and calcium and their mobilization from bone. With a decrease in plasma calcium and 1,25D levels, parathyroid hormone (PTH) secretion is stimulated leading to a further increase in urine Pi excretion but a decrease in calcium excretion. These homeostatic adjustments result in a decrease in extracellular Pi concentration toward normal values, with little change in serum calcium concentration (Figure 6.2).

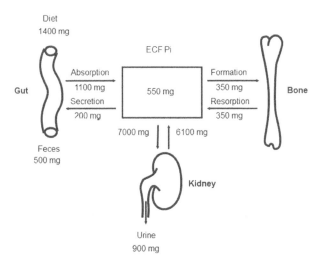

FIGURE 6.1 Phosphorus fluxes between body pools in normal human adult in zero phosphorus balance.

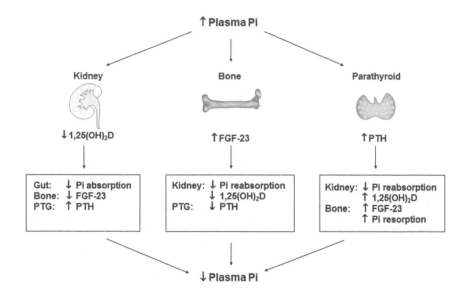

FIGURE 6.2 Homeostatic response to hyperphosphatemia. PTG = parathyroid gland.

An increase in dietary Pi intake and resultant hyperphosphatemia stimulate the production of fibroblast growth factor 23 (FGF23) by bone with increases in the plasma levels, thereby decreasing renal Pi reabsorption and renal 1,25D production. Thus, the concerted interaction of 1,25D, PTH, and FGF23 regulates the flux of Pi from bone, kidney and intestine to maintain plasma Pi concentration and Pi homeostasis. Conversely, in response to a decrease in plasma Pi concentration, production of 1,25D is increased and releases of PTH and FGF23 decreased (12). The effects of hypophosphatemia on bone, kidney, and intestine are opposite to those of hyperphosphatemia; the net result is an increase in Pi concentration toward normal values.

In healthy subjects ingesting typical diets, the serum Pi concentration exhibits a circadian rhythm, characterized by a rapid decrease in early morning to a nadir shortly before noon, a subsequent increase to a plateau in late afternoon, and a small further increase to a peak shortly after midnight (13,14). The amplitude of the rhythm (nadir to peak) is approximately 0.4 mmol/L (1.2 mg/dL) or 30% of the 24-hour mean level. Restriction or supplementation of dietary Pi induces a substantial decrease or increase, respectively, in serum Pi concentrations during the late morning, afternoon, and evening, but induces less or no change in the morning fasting Pi concentration (14).

To minimize the impacts of changes in dietary Pi on serum Pi concentration, one should obtain specimens for analysis in the morning fasting state. Specimens obtained in the afternoon are more affected by diet and thus may be more useful to monitor the effect of dietary Pi on serum Pi concentration, as in patients with renal insufficiency receiving Pi-binding agents to treat hyperphosphatemia.

Other factors can affect the serum Pi concentration. Presumably because of movement of Pi into cells, the serum Pi concentration can be decreased acutely by intravenous infusion of glucose or insulin, ingestion of carbohydrate-rich meals, acute respiratory alkalosis, or infusion or endogenous release of epinephrine. The decrease in Pi concentration induced by acute respiratory alkalosis can be as great as 0.65 mmol/L (2.0 mg/dL) (15). Serum Pi concentration can be increased acutely by metabolic acidosis and by intravenous infusion of calcium (16).

Age exerts substantial effects on the fasting serum Pi concentration. In infants in the first 3 months of life, Pi levels are highest [1.6 to 2.5; mean 2.0 mmol/L (4.8 to 7.4 mg/dL; mean 6.2 mg/dL)] and decrease at ages 1 to 2 years to 1.5 to 1.9; mean 1.6 mmol/L (4.5 to 5.8 mg/dL; mean 5.0 mg/dL) (17). In mid-childhood, values range from 1.1 to 1.9; mean 1.42 mmol/L (3.5 to 5.5mg/dL; mean 4.4 mg/dL) and decrease to adult values by late adolescence (18,19). In adult males, mean serum Pi is ~1.2 mmol/L (3.5 mg/dL) at age 20 and decreases to ~1.0 mmol/L (3.0 mg/dL) at age 70 (19,20). In women, the mean values are similar to those of men until menopause, after which they increase slightly from ~1.1 mmol/L (3.4 mg/dL) at age 50 to ~1.2 mmol/L (3.7 mg/dL) at age 70.

6.2.3 INTESTINAL PHOSPHATE ABSORPTION

Dietary Pi is absorbed in the small intestine, primarily in the duodenum and jejunum, with minimal absorption in the ileum. Pi absorption occurs via two mechanisms: (1) nonsaturable passive diffusion through the paracellular pathway and (2) an active transcellular process localized to the mucosal surface. Under usual conditions of excess dietary intake, Pi absorption occurs primarily via paracellular diffusion which is largely unregulated, whereas when luminal Pi concentration is low, as when dietary Pi is restricted, active transport plays an important role (21–23).

Active transport of Pi across the mucosal membrane is principally mediated by Na/Pi co-transporter type IIb (NPT2b; solute carrier series SLC34A2) (24) and is the rate limiting step in intestinal Pi absorption. Active transport of Pi is up-regulated by 1,25D and low dietary Pi intake (25) via up-regulation of the protein abundance of Npt2b in the intestinal villi. Intestinal Npt2b protein abundance is down-regulated by FGF23, but its effect is indirect and dependent on the action of 1,25D via the vitamin D receptor (26). The cellular and molecular mechanisms of intestinal Pi absorption are reviewed in detail in Chapter 2.

6.3 RENAL PHOSPHATE ABSORPTION

6.3.1 PHYSIOLOGY AND TUBULAR LOCALIZATION

Much of the material discussed here is covered in greater detail in review articles (16,27–30). The proximal tubule is the major site of Pi reabsorption, with approximately 70% of the filtered load reclaimed in the proximal convoluted tubules and about 10% in the proximal straight tubules. In addition, a small but variable portion (<10%) of filtered Pi is reabsorbed in the distal segments of nephrons (16) (Figure 6.3a). Clearance studies in humans and experimental animals show that when the filtered load of Pi is progressively increased, Pi reabsorption increases until a maximum tubular reabsorptive rate for Pi, or TmP, is reached, after which Pi excretion increases in proportion to its filtered load.

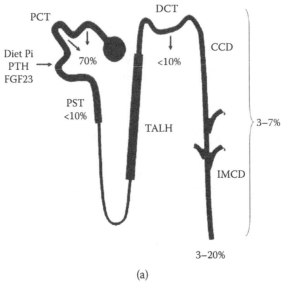

(a)

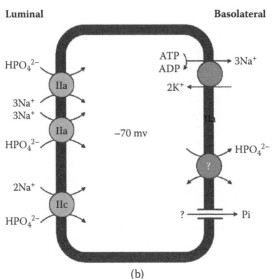

(b)

FIGURE 6.3 (a) Profile of phosphate reabsorption along mammalian nephron, as derived from micropuncture data. PCT = proximal convoluted tubule; PST = proximal straight tubule; TALH = thick ascending limb of Henle's loop; DCT = distal convoluted tubule; CCD = cortical collecting duct; IMCD = inner medullary collecting duct; PTH = parathyroid hormone; FGF23 = fibroblast growth factor 23 (*Source:* Suki WN et al. 2000. In Brenner BM, Ed., *The Kidney*, 6th ed., Philadelphia: W.B. Saunders, pp. 520–574. With permission. (b) Locations of identified and postulated Na$^+$-dependent Pi co-transporters in proximal tubule cells. Data indicate that most proximal tubule Pi reabsorption occurs via type IIa (NPT2a) and type IIc (NPT2c) co-transporters localized to the brush border membranes and are the major targets for physiologic regulation of renal Pi reabsorption (*Source:* Modified from Murer H et al. 1999. *Am J Physiol* 277: F676–F684. With permission.)

The measurement of TmP varies among individuals and within a single individual, due in part to variations in glomerular filtration rate (GFR). Thus, the TmP/GFR ratio or the maximum tubular reabsorption of Pi per unit volume of GFR is the most reliable quantitative estimate of the overall tubular Pi reabsorptive capacity and is considered to reflect the quantity of Na/Pi co-transporters available per unit of kidney mass (21). The serum Pi concentration at which Pi reabsorption is maximal is called the theoretical renal Pi threshold, is equal to the TmP/GFR ratio, and closely approximates the normal fasting serum Pi concentration. Thus, the renal reabsorptive capacity for Pi is the principal determinant of serum Pi concentration.

6.3.1.1   Proximal Tubules

The proximal convoluted tubules (PCTs) reabsorb approximately 70% of the filtered load of Pi. Reabsorption rates in early convolutions (S1 segment) normally are as much as four times greater than those in late convolutions (S2 segment) and the pars recta (S3 segment) (31–33). Due to this axial heterogeneity in Pi transport, most of the Pi reabsorption by the PCT occurs within the first 25% of its length. Inter-nephron heterogeneity in Pi reabsorption also is present in the proximal tubule, with proximal tubules of juxtamedullary nephrons having a greater capacity to both reabsorb Pi (34–37) and adapt to changes in its filtered load (38,39), as compared with proximal tubules of superficial nephrons. In the absence of PTH, the proximal straight tubule (PST) can reabsorb up to an additional 10% of filtered Pi (Figure 6.3a).

6.3.1.2   Henle's Loop, Distal Convoluted Tubules, and Connecting Tubules

Little or no transport of Pi is thought to occur in Henle's Loop except for the PST segment (16). The distal convoluted tubule (DCT) reabsorbs up to 10% of the filtered Pi load in the absence of PTH, with the possibility that segments beyond the accessible late DCT, presumably the connecting tubules, reabsorb an additional 3 to 7% (16).

6.3.1.3   Collecting Tubules

Although some investigators failed to demonstrate Pi reabsorption in isolated perfused cortical collecting tubules, others demonstrated a small but significant net efflux of Pi in this nephron segment (16,40,41).

6.3.2   CELLULAR AND MOLECULAR ASPECTS

Transepithelial Pi transport in the nephron is essentially unidirectional and involves uptake across the brush border membrane, translocation across the cell, and efflux at the basolateral membrane (Figure 6.3b). Pi uptake at the apical cell surface is the rate limiting step in overall Pi reabsorption, the major site of its regulation, and is mediated by Na/Pi co-transporters that depend on the basolateral membrane-associated Na^+/K^+-dependent ATPase.

Na/Pi co-transport is either electrogenic (NPT2a, Pit-2) or electroneutral (NPT2c) and is sensitive to changes in luminal pH, with 10- to 20-fold increases observed when pH is increased from 6 to 8.5. Little is known about the translocation of Pi across cells except that Pi anions rapidly equilibrate with intracellular inorganic and organic Pi pools.

Few data are available regarding the mechanisms involved in the efflux of Pi at the basolateral cell surface. It has been proposed that in proximal tubules, a Na$^+$-dependent electroneutral anion exchanger is at least partially responsible for Pi efflux (42).

Three classes of Na/Pi co-transporters have been identified by expression and homology cloning. The type I Na/Pi co-transporter (NPT1, SLC17A1) is expressed predominantly in brush border membranes of proximal tubule cells (43). The NPT1 transporters are approximately 465 amino acids in length with 7 to 9 membrane spanning segments. NPT1 exhibits broad substrate specificity and mediates the transport of chloride and organic anions as well as high affinity Na/Pi co-transport. Conditions that physiologically regulate proximal tubule Pi transport such as dietary Pi or PTH do not alter type I Na/Pi co-transporter protein or mRNA expression. The human gene encoding the type I transporter is located on chromosome 6p21.3-p23.

The type II family of Na/Pi co-transporters, whose cDNA shares only 20% homology with that of NPT1 (44,45), is comprised of three highly homologous iso-forms: type IIa (NPT2a, SLC34A1) and type IIc (NPT2c, SLC34A3) (46,47) that are expressed exclusively in the brush border membranes of the renal proximal tubules, and type IIb (NPT2b, SLC34A2) expressed in several tissues including small intestine and lung, but not in kidney and is responsible for intestinal absorption of Pi (24).

Human NPT2a and human NPT2c contain 635 and 599 amino acids, respectively; both proteins are predicted to have eight membrane-spanning segments. The human genes encoding NPT2a and NPT2c are located on chromosomes 5q35 and 9q34, respectively (48). NPT2a-mediated Na/Pi co-transport is electrogenic and involves the influx of three Na$^+$ ions and one Pi anion (preferentially divalent) (49). NPT2b-mediated co-transport also is electrogenic, whereas the NPT2c isoform mediates electroneutral transport of two Na$^+$ ions with one divalent Pi anion.

In mice, Npt2a and Npt2c are detected exclusively in the brush border membranes of proximal tubular cells. At the mRNA level, NPT2a is approximately one order of magnitude more abundant than NPT2c. The abundance of Npt2c mRNA and protein are both significantly higher in kidneys of 22 day-old rats than in those of 60-day-old rats, suggesting that Npt2c plays an important role in early postnatal development (46). Several different homozygous and compound heterozygous mutations in the SLC34A3 gene encoding NPT2c have been found in patients affected by hereditary hypophosphatemic rickets with hypercalciuria (HHRH) (50–52), indicating that, at least in humans, this co-transporter has a more prominent role than initially thought. Hybrid depletion studies suggested that Npt2c accounts for approximately 30% of Na/Pi co-transport in kidneys of Pi-deprived adult mice (47).

Type III Na/Pi co-transporters are cell-surface retroviral receptors [gibbon ape leukemia virus (Glvr-1, Pit-1, SLC20A1) and murine amphotropic virus (Ram-1, Pit-2, SLC20A2)] that mediate high affinity electrogenic Na/Pi co-transport when expressed in oocytes and mammalian cells (53,54). Pit-1 and Pit-2 show no sequence similarity to NPT1 or NPT2a. Both Pit-1 and Pit-2 proteins are widely expressed in mammalian tissues including the kidney and have been considered to function as "housekeeping" Na/Pi co-transporters to maintain cellular Pi homeostasis.

Recent studies report immunohistochemical evidence that Pit-2 is localized to the brush border membranes of the rat proximal tubules, and its protein abundance is strongly up-regulated by dietary Pi restriction but with a slower adaptation rate compared to Npt2a (55). Recent studies also found that Pit-2 protein abundance in renal brush border membranes is regulated by PTH and FGF23 (56,57). These studies suggest that Pit-2 is also a mediator of Pi reabsorption in the proximal tubules and that its role in overall renal Pi handling should be re-evaluated.

6.3.2.1 Effect of Npt2a and Npt2c Gene Disruption

The critical role of NPT2a in the maintenance of Pi homeostasis has been clearly demonstrated in mice in which the Npt2a gene was knocked out by targeted mutagenesis (58). Mice that are null for Npt2a exhibited decreased renal Pi reabsorption, about 80% loss of brush border membrane Na/Pi co-transport, hypophosphatemia, an appropriate adaptive increase in renal synthesis and serum concentration of 1,25D (24,58) and associated hypercalcemia, hypercalciuria, and hypoparathyroidism, and an age-dependent skeletal phenotype (58,59). Dietary Pi intake and PTH were without effect on renal brush border membrane Na/Pi co-transport in Npt2a-null mice (60,61), demonstrating that NPT2a is a major regulator of renal Pi handling.

In the brush border membranes of Npt2a-null mice, the abundance of Npt2c protein was increased significantly (62), likely accounting for at least some of the residual Na/Pi co-transport in the mutant mice. Mice that are null for Npt2c exhibit, at different ages, only small increases in blood ionized calcium and some increase in urinary calcium excretion but not hypophosphatemia or increased urinary Pi excretion (63,64), suggesting that Npt2c may be of limited functional significance in rodents. The combined ablation of Npt2a and Npt2c exhibits a more severe phenotype than the ablation of Npt2a or Npt2c alone, suggesting that Npt2c is likely to have a more significant role than suggested by the Npt2c-null animals (64).

6.3.3 REGULATION OF RENAL PHOSPHATE TRANSPORT

The major regulators of renal Pi reabsorption are thought to be dietary Pi intake, PTH, and FGF23, although many hormonal and non-hormonal factors also are known to regulate this process (Table 6.1) (16,27,28). Both NPT2a and NPT2c are the targets of regulation. Dietary Pi, PTH, and FGF23 regulate renal Pi reabsorption primarily by inducing alterations in the abundance of NPT2a protein in the brush border membranes of proximal tubular cells via insertion of existing transporters into the membrane or retrieval of transporters from the membrane with subsequent lysosomal degradation.

Dietary Pi, PTH, and FGF23 also regulate the abundance of NPT2c protein in the brush border membrane (65); however, in contrast to NPT2a, NPT2c does not appear to undergo lysosomal degradation but instead may be recycled and re-inserted into apical membranes. The mechanisms underlying membrane trafficking of NPT2a and NPT2c proteins are complex and involve interaction of the transporters with various scaffolding and signalling proteins such as NHERF1, NHERF2, NHERF3 (PDZK1), NHERF4 (PDZK2), and Shank2E (27,66–69).

TABLE 6.1

Factors Affecting Renal Phosphorus Excretion

Factor	Urine Pi Excretion	Mechanism/Nephron Site
Dietary		
Volume expansion	↑	↑ Filtered load of Pi, ↓ proximal and distal reabsorption
High Pi intake	↑	↓ Proximal reabsorption
Phosphorus restriction	↓	↑ Proximal reabsorption
Metabolic		
Acidosis	↑	↓ Tubular reabsorption
Alkalosis	↓	↑ Tubular reabsorption
Hormones		
PTH	↑	↓ Proximal and distal reabsorption
1,25(OH)$_2$D (chronic)	↓	↑ Proximal reabsorption
FGF-23, FGF-7, sFRP4	↑	↓ Proximal reabsorption
Klotho (phosphatonins)		
Calcitonin	↑	↓ Tubular reabsorption
Growth hormone, IGF-1	↓	↑ Proximal reabsorption, ↑ GFR
Thyroid hormone	↓	↑ Tubular reabsorption
Insulin	↓	↑ Proximal reabsorption
Diuretics		
Mannitol, loop diuretics, thiazides	↑	↓ Tubular reabsorption, sites vary
Other		
Glucose	↑	↓ Osmotic diuresis, ↓ reabsorption PCT
Glucocorticoids	↑	↓ Proximal reabsorption
Immaturity	↓	↑ Proximal and distal reabsorption

6.3.3.1 Dietary Phosphate

Dietary intake of Pi is a key physiologic determinant of renal Pi handling. An increase or decrease in dietary Pi predictably induces an increase or decrease, respectively, in urine Pi excretion; with severe Pi restriction, urine Pi is negligible. This adaptation is independent of changes in the filtered load of Pi, ECF volume, plasma calcium, growth hormone, vitamin D status, or parathyroid activity and appears to reflect changes in the rate of Pi reabsorption by the proximal tubules, specifically, an increase or decrease in the Vmax of Na/Pi co-transport activity.

The adaptation can be demonstrated both in vivo and in isolated perfused PCT segments and brush border membrane vesicles prepared from animals maintained on differing dietary intakes of Pi (70–75). Renal tubular adaptation to changes in Pi intake or plasma Pi concentration occurs rapidly; an increase in brush border membrane vesicle Na/Pi co-transport was observed after 2 to 4 hours of Pi restriction in rats (76–78); conversely a decrease in Pi transport was induced after 1 hour of Pi infusion (79). Similarly, exposure of cultured renal epithelial cells (LLC-PK1) to a low Pi concentration in the medium induced both short-term (minutes) and long-term (hours) adaptations in Na/Pi co-transport (80–82).

Such dietary Pi-induced regulation of Pi reabsorption is achieved primarily by alterations in the abundance of type IIa Na/Pi co-transporter protein in the brush border membranes of proximal tubule cells. Short-term (hours) exposure of rats to a Pi-restricted diet induced increases in both brush border membrane Na/Pi co-transport activity and NPT2a protein abundance, but no change in NPT2a mRNA (83).

Chronic (days) restriction of dietary Pi in mice, rats, and rabbits led to an adaptive increase in brush border membrane Na/Pi co-transport and in the abundance of NPT2a protein and mRNA (84–90). The acute increase in Pi transport induced by Pi deprivation is mediated by microtubule-dependent recruitment of existing NPT2a protein to apical membranes (83). In contrast, exposure to high dietary Pi led to internalization of cell surface NPT2a protein into the endosomal compartments by a microtubule-independent mechanism (83). Internalized NPT2a protein is then delivered to the lysosome by a microtubule-dependent process for degradation (91).

A Pi response element (PRE) was identified in the mouse NPT2a promoter by DNA footprint analysis (92). The PRE was shown to bind a mouse transcription factor known as TFE3. The renal expression of TFE3 is increased in response to Pi deprivation (92). On the basis of these results, it was suggested that TFE3 participates in transcriptional regulation of the NPT2a gene by dietary Pi.

NPT2c also is regulated by dietary Pi. Restriction of dietary Pi induces an increase in NPT2c immunoreactive protein in the apical membranes of proximal tubule cells whereas feeding a high Pi diet induces a decrease (65,93). Internalization of NPT2c was slightly delayed relative to that of NPT2a after acute exposure to high dietary Pi. Internalized NPT2c is, however, not degraded in the lysosomes.

6.3.3.2 Parathyroid Hormone

PTH is a major hormonal regulator of renal Pi reabsorption (16,27). It acts directly on proximal tubular cells to inhibit Na/Pi co-transport through mechanisms that involve rapid internalization of cell surface NPT2a protein (94) and its subsequent lysosomal degradation (95). A prolonged increase in PTH also can induce a decrease in type II Na/Pi co-transporter mRNA abundance (94).

PTH binding to the PTHR1 receptors on the basolateral membranes activates PKA- and/or PKC-dependent signaling pathways, whereas PTH binding to apical receptors activates the PKC pathway (96). The extracellular signal-regulated kinase/mitogen-activated protein kinase (ERK/MAPK) pathway also participates in PTH-induced signaling (97) and the PKA and PKC signaling pathways converge on the ERK/MAPK pathway to internalize NPT2a protein (98).

Although the downstream targets for ERK/MAPK-mediated phosphorylation remain unknown, changes in the phosphorylation state of NPT2a are not associated with its PTH-induced internalization (99). Rather it has been postulated that the phosphorylation of proteins that associate with NPT2a may determine its regulation (27,28).

AKAP79, an A kinase anchoring protein (100) and RAP, a receptor-associated protein (101), were shown to participate in the PTH-mediated retrieval of NPT2a from the plasma membranes of proximal tubular cells. In opossum kidney (OK) cells, AKAP79 associates with NPT2a and the regulatory and catalytic subunits of PKA and this process is necessary for PKA-dependent inhibition of Na/Pi co-transport (100). In RAP-deficient mice, PTH-induced internalization of NPT2a was significantly delayed whereas its regulation by dietary Pi was unaffected (101). Activation of the PKC and PKA pathways also induces phosphorylation of the NHERF1 scaffolding protein that decreases its affinity for Npt2a (27,102–106). In OK cells, NHERF1 phosphorylation increases the lateral mobility of Npt2a; this lateral mobility precedes NPT2a internalization (105).

PTH-dependent regulation of NPT2c is less well understood. In response to PTH, NPT2c disappears from the surfaces of brush border membranes at a much slower rate than does NPT2a, and NPT2c does not seem to undergo lysosomal degradation (29,30,65,107). Indeed, evidence suggests that NPT2c may be recycled and re-inserted into the brush border membranes (108). In rats fed a low Pi diet, NPT2a and NPT2c underwent different regulation by PTH.

PTH (1-34) failed to decrease NPT2a expression in brush border membrane vesicles of rats on a low Pi diet consistent with the blunted phosphaturic effect of PTH observed in hypophosphatemic humans and rodents (109). In contrast, PTH was able to efficiently reduce the expression of NPT2c (107). While NPT2a is expressed in segments S1 through S3 of the proximal tubules, NPT2c is expressed only in the S1 segment.

6.3.3.3   Fibroblast Growth Factor 23

FGF23 is a bone-derived circulating peptide that plays an important role in regulating Pi and vitamin D metabolism. Through a positional cloning approach, FGF23 was first identified as the gene disrupted in patients with autosomal dominant hypophosphatemic rickets (ADHR) (110–112). This disorder is characterized by hypophosphatemia due to renal Pi wasting, inappropriately low or normal serum concentrations of 1,25D, and rickets or osteomalacia (113). Affected patients harbor mutations that alter the FGF23 furin cleavage site (residues 176 through 179), thereby preventing the normal proteolytic processing of FGF23 (114) and causing its accumulation in the plasma.

Excess FGF23 also is implicated in the pathogenesis of two related hypophosphatemic disorders: tumor-induced osteomalacia (115–117) and X-linked hypophosphatemia (XLH) (113). FGF23 is abundantly expressed in tumors that cause tumor-induced osteomalacia (118,119). Serum concentrations of FGF23 are greatly increased in these patients and also in some patients with XLH (120–122). With surgical removal of the tumor, FGF23 concentrations decrease to normal values and the disorder resolves. Extracts from these tumors inhibited Pi transport in renal proximal tubule cells in vitro (123,124), consistent with the notion that FGF23 is responsible for this inhibition.

The human FGF23 gene consists of 3 exons spanning 10 kb of genomic sequence that encode a 251 amino acid precursor protein comprising a hydrophobic amino acid sequence (residues 1 through 24) that likely serves as a leader sequence. Unlike most other fibroblast growth factors but similar to FGF19 and FGF21, FGF23 appears to be secreted efficiently into the circulation. FGF23 binds, albeit with relatively low affinity, to most of the splice variants of the known FGF receptors (125). However, in the presence of klotho, a membrane bound protein with ß-glucuronidase activity, FGF23 can bind with high affinity to FGFR1(IIIc) (126,127). This provides evidence that klotho plays an important role in mediating the actions of FGF23. FGF23 acts on the kidney to impair Pi reabsorption and inhibit the synthesis of 1,25D.

In mice, administration of FGF23 induced a decrease in serum Pi concentration and increased renal Pi excretion by inhibition of brush border membrane Na/Pi co-transport (119,128–131). Mice transplanted with cell lines stably expressing FGF23 and transgenic mice that over-express FGF23 developed hypophosphatemia due to renal Pi wasting, low serum 1,25D concentrations, and abnormal bone development (119,130,132–134). FGF23 suppressed the renal production and serum concentration of 1,25D by suppressing 25-hydroxyvitamin D-1α-hydroxylase (CYP27B1) mRNA and protein expression in vivo and in vitro and stimulating 25-hydroxyvitamin D 24-hydroxylase (CYP24) mRNA expression (119,129,131,134).

Findings opposite to those in FGF23 transgenic animals were observed in mice homozygous for ablation of the FGF23 gene (fgf23-null). These animals developed hyperphosphatemia, increased serum 1,25D concentrations, and abnormal skeleto-genesis and died prematurely, partly due to renal failure secondary to renal calcifi-cation (135–137). The findings in fgf23-null mice overlap significantly with those in klotho-null mice (138–142), even though the klotho-null animals showed greatly increased serum levels of biologically active FGF23 (139). These observations pro-vide further evidence that klotho is an obligatory co-factor that plays an important role in mediating the actions of FGF23.

The cellular and molecular mechanisms by which FGF23 inhibits renal Pi reab-sorption have been studied both in vivo and in vitro (128,130,131,143). In normal mice, a single injection of recombinant human FGF23 rapidly decreased renal brush border membrane Na/Pi co-transport activity and Npt2a mRNA and protein abun-dance as early as 5 hours after treatment (130,131) and this effect was independent of PTH (128).

That FGF23 acts directly on Pi transport was demonstrated in vitro in renal proxi-mal tubule epithelial cells (143,144). In OK cells, FGF23 inhibited sodium-dependent Pi uptake via activation of MAPK signaling pathways in a dose-dependent manner (143,144). Similar to the action of PTH, inhibition of Na/Pi co-transport by FGF23 is dependent on NHERF-1, a scaffolding protein required for retention of Npt2a protein on the apical membranes of proximal tubule cells (144). In the absence of NHERF-1, inhibition of renal Pi co-transport by PTH and FGF23 is blocked.

FGF23 also decreases the abundance of Npt2c mRNA and protein (134) and the abundance of Pit2 protein (56) in the kidney. Inhibition of activity of both of these co-transporters is responsible for the increased renal Pi excretion and resulting hypo-phosphatemia observed in Npt2a-null mice treated with intravenous FGF23 (56). Thus, FGF23 maintains Pi homeostasis by regulating renal Na/Pi co-transport via Npt2a, Npt2c, and Pit-2.

6.3.3.4   Klotho

Klotho has a direct effect on renal Pi reabsorption independent of its role as a co-factor for FGF23 signal transduction (145) as described below. Klotho protein exists in three forms: full length, soluble/cleaved, and secreted. The full-length transmembrane protein is expressed in the kidney, parathyroid gland, choroid plexus, and β-islet cells of the pancreas (146). This form is thought to confer tissue specificity for FGF23 action and convert canonical FGF receptors to FGF23-specific receptors (126). In the kidney, klotho is predominantly expressed in the distal convoluted tubules (147–149).

Initial signaling by FGF23 was demonstrated in distal convoluted tubules (148) but expression of klotho mRNA and protein has also been detected in the proximal tubule epithelia and in tubular fluid obtained from the PCT (145). Therefore, FGF23 may also signal in the proximal tubules to regulate renal Pi transport and vitamin D metabolism. A second form of klotho is a soluble/cleaved protein derived by cleavage of the full-length transmembrane protein by proteases (150,151), which releases the extracellular domain into circulation.

Cleaved klotho is found in plasma, cerebrospinal fluid (152), and urine (153). Treatment with recombinant cleaved klotho protein directly inhibits Na/Pi co-transport in OK cells, in normal rats, and in FGF23-23-null mice in a dose-dependent manner (145). Cleaved klotho inhibits Na/Pi co-transport in isolated renal tubules and brush border membrane vesicles via its enzymatic activity that alters glycosylation of Npt2a and thereby decreases its co-transport activity. However, the exact role of cleaved klotho in the overall maintenance of Pi homeostasis (independent of its function as a co-factor for FGF23 specific-receptor) is unknown. A third form of klotho is the alternate spliced variant also found in circulation; however, it is not well-studied and its function is unknown (154).

6.3.3.5   Other Hormonal Regulators

Administration of 1,25D to vitamin D-deficient rats induced an increase in brush border membrane Na/Pi co-transport accompanied by increases in renal NPT2a mRNA and protein abundance (155). While these results are consistent with direct effects of 1,25D on NPT2a-mediated renal Na/Pi co-transport, they may result from a 1,25D-dependent decrease in PTH levels.

The finding that 1,25D increased the activity of a NPT2a promoter–luciferase reporter gene construct suggests a direct effect of this hormone on NPT2a gene transcription (155). In vitamin D receptor (VDR)-null mice, in which serum levels of PTH and 1,25D are greatly increased, the abundance of NPT2a protein in renal brush border membrane vesicles was significantly decreased, whereas the abundance of NPT2c protein was unaffected (156). This finding suggests that 1,25D has little direct effect on NPT2c expression.

Growth hormone acts directly on the kidney to increase renal Pi reabsorption, independently of PTH (157,158). In growth hormone-deficient subjects, serum Pi concentration and the TmP/GFR are reduced; both increase with administration of growth hormone (159,160). In patients with acromegaly, serum Pi concentrations are increased (161). Growth hormone stimulates proximal tubular Na/Pi co-transport (162–165), which is mediated, at least in part, by increased production and release of insulin-like growth factor 1 (IGF-1) (157,166).

Receptors for growth hormone are present on the basolateral membranes of proximal tubule cells and appear to activate the phospholipase C pathway. Receptors for

IGF-1 also have been identified in proximal tubule membranes and their effects may involve tyrosine kinase activity (157).

Fibroblast growth factor 7 (FGF7), produced by a tumor-induced osteomalacia-causing tumor, was recently shown to inhibit Pi uptake in OK cells, suggesting that it may also cause phosphaturia and may be responsible for tumor-induced osteomalacia in patients in whom circulating FGF23 levels are not increased (167). Secreted frizzled-related protein 4 (sFRP4) which, like FGF23, is highly expressed in tumors from patients with TIO (168), also has been tested for its phosphaturic action. It induced a specific increase in the renal fractional excretion of Pi and hypophosphatemia when infused in rats and inhibited Na/Pi co-transport in vitro when added to OK cells (168).

Other factors that inhibit Pi reabsorption are stanniocalcin, 5-hydroxytryptamine (5-HT), thyroid hormone, PTH-related peptide, calcitonin, atrial natriuretic factor, epidermal growth factor, transforming growth factor-ß, and glucocorticoids (16,27,28,169–174).

6.3.3.6 Non-Hormonal Regulators

Volume status—Expansion of extracellular fluid volume results in an increase and volume contraction causes a decrease in urine Pi excretion (Table 6.1) (16,27,28). The effect may be attributed in part to changes in the filtered load of Pi, rate of Pi reabsorption by the proximal tubules, and changes in plasma ionized calcium, the latter affecting secretion of PTH. A direct effect of volume expansion on tubular Pi reabsorption has also been reported.

Acid–base status—Changes in acid–base status can significantly affect renal handling of Pi (16). Acute respiratory acidosis results in a decrease in renal Pi reabsorption; this effect may depend on an increase in pCO_2 tension but does not depend on an increase in filtered Pi load, expansion of extracellular fluid volume, or change in PTH or blood bicarbonate concentration (175). Conversely, acute respiratory alkalosis induces an increase in renal Pi reabsorption and resistance to the phosphaturic actions of both PTH and cAMP; these effects may depend on changes in pCO_2 tension but are independent of changes in plasma Pi concentration (176).

Although acute metabolic acidosis has minimal effects on urine Pi excretion (177), chronic metabolic acidosis can impair renal Pi reabsorption independently of PTH and even when dietary Pi is severely restricted (178,179). The suppressive effect of metabolic acidosis on Na/Pi co-transport is observed in brush border membrane vesicles and is attributed to a decrease in Vmax of the transporter (179,180). In rats fed ammonium chloride for 10 days, the 60% decrease observed in brush border membrane Na/Pi co-transport activity was associated with a three-fold decrease in brush border membrane Npt2a protein abundance and a two-fold decrease in mRNA (181).

With a shorter duration of acidosis (<24 hours), the changes were of less magnitude and no changes in Npt2a mRNA were observed with very acutely-induced (6 hours) acidosis. The inhibitory effect of metabolic acidosis on Pi transport was independent of endogenous PTH activity but was greatly attenuated in rats fed a low (0.1%) Pi diet (181). In recent studies of mice fed ammonium chloride, the renal abundance of Npt2a mRNA was reduced at 2 but not 7 days of acidosis whereas Npt2c mRNA was reduced at both time points (182). However, the protein abundances of both Npt2a and Npt2c in brush border membranes paradoxically increased (182), suggesting that phosphaturia in acidosis may be induced by direct interactions between protons and the type IIa and IIc Pi co-transporters, thereby reducing transport activity (182).

Acute metabolic alkalosis induced by infusion of sodium bicarbonate reduced Pi reabsorption when the prior dietary intake of Pi was high, but increased it when dietary Pi was normal (183–187). Chronic metabolic alkalosis predictably increased renal Pi reabsorption (188).

Growth and development—As noted above, serum Pi concentrations are considerably higher in newborn infants and young children than in older children and adults. This finding reflects a higher rate of tubular Pi reabsorption in infants and immature animals as demonstrated by their higher values for TmP/GFR compared with adults (189). In newborn animals as compared with adult animals, Pi reabsorption is greater, both in the early proximal convoluted tubules and in more distal nephron segments, presumably the pars recta and segments beyond the distal convoluted tubules. In brush border membrane vesicles, the Vmax for Na/Pi co-transport is higher in newborn than in adult guinea pigs, a finding that cannot be accounted for by differences in plasma Pi concentrations, ionized calcium, PTH, thyroxine, or calcitonin.

The higher capacity for Pi reabsorption by the immature kidney also may reflect its relatively greater number of juxtamedullary nephrons that have higher capacities to reabsorb Pi. Newborn animals demonstrate a blunted phosphaturic response both to Pi loading and to administration of PTH, the latter despite a normal increase in urine cAMP. In Pi-restricted rats, the adaptive increase in Pi reabsorption is much greater in immature than in adult animals. Growth hormone may play an important role in mediating the increased renal reabsorption of Pi during development.

Also, as noted above, the greater abundance of Npt2c mRNA and protein in the kidneys of young rats may contribute to their higher rates of Pi transport as compared to the rates in older animals (46). Thus, through a variety of mechanisms, Pi handling by the immature kidney is regulated such that Pi retention is promoted, presumably to meet the increased needs of the growing organism for Pi (189,190).

Diuretic agents—Although their mechanisms and sites of action differ, certain diuretic agents predictably induce phosphaturia: mannitol, acetazolamide, thiazide diuretics, and loop diuretics. Urine phosphorus excretion is little affected by amiloride, spironolactone, and triamterene (16).

6.4 DISORDERS OF PHOSPHATE HOMEOSTASIS

6.4.1 GENETIC AND ACQUIRED HUMAN DISORDERS

Studies of genetic and acquired disorders of Pi homeostasis in humans and animal models of hypo- and hyper-phosphatemia led to the discovery of several important molecular mechanisms by which Pi homeostasis is maintained by the concerted interactions of circulating 1,25D, FGF23, and PTH. Genetic and human disorders of Pi homeostasis are listed in Table 6.2 and discussed in detail in several recent publications (191–193). Disordered Pi homeostasis in chronic kidney disease (CKD) is described in brief.

6.4.2 Chronic Kidney Disease (CKD)

In early CKD, serum Pi concentrations remain within normal limits until the glomerular filtration rate (GFR) decreases to less than approximately 30ml/min/1.73m^2 (194,195). As GFR declines further, serum Pi levels trend upward with frank hyperphosphatemia [>1.5 mmol/L (4.6 mg/dL)] observed in approximately 40% of pre-dialysis subjects with GFRs below 20 ml/min (194). The maintenance of Pi homeostasis with decreasing GFR is associated with a concomitant progressive increase in fractional urinary excretion of Pi (195). The latter is attributed, at least in part, to the phosphaturic actions of circulating PTH and FGF23 that increase progressively as GFR declines (194–196).

With advanced CKD, disordered mineral metabolism gives rise to CKD-related bone and mineral disorder (CKD-MBD), a systemic disease characterized by biochemical abnormalities of Pi, calcium, 1,25D, PTH, and FGF23 and abnormalities of bone (renal osteodystrophy) including impaired growth in children and vascular soft tissue calcification (197).

The plasma concentration of FGF23 increases early and progressively as GFR declines before the development of hyperphosphatemia (195,196). FGF23 levels are greatly increased in patients with stage V CKD (121,198–200). Patients on dialysis have the highest levels. FGF23 levels remain high in many patients after renal transplantation and contribute to persistent post-transplant hypophosphatemia (201). Deficiency of 1,25D occurs early in the course of progressive CKD in adults (194,202) and recent data suggest that the excess circulating FGF23 is the primary mechanism and thus may be the initiating event in the development of secondary hyperparathyroidism (195,199).

Findings in animal models of CKD are consistent with observations in humans with CKD. Plasma FGF23 levels increase early in rodents with CKD (203) and FGF23 levels are normalized upon treatment with an oral phosphate binder (204). Treatment of CKD in mice with anti-FGF23 neutralizing antibody was associated with decreases in the fractional excretion of Pi and increases in serum Pi concentrations (203). Current data suggest that increased plasma FGF23 is the earliest detectable abnormality in mineral metabolism in CKD. However, the mechanism responsible for the increased bone production and circulation of FGF23 in early CKD remains to be elucidated.

TABLE 6.2
Disorders of Pi Homeostasis

	Gene Mutation	Serum Pi	FEPi	Serum Ca	Urine Ca	Plasma FGF23	Serum PTH	Serum 1,25(OH)$_2$D	Reference
Genetic				Hypophosphatemia					
ADHR	*FGF23*	Low	High	NL	NL/Low	High	NL	Inappropriately NL	111,118
XLH	*Phex*	Low	High	NL	NL/Low	High	NL/High	Inappropriately NL	121,207
ARHR1/ARHP	*Dmp1*	Low	High	NL	NL/Low	High	NL/High	Inappropriately NL	208,209
ARHR2	*ENPP1*	Low	High	NL	NL/Low	High	NL	Inappropriately NL	210,211
OGD	*FGFR1*	Low	High	NL	NL	High	NL/High	Inappropriately NL	212
FD/MAS	*GNAS1*	Low	High	NL/High	NL	High	NL/High	Inappropriately NL	213–217
OSD,	*INPPL1*	Low	High	?	?	High	?	?	218,219
NF1+2	*NF1, NF2*	Low	High	NL/Low	NL/Low	High	NL	Inappropriately NL	193,220
LNSS/ENS	*FGFR3*	Low	High	NL	NL/Low	High	NL	Inappropriately NL	191,221
HHRH	*NPT2a*	Low	Low	NL	High	NL	NL/Low	High	50–52
NPHLOP1	*NPT2c*	Low	High	NL	High	Low/NL	NL/Low	High	222,223
NPHLOP2	*NHERF1*	Low	High	NL	?	?	NL	High	224
Acquired									
TIO	—	Low	High	NL	NL/Low	High	NL/High/Low	Inappropriately NL	121,225,226
Post renal transplant	—	Low	High	NL	NL	High	NL/High	NL	201
Post-hepatectomy	—	Low	High	NL	NL	NL	NL	NL	191,227,228
Burns	—	Low	NL	?	?	NL	?	?	191,229,230

Hyperphosphatemia

Genetic									
FTC	GALNT3, FGF23, Klotho	High	High	High	High	Low/High	Low/High	High	231–236
Acquired									
CKD	—	High	High	NL/Low	NL	High	High	Low	195,199,237

ADHR = autosomal dominant hypophosphatemic rickets.

ARHR1 and ARHR2 = autosomal recessive hypophosphatemic rickets types 1 and 2.

CKD = chronic kidney disease.

ENS = epidermal nevus syndrome.

FD = fibrous dysplasia.

FTC = familial tumoral calcinosis.

HHRH = hereditary hypophosphatemic rickets with hypercalciuria.

LNSS = linear nevus sebaceous syndrome.

MAS = McCune-Albright syndrome.

NF1 and NF2 = neurofibromatosis types 1 and 2.

NL = normal.

NPHLOP1 and NPHLOP2 = nephrolithiasis/osteoporosis, hypophosphatemic types 1 and 2.

OGD = osteoglophonic osteomalacia.

OSD = opsismodysplasia,

TIO = tumor-induced osteomalacia.

XLH = x-linked hypophosphatemia.

REFERENCES

1. Nordin BEC. 1976. Nutritional considerations. In: Nordin BEC, Ed., *Calcium, Phosphate, and Magnesium Metabolism*. New York: Churchill Livingstone, pp. 1–35.
2. Marshall RW. 1976. Plasma fractions. In: Nordin BEC, Ed., *Calcium, Phosphate and Magnesium Metabolism*. London: Churchill Livingston, pp. 162–185.
3. Rowe J et al.1984. Hypophosphatemia and hypercalciuria in small premature infants fed human milk: Evidence for inadequate dietary phosphorus. *J Pediatr* 104: 112–117.
4. Giles MM et al. 1987. Sequential calcium and phosphorus balance studies in preterm infants. *J Pediatr* 110: 591–598.
5. Wilkinson R. 1976. Absorption of calcium, phosphorus, and magnesium. In Nordin BEC, Ed., *Calcium, Phosphate and Magnesium Metabolism*. New York: Churchill Livingstone, pp. 36–112.
6. Tanaka Y et al. 1973. The control of 25-hydroxyvitamin D metabolism by inorganic phosphorus. *Arch Biochem Biophys* 154: 566–574.
7. Baxter LA et al. 1976. Stimulation of 25-hydroxyvitamin D3-1a-hydroxylase by phosphate depletion. *J Biol Chem* 251: 3158–3161.
8. Gray RW et al. 1983. Dietary phosphate deprivation increases 1,25-dihydroxyvitamin D3 synthesis in rat kidney in vitro. *J Biol Chem* 258: 1152–1155.
9. Maierhofer WJ et al. 1984. Phosphate deprivation increases serum 1,25(OH)2-vitamin D concentrations in healthy men. *Kidney Intl* 25: 571–575.
10. Portale AA et al. 1986. Oral intake of phosphorus can determine the serum concentration of 1,25-dihydroxyvitamin D by determining its production rate in humans. *J Clin Invest* 77: 7–12.
11. Portale AA et al. 1989. Physiologic regulation of the serum concentration of 1,25-dihydroxyvitamin D by phosphorus in normal men. *J Clin Invest* 83: 1494–1499.
12. Perwad F et al. 2005. Dietary and serum phosphorus regulate fibroblast growth factor 23 expression and 1,25-dihydroxyvitamin D metabolism in mice. *Endocrinology* 146: 5358–5364.
13. Markowitz M et al. 1981. Circadian rhythms of blood minerals in humans. *Science* 213: 672–674.
14. Portale AA et al. 1987. Dietary intake of phosphorus modulates the circadian rhythm in serum concentration of phosphorus: Implications for the renal production of 1,25-dihydroxyvitamin D. *J Clin Invest* 80: 1147–1154.
15. Mostellar ME et al. 1964. Effects of alkalosis on plasma concentration and urinary excretion of inorganic phosphate in man. *J Clin Invest* 43: 138–149.
16. Bindels RJM, Hoenderop JG, and Biber J. 2011. Transport of calcium, magnesium, and phosphate. In Taal MW et al., Eds., *The Kidney*, 9th ed. Philadelphia: W.B. Saunders, pp. 226–251.
17. Brodehl J et al. 1982. Postnatal development of tubular phosphate reabsorption. *Clin Nephrol* 17: 163–171.
18. Arnaud SB et al. 1973. Serum parathyroid hormone and blood minerals: interrelationships in normal children. *Pediatr Res* 7: 485–493.
19. Greenberg BG et al. 1960. The normal range of serum inorganic phosphorus and its utility as discriminant in the diagnosis of congenital hypophosphatemia. *J Clin Endocrinol* 20: 364–379.
20. Keating FR Jr et al. 1969. The relation of age and sex to distribution of values in healthy adults of serum, calcium inorganic phosphorus, magnesium, alkaline phosphatase, total proteins, albumin, and blood urea. *J Lab Clin Med* 73: 825–834.
21. Lee DBN and Kurokawa K. 1987. Physiology of phosphorus metabolism. In Maxwell MH et al., Eds., *Clinical Disorders of Fluid and Electrolyte Metabolism*, 4th ed. New York: McGraw Hill, pp. 245–295.

22. Favus MJ. 1992. Intestinal absorption of calcium, magnesium, and phosphorus. In Coe FL and Favus MJ, Eds., *Disorders of Bone and Mineral Metabolism.* New York: Raven Press, pp. 57–81.

23. Marks J et al. 2010. Phosphate homeostasis and the renal-gastrointestinal axis. *Am J Physiol Renal Physiol* 299: F285–F296.

24. Hilfiker H et al. 1998. Characterization of a murine type II sodium-phosphate co-transporter expressed in mammalian small intestine. *Proc Natl Acad Sci USA* 95: 14564–14569.

25. Tschope W et al. 1980. Plasma phosphate and urinary calcium in recurrent stone formers. *Miner Electrolyte Metabol* 4: 237–245.

26. Inoue Y et al. 2005. Role of the vitamin D receptor in FGF23 action on phosphate metabolism. *Biochem J* 390: 325–331.

27. Biber J et al. 2013. Phosphate transporters and their function. *Annu Rev Physiol* 75: 535–550.

28. Biber J et al. 2009. Regulation of phosphate transport in proximal tubules. *Pflugers Arch* 458: 39–52.

29. Virkki LV et al. 2007. Phosphate transporters: a tale of two solute carrier families. *Am J Physiol Renal Physiol* 293: F643–F654.

30. Tenenhouse HS. 2007. Phosphate transport: molecular basis, regulation and pathophysiology. *J Steroid Biochem Mol Biol* 103: 572–577.

31. Baumann K et al. 1975. Renal phosphate transport: inhomogeneity of local proximal transport rates and sodium dependence. *Pflugers Arch* 356: 287–297.

32. Ullrich KJ et al. 1977. Phosphate transport in the proximal convolution of the rat kidney. *Pflugers Arch* 372: 269–274.

33. McKeown JW et al. 1979. Intrarenal heterogeneity for fluid, phosphate and glucose absorption in the rabbit. *Am J Physiol* 237: F312–F318.

34. Haas JA et al. 1978. Nephron heterogeneity of phosphate reabsorption. *Am J Physiol* 234: F287–F290.

35. Haramati A et al. 1984. Nephron heterogeneity of phosphate reabsorption: effect of parathyroid hormone. *Am J Physiol* 246: F155–F158.

36. Goldfarb S. 1980. Juxtamedullary and superficial nephron phosphate reabsorption in the cat. *Am J Physiol* 239: F336–F342.

37. deRouffignac C et al. 1973. Micropuncture study of water and electrolyte movements along the loop of Henle in Psammomys with special reference to magnesium, calcium, and phosphorus. *Pflugers Arch* 344: 309–326.

38. Knox FG et al. 1977. Phosphate transport in superficial and deep nephrons in phosphate-loaded rats. *Am J Physiol* 233: F150–F153.

39. Muhlbauer RC et al. 1977. Tubular localization of adaptation to dietary phosphate in rats. *Am J Physiol* 233: F342–F348.

40. Shareghi GA et al. 1982. Phosphate transport in the light segment of the rabbit cortical collecting tubule. *Am J Physiol* 242: F379–F384.

41. Peraino RA et al. 1980. Phosphate transport by isolated rabbit cortical collecting tubule. *Am J Physiol* 238: F358–F362.

42. Barac-Nieto M et al. 2002. Basolateral phosphate transport in renal proximal-tubule-like OK cells. *Exp Biol Med* 227: 626–631.

43. Custer M et al. 1993. Localization of NaPi-1, a Na/Pi co-transporter, in rabbit kidney proximal tubules I: mRNA localization by reverse transcription/polymerase chain reaction. *Pflugers Arch* 424: 203–209.

44. Werner A et al. 1991. Cloning and expression of cDNA for a Na/Pi co-transport system of kidney cortex. *Proc Natl Acad Sci USA* 88: 9608–9612.

45. Magagnin S et al. 1993. Expression cloning of human and rat renal cortex Na/Pi co-transport. *Proc Natl Acad Sci USA* 90: 5979–5983.

46. Segawa H et al. 2002. Growth-related renal type II Na/Pi co-transporter. *J Biol Chem* 277: 19665–19672.

47. Ohkido I et al. 2003. Cloning, gene structure and dietary regulation of the type-IIc Na/Pi co-transporter in the mouse kidney. *Pflugers Arch* 446: 106–115.

48. Hartmann CM et al. 1996. Structure of murine and human renal type II Na+-phosphate co-transporter genes (Npt2 and NPT2). *Proc Natl Acad Sci USA* 93: 7409–7414.

49. Forster IC et al. 1999. Stoichiometry and Na+ binding cooperativity of rat and flounder renal type II Na + Pi co-transporters. *Am J Physiol* 276: F644–F649.

50. Bergwitz C et al. 2006. SLC34A3 mutations in patients with hereditary hypophosphatemic rickets with hypercalciuria predict a key role for the sodium–phosphate co-transporter NaPi-IIc in maintaining phosphate homeostasis. *Am J Hum Genet* 78: 179–192.

51. Lorenz-Depiereux B et al. 2006. Hereditary hypophosphatemic rickets with hypercalciuria caused by mutations in the sodium–phosphate co-transporter gene SLC34A3. *Am J Hum Genet* 78: 193–201.

52. Ichikawa S et al. 2006. Intronic deletions in the SLC34A3 gene cause hereditary hypophosphatemic rickets with hypercalciuria. *J Clin Endocrinol Metabol* 91: 4022–4027.

53. Collins JF et al. 2004. The SLC20 family of proteins: dual functions as sodium–phosphate co-transporters and viral receptors. *Pflugers Arch* 447: 647–652.

54. Kavanaugh MP et al. 1994. Cell-surface receptors for gibbon ape leukemia virus and amphotropic murine retrovirus are inducible sodium-dependent phosphate symporters. *Proc Natl Acad Sci USA* 91: 7071–7075.

55. Villa-Bellosta R et al. 2008. The Na+/Pi co-transporter PiT-2 (SLC20A2) is expressed in the apical membrane of rat renal proximal tubules and regulated by dietary Pi. *Am J Physiol Renal Physiol* 296: F691–699.

56. Tomoe Y et al. 2010. Phosphaturic action of fibroblast growth factor 23 in Npt2 null mice. *Am J Physiol Renal Physiol* 298: F1341–F1350.

57. Picard N et al. 2010. Acute parathyroid hormone differentially regulates renal brush border membrane phosphate co-transporters. *Pflugers Arch* 460: 677–687.

58. Beck L et al. 1998. Targeted inactivation of Npt2 in mice leads to severe renal phosphate wasting, hypercalciuria, and skeletal abnormalities. *Proc Natl Acad Sci USA* 95: 5372–5377.

59. Thiede MA et al. 1988. Expression of a calcium-mobilizing parathyroid hormone-like peptide in lactating mammary tissue. *Science* 242: 278–280.

60. Kanis JA et al. 1981. The role of vitamin D metabolites in the osteomalacia of renal disease. *Curr Med Res Opin* 7: 294–315.

61. Hoag HM et al. 1999. Effects of Npt2 gene ablation and low-phosphate diet on renal Na(+)/phosphate co-transport and co-transporter gene expression. *J Clin Invest* 104: 679–686.

62. Tenenhouse HS et al. 2003. Differential effects of Npt2a gene ablation and X-linked Hyp mutation on renal expression of Npt2c. *Am J Physiol Renal Physiol* 285: F1271–F1278.

63. Segawa H et al. 2009. Type IIc sodium-dependent phosphate transporter regulates calcium metabolism. *J Am Soc Nephrol* 20: 104–113.

64. Segawa H et al. 2009. Npt2a and Npt2c in mice play distinct and synergistic roles in inorganic phosphate metabolism and skeletal development. *Am J Physiol Renal Physiol* 297: F671–F678.

65. Miyamoto K et al. 2007. New aspect of renal phosphate reabsorption: the type IIc sodium-dependent phosphate transporter. *Am J Nephrol* 27: 503–515.

66. Forster IC et al. 2006. Proximal tubular handling of phosphate: a molecular perspective. *Kidney Intl* 70: 1548–1559.

67. Villa-Bellosta R et al. 2008. Interactions of the growth-related, type IIc renal sodium/phosphate co-transporter with PDZ proteins. *Kidney Intl* 73: 456–464.

68. Ardura JA et al. 2011. Regulation of G protein-coupled receptor function by Na+/H+ exchange regulatory factors. *Pharmacol Rev* 63: 882–900.

69. Cunningham R et al. 2010. Role of NHERF and scaffolding proteins in proximal tubule transport. *Urol Res* 38: 257–262.

70. Stoll R et al. 1979. Effect of dietary phosphate intake on phosphate transport by isolated rat renal brush border vesicles. *Biochem J* 180: 465–470.

71. Kempson SA et al. 1979. Phosphate transport across renal cortical brush border membrane vesicles from rats stabilized on a normal, high or low phosphate diet. *Life Sci* 24: 881–888.

72. Tenenhouse HS et al. 1979. Renal brush border membrane adaptation to phosphorus deprivation in the Hyp/Y mouse. *Nature* 281: 225–227.

73. Brazy PC et al. 1980. Comparative effects of dietary phosphate, unilateral nephrectomy, and parathyroid hormone on phosphate transport by the rabbit proximal tubule. *Kidney Intl* 17: 788–800.

74. Barrett PQ et al. 1980. Effect of dietary phosphate on transport properties of pig renal microvillus vesicles. *Am J Physiol* 239: F352–F359.

75. Cheng L et al. 1983. Phosphate uptake by renal membrane vesicles of rabbits adapted to high and low phosphorus diets. *Am J Physiol* 245: F175–F180.

76. Levine BS et al. 1984. Early renal brush border membrane adaptation to dietary phosphorus. *Miner Electrolyte Metabol* 10: 222–227.

77. Levine BS et al. 1986. Renal adaptation to phosphorus deprivation: characterization of early events. *J Bone Miner Res* 1: 33–40.

78. Caverzasio J et al. 1985. Mechanism of rapid phosphate (Pi) transport adaptation to a single low Pi meal in rat renal brush border membrane. *Pflugers Arch* 404: 227–231.

79. Cheng L et al. 1984. Renal adaptation to phosphate load in the acutely thyroparathyroidectomized rat: rapid alteration in brush border membrane phosphate transport. *Am J Physiol* 246: F488–F494.

80. Biber J et al. 1985. Na/Pi co-transport in LLC-PK cells: fast adaptive response to Pi deprivation. *Am J Physiol* 249: C430–C434.

81. Caverzasio J et al. 1985. Adaptation of phosphate transport in phosphate-deprived LLC-PK cells. *Am J Physiol* 248: F122–F127.

82. Escoubet B et al. 1989. Adaptation to Pi deprivation of cell Na-dependent Pi uptake: a widespread process. *Am J Physiol* 256: C322–C328.

83. Lotscher M et al. 1997. Role of microtubules in the rapid regulation of renal phosphate transport in response to acute alterations in dietary phosphate content. *J Clin Invest* 99: 1302–1312.

84. Werner A et al. 1994. Increase of Na/Pi co-transport encoding mRNA in response to low Pi diet in rat kidney cortex. *J Biol Chem* 269: 6637–6639.

85. Levi M et al. 1994. Cellular mechanisms of acute and chronic adaptation of rat renal P(i) transporter to alterations in dietary P(i). *Am J Physiol* 267: F900–F9008.

86. Tenenhouse HS et al. 1995. Effect of P(i) restriction on renal Na(+)-P(i) co-transporter mRNA and immunoreactive protein in X-linked Hyp mice. *Am J Physiol* 268: F1062–F1069.

87. Verri T et al. 1995. Cloning of a rabbit renal Na/Pi co-transporter regulated by dietary phosphate. *Am J Physiol* 268: F626–F633.

88. Beck L et al. 1996. Renal expression of Na+ phosphate co-transporter mRNA and protein: effect of the Gy mutation and low phosphate diet. *Pflugers Arch* 431: 936–941.

89. Katai K et al. 1997. Acute regulation by dietary phosphate of the sodium-dependent phosphate transporter (NaP(i)-2) in rat kidney. *J Biochem (Tokyo)* 121: 50–55.

90. Takahashi F et al. 1998. Effects of dietary Pi on the renal Na+-dependent Pi transporter NaPi-2 in thyroparathyroidectomized rats. *Biochem J* 333: 175–181.

91. Pfister MF et al. 1998. Cellular mechanisms involved in the acute adaptation of OK cell Na/Pi-co-transport to high- or low-Pi medium. *Pflugers Arch* 435: 713–719.

92. Kido S et al. 1999. Identification of regulatory sequences and binding proteins in the type II sodium/phosphate co-transporter NPT2 gene responsive to dietary phosphate. *J Biol Chem* 274: 28256–28263.

93. Segawa H et al. 2005. Internalization of renal type IIc Na-Pi co-transporter in response to a high-phosphate diet. *Am J Physiol Renal Physiol* 288: F587–F596.

94. Kempson SA et al. 1995. Parathyroid hormone action on phosphate transporter mRNA and protein in rat renal proximal tubules. *Am J Physiol* 268: F784–F791.

95. Pfister MF et al. 1997. Parathyroid hormone-dependent degradation of type II Na+/Pi co-transporters. *J Biol Chem* 272: 20125–20130.

96. Traebert M et al. 2000. Luminal and contraluminal action of 1-34 and 3-34 PTH peptides on renal type IIa Na-P(i) co-transporter. *Am J Physiol Renal Physiol* 278: F792–F798.

97. Lederer ED et al. 2000. Parathyroid hormone stimulates extracellular signal-regulated kinase (ERK) activity through two independent signal transduction pathways: role of ERK in sodium–phosphate co-transport. *J Am Soc Nephrol* 11: 222–231.

98. Bacic D et al. 2003. Involvement of the MAPK-kinase pathway in the PTH-mediated regulation of the proximal tubule type IIaNa(+)/P(i) co-transporter in mouse kidney. *Pflugers Arch* 446: 52–60.

99. Jankowski M et al. 2001. The opossum kidney cell type IIa Na/P(i) co-transporter is a phosphoprotein. *Kidney Blood Press Res* 24: 1–4.

100. Khundmiri SJ et al. 2003. Parathyroid hormone regulation of type II sodium–phosphate co-transporters is dependent on an A kinase anchoring protein. *J Biol Chem* 278: 10134–10141.

101. Bacic D et al. 2003. Impaired PTH-induced endocytotic down-regulation of the renal type IIa Na+/Pi co-transporter in RAP-deficient mice with reduced megalin expression. *Pflugers Arch* 446: 475–484.

102. Deliot N et al. 2005. Parathyroid hormone treatment induces dissociation of type IIa Na+-P(i) co-transporter-Na+/H+ exchanger regulatory factor-1 complexes. *Am J Physiol Cell Physiol* 289: C159–C167.

103. Voltz JW et al. 2007. Phosphorylation of PDZ1 domain attenuates NHERF-1 binding to cellular targets. *J Biol Chem* 282: 33879–33887.

104. Weinman EJ et al. 2007. Parathyroid hormone inhibits renal phosphate transport by phosphorylation of serine 77 of sodium-hydrogen exchanger regulatory factor-1. *J Clin Invest* 117: 3412–3420.

105. Weinman EJ et al. 2011. Dynamics of PTH-induced disassembly of Npt2a/NHERF-1 complexes in living OK cells. *Am J Physiol Renal Physiol* 300: F231–F235.

106. Weinman EJ et al. 2010. Cooperativity between the phosphorylation of Thr95 and Ser77 of NHERF-1 in the hormonal regulation of renal phosphate transport. *J Biol Chem* 285: 25134–25138.

107. Segawa H et al. 2007. Parathyroid hormone-dependent endocytosis of renal type IIc Na/Pi co-transporter. *Am J Physiol Renal Physiol* 292: F395–F403.

108. Blaine J et al. 2007. Differential regulation of renal NaPi-IIa and NaPi-IIc trafficking by PTH. *J Am Soc Nephrol* 18: 56A.

109. Marcinkowski W et al. 1971. Renal mRNA of PTH-PTHrP receptor, [Ca²⁺]i and phosphaturic response to PTH in phosphate depletion. *Miner Electrolyte Metabol* 1997. 23: 48–57.

110. Bianchine JW et al. Familial hypophosphatemic rickets showing autosomal dominant inheritance. *Birth Defects Orig Artic Ser* 7: 287–295.

111. Econs MJ et al. 1997. Autosomal dominant hypophosphatemic rickets/osteomalacia: clinical characterization of a novel renal phosphate-wasting disorder. *J Clin Endocrinol Metabol* 82: 674–681.
112. ADHR Consortium. 2000. Autosomal dominant hypophosphataemic rickets is associated with mutations in FGF23. *Nat Genet* 26: 345–348.
113. Tenenhouse HS and Econs MJ. 2001. Mendelian hypophosphatemias. In Scriver CR et al., Eds., *The Metabolic and Molecular Basis of Inherited Disease*. New York: McGraw Hill, pp. 5039–5068.
114. White KE et al. 2001. Autosomal-dominant hypophosphatemic rickets (ADHR) mutations stabilize FGF-23. *Kidney Intl* 60: 2079–2086.
115. Sweet RA et al. 1980. Vitamin D metabolite levels in oncogenic osteomalacia. *Ann Intern Med* 93: 279–280.
116. Econs MJ et al. 1994. Tumor-induced osteomalacia: unveiling a new hormone. *New Engl J Med* 330: 1679–1681.
117. Rasmussen H and Tenenhouse HS. 1998. Mendelian hypophosphatemias. In Scriver CR et al., Eds., *The Metabolic Basis of Inherited Disease*. New York: McGraw Hill.
118. White KE et al. 2001. The autosomal dominant hypophosphatemic rickets (ADHR) gene is a secreted polypeptide over-expressed by tumors that cause phosphate wasting. *J Clin Endocrinol Metabol* 86: 497–500.
119. Shimada T et al. 2001. Cloning and characterization of FGF23 as a causative factor of tumor-induced osteomalacia. *Proc Natl Acad Sci USA* 98: 6500–6505.
120. Yamazaki Y et al. 2002. Increased circulatory level of biologically active full-length FGF-23 in patients with hypophosphatemic rickets/osteomalacia. *J Clin Endocrinol Metabol* 87: 4957–4960.
121. Jonsson KB et al. 2003. Fibroblast growth factor 23 in oncogenic osteomalacia and X-linked hypophosphatemia. *New Engl J Med* 348: 1656–1663.
122. Imel EA et al. 2010. Treatment of X-linked hypophosphatemia with calcitriol and phosphate increases circulating fibroblast growth factor 23 concentrations. *J Clin Endocrinol Metabol* 95: 1846–1850.
123. Cai Q et al. 1994. Brief report: inhibition of renal phosphate transport by a tumor product in a patient with oncogenic osteomalacia. *New Engl J Med* 330: 1645–1649.
124. Jonsson KB et al. 2001. Extracts from tumors causing oncogenic osteomalacia inhibit phosphate uptake in opossum kidney cells. *J Endocrinol* 169: 613–620.
125. Yu X et al. 2005. Analysis of the biochemical mechanisms for the endocrine actions of fibroblast growth factor-23. *Endocrinology* 146: 4647–4656.
126. Urakawa I et al. 2006.Klotho converts canonical FGF receptor into a specific receptor for FGF23. *Nature* 444: 770–774.
127. Kurosu H et al. 2006. Regulation of fibroblast growth factor-23 signaling by klotho. *J Biol Chem* 281: 6120–6123.
128. Saito II ct al. 2003. Human fibroblast growth factor 23 mutants suppress Na+-dependent phosphate co-transport activity and 1a,25-dihydroxyvitamin D3 production. *J Biol Chem* 278: 2206–2211.
129. Bai XY et al. 2003. The autosomal dominant hypophosphatemic rickets R176Q mutation in FGF23 resists proteolytic cleavage and enhances in vivo biological potency. *J Biol Chem* 278: 9843–9849.
130. Shimada T et al. 2004. FGF-23 is a potent regulator of vitamin D metabolism and phosphate homeostasis. *J Bone Miner Res* 19: 429–435.
131. Perwad F et al. 2007. Fibroblast growth factor 23 impairs phosphorus and vitamin D metabolism in vivo and suppresses 25-hydroxyvitamin D-1α-hydroxylase expression in vitro. *Am J Physiol Renal Physiol* 293: F1577–F1583.

132. Shimada T et al. 2002. Mutant FGF-23 responsible for autosomal dominant hypo-phosphatemic rickets is resistant to proteolytic cleavage and causes hypophosphatemia in vivo. *Endocrinology* 143: 3179–3182.

133. Bai X et al. 2004. Transgenic mice over-expressing human fibroblast growth factor 23 (R176Q) delineate a putative role for parathyroid hormone in renal phosphate wasting disorders. *Endocrinology* 145: 5269–5279.

134. Larsson T et al. 2004. Transgenic mice expressing fibroblast growth factor 23 under the control of the α1(I) collagen promoter exhibit growth retardation, osteomalacia, and disturbed phosphate homeostasis. *Endocrinology* 145: 3087–3094.

135. Sitara D et al. 2004. Homozygous ablation of fibroblast growth factor-23 results in hyper-phosphatemia and impaired skeletogenesis, and reverses hypophosphatemia in Phex-deficient mice. *Matrix Biol* 23: 421–432.

136. Liu S et al. 2006. Pathogenic role of Fgf23 in Hyp mice. *Am J Physiol Endocrinol Metabol* 291: E38–E49.

137. Shimada T et al. 2002. Targeted ablation of Fgf23 demonstrates an essential physiologi-cal role of FGF23 in phosphate and vitamin D metabolism. *J Clin Invest* 2004. 113: 561–568.

138. Yoshida T et al. 2003. Mediation of unusually high concentrations of 1,25-dihydroxyvitamin D in homozygous klotho mutant mice by increased expression of renal 1α-hydroxylase gene. *Endocrinology* 143: 683–689.

139. Segawa H et al. 2007. Correlation between hyperphosphatemia and type II Na/Pi co-transporter activity in klotho mice. *Am J Physiol Renal Physiol* 292: F769–F779.

140. Razzaque MS et al. 2007. The emerging role of the fibroblast growth factor-23–klotho axis in renal regulation of phosphate homeostasis. *J Endocrinol* 194: 1–10.

141. Kuro M. 2006. Klotho as a regulator of fibroblast growth factor signaling and phosphate–calcium metabolism. *Curr Opin Nephrol Hypertens* 15: 437–441.

142. Liu S et al. 2007. Emerging role of fibroblast growth factor 23 in a bone–kidney axis regulating systemic phosphate homeostasis and extracellular matrix mineralization. *Curr Opin Nephrol Hypertens* 16: 329–335.

143. Yamashita T et al. 2002. Fibroblast growth factor (FGF)-23 inhibits renal phosphate reabsorption by activation of the mitogen-activated protein kinase pathway. *J Biol Chem* 277: 28265–28270.

144. Weinman EJ et al. 2011. Fibroblast growth factor-23-mediated inhibition of renal phosphate transport in mice requires sodium–hydrogen exchanger regulatory factor-1 (NHERF-1) and synergizes with parathyroid hormone. *J Biol Chem* 286: 37216–37221.

145. Hu MC et al. 2010. Klotho: a novel phosphaturic substance acting as an autocrine enzyme in the renal proximal tubule. *FASEB J* 24: 3438–3450.

146. Hu MC et al. 2013. Fibroblast growth factor 23 and klotho: physiology and pathophysi-ology of an endocrine network of mineral metabolism. *Annu Rev Physiol* 75: 503–533.

147. Kuro M et al. 1997. Mutation of the mouse klotho gene leads to a syndrome resembling ageing. *Nature* 390: 45–51.

148. Farrow EG et al. 2009. Initial FGF23-mediated signaling occurs in the distal convoluted tubule. *J Am Soc Nephrol* 20: 955–960.

149. Farrow EG et al. 2010. Altered renal FGF23-mediated activity involving MAPK and Wnt: effects of the Hyp mutation. *J Endocrinol* 207: 67–75.

150. Bloch L et al. 2009. Klotho is a substrate for alpha-, beta- and gamma-secretase. *FEBS Lett* 583: 3221–3224.

151. Chen CD et al. 2007. Insulin stimulates the cleavage and release of the extracel-lular domain of klotho by ADAM10 and ADAM17. *Proc Natl Acad Sci USA* 104: 19796–19801.

152. Imura A et al. 2004.Secreted klotho protein in sera and CSF: implication for post-translational cleavage in release of klotho protein from cell membrane. *FEBS Lett* 565: 143–147.

153. Hu MC et al. 2011. Klotho deficiency causes vascular calcification in chronic kidney disease. *J Am Soc Nephrol* 22: 124–136.

154. Shiraki-Iida T et al. 1998. Structure of the mouse klotho gene and its two transcripts encoding membrane and secreted protein. *FEBS Lett* 424: 6–10.

155. Taketani Y et al. 1998. Regulation of type II renal Na+-dependent inorganic phosphate transporters by 1,25-dihydroxyvitamin D3: identification of a vitamin D-responsive element in the human NAPi-3 gene. *J Biol Chem* 273: 14575–14581.

156. Segawa H et al. 2004. Intestinal Na/P(i) co-transporter adaptation to dietary P(i) content in vitamin D receptor-null mice. *Am J Physiol Renal Physiol* 287: F39–F47.

157. Hammerman MR. 1989. The growth hormone-insulin-like growth factor axis in kidney. *Am J Physiol* 257: F503–F514.

158. Murer H et al. 1991. Cellular mechanisms in proximal tubular reabsorption of inorganic phosphate. *Am J Physiol* 260: C885–C899.

159. Gertner JM et al. 1979. Parathyroid function and vitamin D metabolism during human growth hormone replacement. *J Clin Endocrinol Metabol* 49: 185–188.

160. Gertner JM et al. 1981. The effects on mineral metabolism of overnight growth hormone infusion in growth hormone deficiency. *J Clin Endocrinol Metabol* 53: 818–822.

161. McMillan DE et al. 1968. Evaluation of clinical activity of acromegaly by observation of the diurnal variation of serum inorganic phosphate. *Metabolism* 17: 966–976.

162. Hammerman MR et al. 1980. Regulation of canine renal vesicle Pi transport by growth hormone and parathyroid hormone. *Biochim Biophys Acta* 603: 322–335.

163. Mulroney SE et al. 1989. Antagonist to GH-releasing factor inhibits growth and renal Pi reabsorption in immature rats. *Am J Physiol* 257: F29–F34.

164. Caverzasio J et al. 1990. Stimulatory effect of insulin-like growth factor-1 on renal Pi transport and plasma 1,25-dihydroxyvitamin D3. *Endocrinology* 127: 453–459.

165. Quigley R et al. 1991.Effects of growth hormone and insulin-like growth factor I on rabbit proximal convoluted tubule transport. *J Clin Invest* 88: 368–374.

166. Caverzasio J et al. 1989. Insulin-like growth factor I stimulates Na-dependent Pi transport in cultured kidney cells. *Am J Physiol* 257: F712–F717.

167. Carpenter TO et al. 2005. Fibroblast growth factor 7: an inhibitor of phosphate transport derived from oncogenic osteomalacia-causing tumors. *J Clin Endocrinol Metabol* 90: 1012–1020.

168. Berndt T et al. 2003. Secreted frizzled-related protein 4 is a potent tumor-derived phosphaturic agent. *J Clin Invest* 112: 785–794.

169. Wagner GF et al. 1997. Human stanniocalcin inhibits renal phosphate excretion in the rat. *J Bone Miner Res* 12: 165–171.

170. Hafdi Z et al. 1996. Locally formed 5-hydroxytryptamine stimulates phosphate transport in cultured opossum kidney cells and in rat kidney. *Biochem J* 320: 615–621.

171. Alcalde AI et al. 1999. Role of thyroid hormone in regulation of renal phosphate transport in young and aged rats. *Endocrinology* 140: 1544–1551.

172. Arar M et al. 1999. Epidermal growth factor inhibits Na/Pi co-transport in weaned and suckling rats. *Am J Physiol* 276: F72–F78.

173. Levi M et al. 1995. Dexamethasone modulates rat renal brush border membrane phosphate transporter mRNA and protein abundance and glycosphingolipid composition. *J Clin Invest* 96: 207–216.

174. Hilfiker H et al. 1998. Characterization of the 5′-flanking region of OK cell type II Na/Pi co-transporter gene. *Am J Physiol* 274: F197–F204.

175. Webb RK et al. 1977. Relationship between phosphaturia and acute hypercapnia in the rat. *J Clin Invest* 60: 829–837.
176. Hoppe A et al. 1982. Effect of respiratory alkalosis on renal phosphate excretion. *Am J Physiol* 243: F471–F475.
177. Beck N. 1975. Effect of metabolic acidosis on renal action of parathyroid hormone. *Am J Physiol* 228: 1483–1488.
178. Beck N. 1981. Effect of metabolic acidosis on renal response to parathyroid hormone in phosphorus deprived rats. *Am J Physiol* 241: F23–F27.
179. Kempson SA. 1982. Effect of metabolic acidosis on renal brush border membrane adaptation to low phosphorus diet. *Kidney Intl* 22: 225–233.
180. Levine BS et al. 1983. Effect of metabolic acidosis on phosphate transport by the renal brush border membrane. *Biochim Biophys Acta* 727: 7–12.
181. Ambuhl PM et al. 1998. Regulation of renal phosphate transport by acute and chronic metabolic acidosis in the rat. *Kidney Intl* 53: 1288–1298.
182. Nowik M et al. 2008. Renal phosphaturia during metabolic acidosis revisited: molecular mechanisms for decreased renal phosphate reabsorption. *Pflugers Arch* 457: 539–549.
183. Yanagawa N and Lee DBN. 1992. Renal handling of calcium and phosphorus. In Coe FL and Favus MJ, Eds., *Disorders of Bone and Mineral Metabolism*. New York: Raven Press, pp. 3–40.
184. Kuntziger H et al. 1980. Localization of parathyroid hormone-independent sodium bicarbonate inhibition of tubular phosphate reabsorption. *Kidney Intl* 17: 749–755.
185. Zilenovski AM et al. Effect of sodium bicarbonate on phosphate excretion in acute and chronic PTX rats. *Am J Physiol* 236: F184–F191.
186. Quamme GA. 1985. Effects of metabolic acidosis, alkalosis, and dietary hydrogen ion intake on phosphate transport in the proximal convoluted tubule. *Am J Physiol* 249: F769–F779.
187. Steele TH. Bicarbonate induced phosphaturia dependence upon the magnitude of phosphate reabsorption. *Pflugers Arch* 370: 291–294.
188. Mizgala CL et al. 1985. Renal handling of phosphate. *Physiol Rev* 65: 431–466.
189. Stewart CL et al. 1992. Transport of calcium and phosphorus. In Polin R and Fox WW, Eds., *Fetal and Neonatal Physiology*. Philadelphia: W.B. Saunders, pp. 1223–1231.
190. Spitzer A et al. 1983. Renal regulation of phosphate homeostasis during growth. *Semin Nephrol* 3: 87–93.
191. Bergwitz C et al. 2012. FGF23 and syndromes of abnormal renal phosphate handling. *Adv Exp Med Biol* 728: 41–64.
192. Martin A et al. 2012. Regulation and function of the FGF23/klotho endocrine pathways. *Physiol Rev* 92: 131–155.
193. Carpenter TO, 2012. The expanding family of hypophosphatemic syndromes. *J Bone Miner Metabol* 30: 1–9.
194. Levin A et al. 2007. Prevalence of abnormal serum vitamin D, PTH, calcium, and phosphorus in patients with chronic kidney disease: results of the study to evaluate early kidney disease. *Kidney Intl* 71: 31–38.
195. Isakova T et al. 2011. Fibroblast growth factor 23 is elevated before parathyroid hormone and phosphate in chronic kidney disease. *Kidney Intl* 79: 1370–1378.
196. Portale AA et al. 2012. Fibroblast growth factor 23 is a risk factor for left ventricular hypertrophy in chronic kidney disease in children (CKiD) cohort. *J Am Soc Nephrol* 23: 920A.
197. Moe S et al. 2006. Definition, evaluation, and classification of renal osteodystrophy: a position statement from Kidney Disease: Improving Global Outcomes (KDIGO). *Kidney Intl* 69: 1945–1953.

198. Larsson T et al. 2003. Circulating concentration of FGF-23 increases as renal function declines in patients with chronic kidney disease, but does not change in response to variation in phosphate intake in healthy volunteers. *Kidney Intl* 64: 2272–2279.

199. Gutierrez O et al. 2005. Fibroblast growth factor-23 mitigates hyperphosphatemia but accentuates calcitriol deficiency in chronic kidney disease. *J Am Soc Nephrol* 16: 2205–2215.

200. Imanishi Y et al. 2004. FGF-23 in patients with end-stage renal disease on hemodialysis. *Kidney Intl* 65: 1943–1946.

201. Bhan I et al. 2006. Post-transplant hypophosphatemia: tertiary hyperphosphatoninism? *Kidney Intl* 70:1486–1494.

202. Pitts TO et al. 1988. Hyperparathyroidism and 1,25-dihydroxyvitamin D deficiency in mild, moderate, and severe renal failure. *J Clin Endocrinol Metabol* 67: 876–881.

203. Hasegawa H et al. 2010. Direct evidence for a causative role of FGF23 in the abnormal renal phosphate handling and vitamin D metabolism in rats with early-stage chronic kidney disease. *Kidney Intl* 78: 975–980.

204. Nagano N et al. 2006. Effect of manipulating serum phosphorus with phosphate binder on circulating PTH and FGF23 in renal failure rats. *Kidney Intl* 69: 531–537.

205. Suki WN, Lederer ED, and Rouse D. 2000. Renal transport of calcium, magnesium, and phosphate. In: Brenner BM, Ed., *The Kidney*, 6th ed. Philadelphia: W.B. Saunders, pp. 520–574.

206. Murer H et al. 1999. Posttranscriptional regulation of the proximal tubule NaPi-II transporter in response to PTH and dietary Pi. *Am J Physiol* 277: F676–F684.

7 Vitamin D: Activities for Bone Health

Howard A. Morris, Paul H. Anderson,
and B.E. Christopher Nordin

CONTENTS

7.1 INTRODUCTION

Vitamin D was identified as a key nutrient for bone health nearly 100 years ago [1]. Since then, the highest levels of clinical evidence confirm that adequate vitamin D status reduces the risks of musculoskeletal diseases including rickets in children, osteomalacia in adults, and osteoporosis in the frail elderly and also reduces the risks of falls, fractures, and premature death. Considerable controversy still surrounds the molecular actions of vitamin D in the skeleton, the levels required for musculoskeletal health, and the interaction of the vitamin with dietary calcium intake [2,3].

The identification in the 1970s of 1,25-dihydroxyvitamin D (1,25D), synthesized in the kidney as a biologically active metabolite, and its action as a ligand for the vitamin D receptor (VDR) nuclear transcription factor largely elucidated the endocrine mode of action of vitamin D [4]. In recent years, expansion of our knowledge of vitamin D indicates it is metabolized within a wide range of non-renal tissues to synthesize 1,25D and activate the VDRs within the tissues of synthesis [5].

In bone tissue, each major bone cell responds to the vitamin D pro-hormone known as 25-hydroxyvitamin D (25D) via the local synthesis of 1,25D to exert paracrine or autocrine biological effects. This new knowledge reveals plausible physiological and molecular mechanisms for activities and tissue responses to vitamin D under conditions when renal synthesis of 1,25D is low. It may also help resolve the controversy regarding the level of serum 25D required to maintain bone health [6].

The ability of the kidney to markedly increase expression of the gene coding for the key synthetic enzyme for 1,25D, the 25-hydroxyvitamin D 1α-hydroxylase (CYP27B1) is well described [7]. However, the regulation of expression and the degree of up-regulation of its expression is quite different from the processes in bone cells [8]. Based on principles of enzyme kinetics, it is feasible that the high level of CYP27B1 activity induced in renal cells under specific conditions allows the synthesis of adequate plasma 1,25D at levels of 25D that are inadequate for bone cells because of lower CYP27B1 activity. It is plausible therefore that different critical levels of serum 25D for renal and skeletal tissues are required to provide adequate synthesis of 1,25D under various environmental conditions.

7.2　VITAMIN D AND METABOLIC BONE DISORDERS

7.2.1　Genetic Disorders

Although vitamin D was identified as an essential physiological regulator through observations of nutritional deficiencies, much information has arisen from investigation of genetic disorders in humans and more recently in mouse models.

The first genetic disorder to be recognized is known as hereditary 1,25-dihydroxy vitamin-D-resistant rickets (HVDRR) although a variety of terms were used previously [9]. Albright and colleagues alluded to end-organ resistance to vitamin D in a 1937 report but the first patients with HVDRR were reported in 1978 by two groups [10,11]. Since then, numerous case reports of HVDRR patients have been published [12]. The characterization of the molecular basis of HVDRR was markedly simplified when skin cells were identified as expressing the VDR [13]. Subsequently a variety of mutant VDR molecules have been identified with pathologies including inability of 1,25D to bind to VDR and ablation of vitamin D biological activities. Thus, HVDRR includes a spectrum of abnormalities in the VDR arising from partial or total resistance to 1,25D. Genomic sequencing identified a wide range of mutations within the VDR associated with these pathologies [9].

HVDRR patients mainly present with hypocalcemia, hypophosphatemia, hyperparathyroidism, and/or rickets in childhood or osteomalacia in adulthood. Treatment is largely focused on raising plasma calcium levels with calcium supplementation and 1,25D (calcitriol) therapy; responses vary widely. Measurements of serum vitamin D metabolites usually indicate normal 25D levels with markedly elevated 1,25D levels.

Clinical experience indicates that after puberty and into adulthood many of these patients are able to maintain normal plasma calcium and phosphate homeostasis with modest oral calcium supplements or sometimes none. Normalization of plasma calcium and phosphate levels appears to be all that is necessary to correct the mineralization defect of rickets or osteomalacia. Calcium supplementation also corrects the hyperparathyroidism that appears to correct hypophosphatemia. No other pathologies attributable to inactivation of vitamin D have been detected in these patients to date except alopecia, which is unaffected by normalization of plasma calcium [9].

Mice in which the gene for VDR has been ablated throughout the body (global VDRKO) were initially developed in 1997. All the various lines developed since then mimic the pathology of HVDRR patients demonstrating a rachitic phenotype with hypocalcemia, hyperparathyroidism, and alopecia when fed a normal laboratory chow diet [14–16]. Interestingly when these mice are fed a "rescue diet" containing high levels of calcium and phosphate and lactose from weaning, their plasma calcium and phosphate homeostasis is restored and parathyroid hormone (PTH) levels are reduced [17]. Under this feeding regimen, bone mineral status of global VDRKO mice including bone volumes and strength at 10 weeks of age were equal to wild type mice fed the same diet [18]. Such data support the concept that vitamin D activities to maintain bone mineral status are limited to those required to maintain plasma calcium and phosphate homeostasis.

A later study in older mice investigated the bone mineral status of global VDRKO mice fed the rescue diet from weaning until 17 weeks of age [19]. Their bone mineral status was significantly reduced compared with wild type mice. Furthermore, these VDRKO mice demonstrated reduced osteoclast numbers and expression of the gene coding for receptor activator of nuclear factor-B ligand (RANKL) in bone tissue, indicating that reduced bone volume was not the result of increased bone resorption. These mice demonstrated reduced osteoblast numbers and mineral apposition rates, prompting the authors to state that "bone formation may be more vitamin D-dependent as the animals age" [19]. Such effects must be confirmed in other experimental models before general conclusions can be drawn.

Another rare form of rickets arising from an in-born error of vitamin D metabolism was identified when 1,25D (calcitriol) became available as a therapeutic agent in 1973 [20]. It was evident that this pathology arose from the inability to convert 25D to 1,25D and is termed pseudo-vitamin D deficiency rickets (PDDR). Patients with PDDR usually present during their first year of life with signs of marked hypocalcemia such as neurological signs or even hypocalcemic seizures, with radiological examinations revealing classical changes of rickets [21]. Unlike HDDR, PDDR patients do not exhibit signs of alopecia. Biochemical investigations indicate profound hypocalcemia and hyperparathyroidism with either normal or low plasma phosphate levels.

Measurement of vitamin D metabolites provides the key indicators for diagnosis of PDDR where serum levels of 1,25D are very low or undetectable while 25D levels are normal. This pattern is clearly different from that seen with HVDRR. Current treatment is replacement with calcitriol to achieve normocalcemia and normal PTH levels. Calcium supplements may be required initially to heal bone.

Cloning of the human CYP27B1 gene in 1997 allowed considerable progress in elucidating the molecular etiology of PDDR [22]. Many mutations in this gene have been identified, demonstrating various mechanisms of disruption of the gene product and are dispersed across all exons [21]. Most mutations result in total loss of CYP27B1 activity, although some mutations appear to retain partial activity [23].

Independent reports of the characterization of two mouse models of PDDR (global CYP27B1KO) appeared in 2001 [19,24]. These mice demonstrated a similar phenotype to the global VDRKO mice with hypocalcemia, hypophosphatemia, hyperparathyroidism, and rickets when fed diets with normal levels of calcium and phosphate. As with PDDR patients, these mice are not alopecic. When CYP27B1KO mice were fed the rescue diet with high calcium, phosphate, and lactose, resolution of the rickets phenotype was observed with normalization of plasma calcium and phosphate levels. Another difference between the VDRKO and CYP27B1KO mouse lines that persisted with the rescue diet is that the growth plate in the CYP27B1KO mice remained enlarged and distorted in contrast to VDRKO mice in which it was normalized.

7.2.2 Nutritional Deficiency, Rickets, and Osteomalacia

We have known since the early 1900s that severe vitamin D deficiency results in metabolic bone diseases known as rickets in children and osteomalacia in adults [1]. Very low plasma 25D levels are insufficient to provide substrate for the renal CYP27B1 enzyme to generate adequate plasma 1,25D levels. As observed when vitamin D activity is genetically ablated, the most obvious phenotype of vitamin D deficiency is disruption of plasma calcium and phosphate homeostasis [4].

There is no evidence of alopecia with nutritional vitamin D deficiency. The kidney is capable of markedly up-regulating expression of CYP27B1 by some 40-fold under the combined influence of PTH and hypocalcemia [7]. This marked up-regulation of renal CYP27B1 enzyme activity allows for production of 1,25D to be maintained at relatively low plasma levels of the 25D substrate. Clinical [25] and rodent model data [26] indicate that under these conditions adequate serum 1,25D levels can be maintained with serum 25D levels at 20 nmol/L (8 ng/mL) or greater. These serum 1,25D levels are adequate to maintain intestinal calcium absorption and actions at the kidney to maximize renal tubular reabsorption of calcium and on bone to stimulate calcium and phosphate flow into the plasma pool by stimulating bone resorption such that normocalcemia is maintained [25].

7.2.3 Osteoporosis, Falls, and Fractures

Since the 1970s significant clinical evidence demonstrated that low vitamin D status contributes to the risk of hip fractures in the elderly [27,28]. Meta-analyses of case control studies conducted over some 30 years clearly demonstrate a strong association between decreased serum 25D levels and increased risk of hip fracture in this age group [29]. In many studies, the level of serum 25D associated with an increase in the risk of hip fracture in the elderly was less severe (approximately 40 nmol/L (16 ng/mL)) [28,30] than that identified as critical for osteomalacia (20 nmol/L or 8 ng/mL) [25,31].

The causal relationship between low vitamin D status and hip fracture was established through randomized, placebo-controlled clinical trials (RCTs) of vitamin D supplementation, usually in combination with a calcium supplement, to assess the effects on risk of fracture. The first trial conducted by Chapuy et al. in 1992 [32] provided strong evidence that vitamin D and calcium supplementation reduced the risk of hip and non-vertebral fractures in the elderly. Subsequent trials produced conflicting results, with their quality varying markedly, particularly with regard to doses of vitamin D, compliance with the study treatment, and confounding by uncontrolled dietary supplements [33].

Various meta-analyses of the outcomes of these RCTs provided conflicting interpretations. However, when vitamin D dose is considered, a significant benefit of vitamin D at a dosage between 800 and 2000 IU per day and calcium (1000 mg per day) has been consistently established [33]. Re-analyses of the Women's Health Trial excluding subjects taking their own supplements demonstrated positive results for vitamin D and calcium supplementation in reducing the risk of hip fracture over 5 years of study, even at levels of 400 IU vitamin D combined with 1000 mg calcium daily [34]. In contrast meta-analysis of fracture prevention trials when 1,25D (calcitriol) was administered as a single treatment found no reduction in fracture risk [35]. An alternative strategy is using low dose calcitriol therapy in combination with calcium supplementation to correct intestinal calcium malabsorption, which is common among postmenopausal osteoporosis patients [36]. This regimen reduces bone resorption [37].

All these data support the view that decreased vitamin D status increases the risk of hip fracture in the elderly, which is related to the serum level of the 25D metabolite and not to the serum 1,25D level. The level of serum 25D at which the risk of fracture is increased is not as low as that required to cause osteomalacia. Therefore, a major question is whether hip fracture patients suffer from osteomalacia or osteoporosis. Bone histology studies demonstrated that only a small minority of hip fracture patients exhibited signs of osteomalacia [38-41]. A significant minority of hip fracture patients revealed osteoporosis, others had osteopenia, and some patients may have had both conditions.

7.3   METABOLISM AND MOLECULAR MODES OF ACTION

Vitamin D_3 (also known as cholecalciferol) arises from sunlight exposure of the skin. The ultraviolet B (UVB) radiation converts 7-dehydrocholesterol to pre-vitamin D_3 which at body temperature isomerizes to vitamin D_3 [4]. Vitamin D sources in the diet from both animal (vitamin D_3) and plant sources (vitamin D_2 also known as ergocalciferol) and their absorption at the intestine were discussed in Chapters 1 and 2.

In the circulation, vitamin D and its metabolites are largely bound to the vitamin D binding protein (DBP). Vitamin D is activated by two consecutive hydroxylation reactions catalyzed by specific P450 enzymes (Figure 7.1) [42]. The first

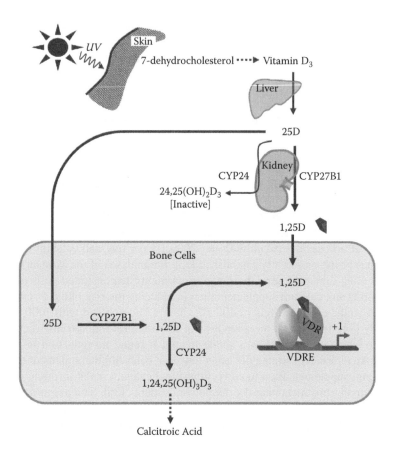

FIGURE 7.1 Vitamin D metabolism involves hydroxylation of 25D by the CYP27B1 enzyme in renal proximal tubule cells. This step yields the active form of vitamin D in plasma known as 1,25D. Alternatively 25D can be 24-hydroxylated by the 25-hydroxyvitamin D-24-hydroxylase (CYP24) enzyme in the first step of vitamin D catabolism into calcitroic acid. The 1,25D binds to the VDR in the nuclei of target cells where it can alter gene transcription of vitamin D-responsive genes such as those involved in calcium homeostasis, bone cell activity, and cellular differentiation. Bone cells also express CYP27B1 and can synthesize 1,25D. CYP24 is also present and can deactivate these vitamin D metabolites in bone cells. The regulation and importance of the bone CYP27B1 enzyme, however, remain unclear.

hydroxylation at the carbon 25 position is catalyzed by the vitamin D-25 hydroxylase enzyme (CYP2R1) to form the pro-hormone 25D [43]. This enzyme is expressed in the liver, which appears to be the major site of synthesis for plasma 25D [44]. However, many tissues also express CYP2R1 and therefore synthesis of 25D can occur locally throughout the body [45]. Furthermore, a number of enzymes can catalyze this 25-hydroxylation reaction although with lower affinity than the CYP2R1 enzyme [43]. The level of 25D in serum best reflects vitamin D status because of its properties with regard to solubility and binding to vitamin D binding protein [46].

The second hydroxylation in this pathway occurs at the carbon 1 position and is responsible for synthesis of the biologically active 1,25D metabolite that has the highest affinity of all the vitamin D metabolites for the nuclear VDR [42]. The renal activity of CYP27B1 was identified as responsible for synthesizing plasma 1,25D as the active metabolite of vitamin D in 1970 [47]. In a healthy state, renal synthesis is the sole source of plasma 1,25D [8] except during pregnancy where some consider that the placenta makes a contribution [48].

Various disease states can increase plasma 1,25D levels through synthesis at extrarenal sites. This synthesis can occur with increased numbers of plasma cells including macrophages and white blood cells that express the CYP27B1 gene. Such levels of plasma 1,25D levels may be responsible for the development of hypercalcemia [49]. Again, just as for CYP2R1, many tissues express the CYP27B1 gene which, under particular physiological states, may be at a higher level than production by the kidney [50]. For example, in young male mice fed normal dietary calcium, the highest levels of CYP27B1 expression were in the testes and brain.

A third step in vitamin D metabolism is hydroxylation at the carbon 24 position by the 25-hydroxyvitamin D-24-hydroxylase (CYP24) enzyme. This enzyme is largely responsible for catabolism of vitamin D metabolites through its multi-catalytic activity with hydroxylation, preferably at carbon 23 in humans but may occur at carbon 24 in humans and other species [42]. This is the first step in a series of reactions involving the sequential cleavage of four aliphatic hydrocarbons to synthesize calcitroic acid which is eliminated via the kidneys.

The renal CYP24 activity is responsible for synthesis of plasma 24,25-dihydroxyvitamin D (24,25D) and also contributes to plasma 1,25D levels by regulating the clearance of vitamin D metabolites including 1,25D [8]. The combination of renal CYP27B1 and CYP24 messenger RNA (mRNA) levels accounts for some 85% of the variance of plasma 1,25D levels in rats. Biological activity for 24,25D has been proposed by way of a specific membrane-associated receptor involved in bone fracture repair [51].

7.3.1 Regulation of Plasma 1,25D Levels

Regulation of renal CYP27B1 and CYP24 gene expression plays key roles in plasma calcium and phosphate homeostasis by regulating plasma 1,25D levels. Renal CYP27B1 expression is regulated by each of the calcium- and phosphate-regulating hormones. Many of these regulatory factors including localization of gene expression to the renal proximal tubular cells of the kidney are contained within the proximal 1503 base pairs (bp) upstream of the human CYP27B1 gene [50].

PTH markedly stimulates renal CYP27B1 expression in these cells. Two mechanisms have been described for PTH stimulation. One acts through a vitamin D inhibitory receptor (VDIR) that binds to a site approximately –500 bp upstream of the CYP27B1 promoter region [52]. A second mechanism acts through a cyclic-AMP dependent protein kinase A activity by way of a CCAAT box site within the proximal –305 bp upstream of the CYP27B1 promoter region [53]. These actions occur under conditions of hypocalcemia, when plasma PTH levels are highest.

Interestingly, calcitonin also stimulates expression of CYP27B1 but in the distal convoluted tubules of the kidneys. This occurs under conditions of normocalcemia through stimulation of a protein kinase C pathway by the activated calcitonin receptor [54]. The physiological relevance of this action of calcitonin is unknown as plasma calcitonin levels are low when plasma calcium is normal.

Inhibition of CYP27B1 expression also plays a critical role in regulating plasma 1,25D levels. We know that 1,25D is a negative regulator of renal CYP27B1 expression via a novel mechanism involving the VDIR located around −500 bp within the proximal promoter [52]. This mechanism has been demonstrated only in kidney cells. Another important inhibitor of renal CYP27B1 expression is fibroblast growth factor 23 (FGF23), a plasma hormone produced largely by mature osteocytes. These activities are discussed in greater detail in Chapters 5 and 6.

As mentioned above, the regulation of catabolism of 1,25D through expression of CYP24 in the renal proximal convoluted tubules is also critical for regulating plasma 1,25D levels as demonstrated by the phenotype of the CYP24-null mouse [55]. The inverse relationship between CYP24 and CYP27B1 expression in the kidney is unusual and appears limited to renal tissue [8]. CYP24 is considered to be expressed in all cells expressing VDR [42]. In extrarenal cells, a positive relationship between CYP27B1 and CYP24 expression has been demonstrated [8]. This inverse relationship in renal cells lends support to the concept that the renal proximal tubules metabolize 25D for synthesis of plasma 1,25D and subsequent endocrine activities. In extrarenal tissues, the positive relationship between expression of these genes suggests that such local synthesis of 1,25D promotes autocrine or paracrine activities.

In the kidney, the reciprocal relationship between CYP27B1 and CYP24 mRNA levels is largely the product of reciprocal actions of the calciotropic hormones on the expression of these genes. For example, the major stimulator for CYP24 expression is 1,25D which, as discussed above, directly inhibits renal CYP27B1 expression. CYP24 induction by 1,25D involves activation of VDR through binding to tandem vitamin D-responsive elements (VDREs) in the proximal CYP24 promoter [56], although variations of regulation occur among humans, rats, and other species [57].

Also, 1,25D stimulates intracellular signaling (non-genomic) pathways to activate transcription factors that depend on VDR signaling to further enhance CYP24 transcriptional activity [58]. Activation of these pathways ultimately results in phosphorylation of a transcription factor such as one of the E26 (Ets) family members that binds to the gene promoter region in the area of the VDREs to further stimulate transcription. Each of these mechanisms is dependent on a liganded VDR and interacts to markedly increase CYP24 enzyme levels in the presence of 1,25D. Such increases of CYP24 enzyme activity presumably minimize toxic activities by rapidly reducing plasma 1,25D levels.

Increased PTH levels decrease CYP24 activity in kidney cells although the mechanism of this effect remains controversial. PTH has been reported to destabilize CYP24 mRNA and reduce CYP24 enzyme activity [59]. Calcitonin induces CYP24 expression in a human embryonic kidney cell line through a combination of protein kinase A and protein kinase C activities that may be physiologically relevant under conditions of hypercalcemia when calcitonin levels are elevated and it would be advantageous to reduce plasma 1,25D levels [60]. FGF23 actions to lower plasma 1,25D levels also depend on stimulation of CYP24 expression in addition to inhibition of CYP27B1 expression (see Chapter 6). The stimulation of CYP24 expression depends mainly on VDR actions through a VDRE, unlike the inhibition of CYP27B1.

7.3.2 Regulation of Gene Transcription

Vitamin D exerts its biological activity through the binding of the metabolite 1,25D to a protein receptor in a similar manner to other steroid hormones. The best described vitamin D receptor (VDR) is a member of the nuclear steroid hormone receptor superfamily acting to stimulate gene transcription after binding 1,25D and forming a heterodimer with the retinoid-X receptor (RXR) protein [61]. Vitamin D-responsive genes are defined by the genetic coding of a specific control element known as the vitamin D response element (VDRE) in the regulatory region of the genome.

Often but not always, VDREs are situated in physical proximity to the transcriptional start site for a vitamin D-responsive gene. The binding of the 1,25D-VDR-RXR complex to the VDRE initiates the recruitment and assembly of a very large complex of proteins known as co-activators. This complex has at least two functions. It remodels the locally condensed chromatin through the presence of various enzymes that either add moieties such as acetyl or methyl groups to histones or remove them. It also communicates with the RNA polymerase II enzyme that is responsible for transcription of the vitamin D-responsive genes through mRNA synthesis.

The totality of such transcriptional complexes defines the specificity and sensitivity of steroid hormones such as vitamin D to regulate a multiplicity of biological responses through a wide range of tissues. We currently understand the contributions of at least four elements of the transcriptional complex [62]. In the case of vitamin D, the 1,25D nuclear receptor ligand identifies the physiological specificity of the response. The VDRE identifies the genetic specificity of the response. The various co-activators and other proteins complexing to the liganded VDR-RXR heterodimer bound to the VDRE identify the cell specificity. Finally, the specific gene identifies the biological response.

7.3.3 Regulation of Intracellular Signaling and Non-Genomic Actions

It has been recognized for some 30 years that 1,25D exerts biological activities over significantly shorter times than those required for regulation of gene transcription as described above. These activities take place over minutes while the genomic synthesis of mRNA and translation into proteins following 1,25D activation requires some 5 to 10 hours before detectable protein levels can be measured. These rapid activities include modulation of intracellular calcium levels and activation of intracellular signaling through phosphate kinases and phosphatases. These rapid activities appear to activate different intracellular signaling pathways in different cell types [58,63]. The end result of many of these activities is an alteration of gene transcription [58].

Evidence indicates that 1,25D acts through a distinct membrane-associated rapid response steroid binding receptor (MARRS) [64] to initiate such rapid activities. This protein belongs to a superfamily of multifunctional glucose-regulated and redox-sensitive proteins implicated in binding thyroid hormones and estrogens in glycoprotein biosynthesis and in immune responses [65]. The well-characterized nuclear VDR has also been found to elicit similar rapid responses, presumably in association with plasma cell membrane constituents [58,66].

When primary osteoblasts isolated from calvaria from both wild type and global VDRKO mice were incubated with 1,25D, intracellular calcium was increased within 1 minute and the protein kinase C pathway was activated within 5 minutes in cells from both mouse lines, indicating that the nuclear VDR was unnecessary for these actions [67]. In another model of osteoblasts, the ROS17/2.8 rat osteosarcoma cell line, the expression of the nuclear VDR was demonstrated to be essential for 1,25D to increase intracellular calcium ions within 3 minutes [66]. Thus, it appears that at least two forms of the VDR are capable of eliciting rapid responses in osteoblast-like cells although the physiological context for the selection of the specific receptor for activity is currently not understood.

7.3.4 ACTIONS OF RECEPTOR THROUGH BINDING TO INTRACELLULAR PROTEINS

A further mechanism of action for vitamin D is direct binding of VDR to intracellular proteins. Many of the proteins that bind with VDR have been identified as either transcriptional co-activators or co-repressors that constitute the transcriptional complex necessary for genomic actions as described above or act on their own as transcription factors.

One of the most intriguing activities described for VDR in this context is its role in hair follicle cycling. It is well known that humans and mice in which the nuclear VDR gene is inactivated develop alopecia along with other disorders, most particularly hypocalcemia and hypophosphatemia [14]. In contrast, humans and mice in which the CYP27B1 gene is inactivated do not develop alopecia despite sharing disordered plasma calcium and phosphate homeostasis [24].

The action of the β-catenin protein normally located within the cell cytoplasm is critical for maintenance of hair follicle growth in hair follicle stem cells [68]. Activation of β-catenin occurs through the well characterized-Wnt signaling pathway that stimulates the translocation of β-catenin from the cytoplasm to the nucleus where it binds to transcription factors of the T cell factor (TCF) and lymphoid enhancer factor (LEF) families. In hair follicle stem cells, these transcription factors stimulate expression of genes coding for specific keratins that make up the structural proteins of hair and therefore are critical for hair growth [68]. The binding of VDR to β-catenin in these cells is a critical stage for the activation of β-catenin to stimulate transcription of the keratin genes. There is no requirement for 1,25D binding to VDR for this activity. Whether there is a requirement for the VDR to bind another ligand is unresolved at this time.

VDR binds directly to β-catenin in a number of cell systems modulating β-catenin-responsive genes in some cell types while modulating vitamin D-responsive genes in others [69]. Importantly for skeletal physiology, the Wnt signaling pathway and β-catenin regulate bone formation as indicated by the actions of sclerostin, the Wnt signaling pathway antagonist. Sclerostin binds to the LRP5/6 proteins. In a complex with the frizzled receptor (the first component of the Wnt signaling pathway), it markedly inhibits bone formation. Inhibitors of sclerostin are currently undergoing trials as treatments for postmenopausal osteoporosis [70].

Do VDR and β-catenin interact in osteoblasts to modulate bone formation and is this activity dependent on 1,25D as a VDR ligand? Preliminary evidence from in vitro experimentation with a human osteoblast-like osteosarcoma cell line indicates that VDR does stimulate β-catenin activity in this cell line. This osteoblast-like activity appears to be independent of 1,25D [71] and contrasts with results from similar experimentation with a colon cancer cell line; the authors reported that the β-catenin–VDR interaction inhibited β-catenin activity.

Most interesting are data identifying VDR antagonists that inactivate the VDR through a VDRE by blocking recruitment of the classical transcriptional complex. Mutations identified within the VDR gene allow the antagonist–VDR complex to interact with β-catenin, stimulating biological activities by way of this pathway [72]. Thus, specific amino acid residues in the VDR can discriminate between classical genomic activities of VDR through a VDRE and its ability to interact with β-catenin.

A mutation in one such amino acid of the VDR that inactivates the classical genomic pathway acting through a VDRE but maintains the β-catenin–VDR pathway has been identified in a patient with hereditary vitamin D-dependent rickets. The patient exhibits manifestations of rickets but is not alopecic [73].

7.4 CELLULAR REGULATION OF BONE MINERAL HOMEOSTASIS

7.4.1 BASIC MULTICELLULAR UNIT OF BONE REMODELING AND RESORPTION

Skeletal architecture is dependent on the activities of three major bone cell types as well as interaction with the hemopoietic system within the bone marrow. Osteoblasts are bone-forming cells derived from a mesenchymal lineage. Osteocytes are the most numerous cell types embedded in bone mineral and arise from the terminal differentiation of osteoblasts. Osteoclasts are bone-resorbing cells derived from the hemopoietic lineage. Bone architecture is modified through the coordinated activities of these cells located at a common anatomical site, the basic multicellular unit of bone remodeling. Each of these cell types expresses the VDR and demonstrates vitamin D biological activities. Also, each cell type is capable of metabolizing vitamin D, particularly 25D to form the 1,25D active metabolite to exert biological activities [74].

The best characterized direct activity of vitamin D on bone cells is the action of 1,25D on osteoblasts to increase osteoclastogenesis and bone resorption [75]. This action plays a key role in maintaining plasma calcium and phosphate homeostasis. The 1,25D activates the VDR in osteoblast cells to increase expression of the gene coding for RANKL. The RANKL protein is localized to the external surface membranes of osteoblasts and binds to receptor activator of nuclear factor κ (RANK) expressed on the surfaces of osteoclast progenitor cells to stimulate osteoclastogenesis and bone resorption. This pathway of activation of bone resorption depends on osteoblastic expression of VDR [76].

A report indicates that 1,25D acting through the VDR exerts a wide range of activities in osteoclast precursors and osteoclasts [77]. Preliminary in vitro data show that 25D can be metabolized to 1,25D by osteoclasts to modulate a variety of activities including increasing osteoclast number and size while suppressing their bone resorptive action [78,79]. The ability of osteoclasts to adhere to and migrate across the bone surface is inhibited by metabolism of 25D [80]. The current challenge is reconciling such in vitro findings with in vivo responses.

7.4.2 Mechanisms of Bone Formation

Bone formation involves the coordinated synthesis of osteoid matrix followed by mineralization. The osteoid is composed largely of type I collagen with other proteins including osteocalcin, osteopontin, osteonectin, bone sialoprotein-1, and proteoglycans present [81]. Mineralization occurs at discrete sites, particularly along collagen fibrils incorporating calcium and phosphate to form hydroxyapatite crystals and a mature bone matrix. The life cycles of osteoblasts and their maturation into osteocytes are tightly linked to the mineralization process.

The first activity requires osteoblast cell proliferation followed by cell maturation, initially involving the synthesis and secretion of proteins of osteoid including type I collagen. These steps are followed by mineralization accompanied by the maturation of some osteoblasts to pre-osteocytes that are embedded in unmineralized osteoid. Upon completion of mineralization, most of the osteoblasts undergo apoptosis while the pre-osteocytes mature into osteocytes embedded in mineralized tissue. A small number of osteoblasts transform into lining cells localized to bone surfaces. Mineralization is tightly controlled by the synthesis of stimulating and inhibitory factors by osteoblasts, osteocytes, and osteoclasts at various stages of maturation.

7.4.3 Vitamin D Activities within Osteoblasts and Osteocytes

In vitro experimentation with primary bone cells isolated from rodents and humans demonstrates that inclusion of 1,25D in culture media inhibits osteoblast proliferation and enhances osteoblast maturation and mineral deposition [74,81,82]. The expression of many genes key to osteoblast maturation and mineral deposition is modulated by 1,25D. The process includes increased gene expression of type I collagen; alkaline phosphatase; matrix gla protein, an inhibitor of aberrant calcification of cartilage and arteries; osteopontin, another inhibitor of mineralization; bone sialoprotein, and osteocalcin.

Osteocytes in culture respond to 1,25D with induction of fibroblast growth factor-23 (FGF23), coding for the major phosphate-regulating hormone and dentin matrix protein 1 (DMP1), a source of inhibitors of mineralization [77]. Modulation of expression of some of these genes may be the result of a direct genomic action of 1,25D-VDR through interaction with a VDRE. However, the expression of other genes may be stimulated indirectly through the action of 1,25D to enhance maturation of the osteoblast phenotype [81].

The stage of maturation appears to influence the genetic response of osteoblasts to 1,25D. Induction of RANKL expression by 1,25D is increased in immature primary normal human bone-like cells compared to their more mature counterparts [83]. Similarly, mouse osteoblasts derived from calvaria that demonstrate a more immature osteoblast phenotype expressed RANKL some 1000-fold more than cells isolated from mouse long bones that showed a more mature phenotype. After incubation with 1,25D, the immature calvarial cells increased RANKL expression a further five-fold while 1,25D did not increase RANKL expression in the more mature long bone cells [84].

7.5   ENDOCRINE ACTIVITIES

7.5.1   REGULATION OF PLASMA CALCIUM AND PHOSPHATE HOMEOSTASIS

Vitamin D exerts endocrine activity to maintain plasma calcium and phosphate homeostasis via the actions of plasma 1,25D and the VDR on at least three organs (kidney, small intestine, and bone) as presented in Chapters 2, 3, and 6. In a healthy and non-pregnant state, plasma 1,25D arises from synthesis by the kidney and the regulation of the renal synthesis plays a key role in maintaining calcium and phosphate homeostasis [42].

Endocrine activity is defined by a relationship between plasma levels of a hormone, in this case 1,25D, and a biological activity at a distant organ. Plasma levels of 1,25D clearly demonstrate a positive relationship with intestinal absorption of calcium in humans and rodent models [85,86]. In patients with mild renal disease, oral administration of 1,25D stimulated urinary calcium excretion and normalized plasma ionized calcium levels [87].

Plasma 1,25D levels are positively related to rodent renal mRNA levels of calbindin 28K, a gene coding for a key protein for the renal tubular reabsorption of calcium [88]. Increasing plasma levels of 1,25D through feeding a low calcium diet or direct injection increases osteoclastic bone resorption by increasing RANKL expression by osteoblast cells in bone [89]. Thus, the endocrine actions of 1,25D have been well demonstrated with regard to the regulation of plasma calcium homeostasis.

7.5.2   ENDOCRINE ACTIVITIES: STIMULATION OF BONE RESORPTION AND INHIBITION OF BONE FORMATION

In vitro and in vivo studies indicate that vitamin D activity promotes bone mineral retention and bone mineral loss. The duality of these actions on bone can be considered as a mechanism to maintain plasma calcium homeostasis under various physiological states although this concept has yet to be unequivocally proven.

As discussed above, global VDRKO mice at 17 weeks of age showed reduced capacity for RANKL expression and possibly defects in mineral apposition, suggesting that VDR activity is necessary for optimal mineral apposition as animals age [19]. Impaired RANKL expression and activity in an osteoblast-specific *VDR* knockout mouse model recently confirmed the essential role for VDR in regulating osteoclastogenesis [90]. However, no changes in bone formation parameters were detectable in these 16-week old mice, confirming that a major role for VDR activity in osteoblasts is stimulating bone resorption.

The role of VDR has also been examined in osteocytes with a mouse model in which the VDR gene is specifically deleted in osteocytes by utilizing the promoter region of the DMP1 gene. Under normal dietary conditions, neither bone mineral status nor plasma calcium or phosphate homeostasis was different in osteocyte-VDRKO mice compared to wild type mice [91]. When supra-physiological doses of 1,25D were administered to wild type mice, marked up-regulation of genes involved with the inhibition of mineralization was observed. In contrast, no effects were detected in osteocyte-VDRKO mice. These genes regulate the synthesis and transport of pyrophosphate, a major inhibitor of mineral deposition. Such effects in wild type mice were associated with localized regions of under-mineralized bone associated with osteocyte lacunae. The results from this mouse model suggest that in, addition to stimulation of bone catabolism, in the presence of high plasma 1,25D levels, osteocyte VDR-mediated activity inhibits calcium deposition. This activity would help maintain plasma calcium homeostasis under conditions when dietary calcium intake is low and plasma 1,25D levels are raised.

Unlike the catabolic and anti-mineralization effects of vitamin D in bone, osteoblast VDR also mediates an anabolic activity within bone under conditions of adequate dietary calcium intake. The over-expression of VDR specifically in mature osteoblast lineage cells (OSVDR mice) demonstrates increased mineral apposition and decreased bone resorption activity resulting in increased cortical and trabecular bone volumes [92]. However, OSVDR mice fed low dietary calcium lost their increased bone volume phenotype [93]. Therefore, increased bone volume in OSVDR mice depends on the adequacy of dietary calcium and possibly low plasma 1,25D levels.

Data from this model suggest that increased levels of VDR in mature osteoblast cells render bone tissue more sensitive to regulators of plasma calcium homeostasis, presumably plasma 1,25D. These data are consistent with the observation described above arising from the osteoblast-specific VDRKO mouse model that demonstrated insensitivity to 1,25D actions on bone with decreased expression of RANKL, decreased osteoclast activity, and increased bone volume [90].

7.6   AUTOCRINE AND PARACRINE ACTIVITIES

7.6.1   SYNTHESIS OF 1,25D BY MESENCHYMAL STEM CELLS, OSTEOBLASTS, OSTEOCYTES, AND OSTEOCLASTS

As discussed, a body of clinical literature describes the relationship of serum 25D levels and fracture risk, which is not evident with serum 1,25D levels. The findings that each of the bone cell types in both human and rodents has the capability to metabolize vitamin D with emphasis on the conversion of 25D to 1,25D provides a physiological context for this clinical observation (Figure 7.1) [94].

Incubation with physiological levels of 25D elicits effects from osteoblast-like cells in culture biological cells, for which expression of CYP27B1 is essential; incubation with 1,25D produced the same effects [79,95]. When mice were fed a standard chow diet containing about 1% dietary calcium, the expression of CYP27B1 in the skeleton was approximately equal to that in the kidney [96]. As discussed above, the regulation of renal CYP27B1 is very different from expression in bone. Renal expression is specifically and markedly up-regulated by hypocalcemia associated with hyperparathyroidism and low 25D levels [7,8]. Bone expression of CYP27B1 is up-regulated in mice fed adequate dietary calcium. Adequate dietary calcium suppresses renal CYP27B1 expression [97].

7.6.2   IN VITRO AND IN VIVO ACTIVITIES OF LOCALLY SYNTHESIZED 1,25D

Through conversion to 1,25D and activation of VDR within bone cells, 25D can stimulate maturation of mesenchymal stem cells, osteoblasts, and osteoclasts. It enhances maturation of osteoblast-like cells and mineral deposition in vitro [95]. Whether the local conversion of 25D to 1,25D elicits different actions on bone cells compared to 1,25D available from plasma remains unclear. However, both in vitro and in vivo studies found that the levels of 25D required to stimulate these responses are closer to physiological serum levels than those required for 1,25D. Such observations may be explained by limitations of the systems used to conduct these studies. For example, the induction of CYP24 mRNA levels is usually more subdued with 25D than with 1,25D in culture media [79,95].

Preliminary data from a transgenic mouse model that increases CYP27B1 expression five-fold, specifically in osteoblasts and osteocytes, demonstrated increases in trabecular and cortical bone volumes [98]. Notably, this increase in bone volume results from a modest increase in bone formation rather than a reduction in osteoclast activity [99].

7.7   CONCLUSIONS

Vitamin D contributes to regulation of plasma calcium and phosphate homeostasis with consequent actions on the skeleton, through the actions of the VDR largely when liganded with 1,25D. While adequate vitamin D status can clearly benefit bone mineral status, all current evidence suggests that such outcomes arise in the presence of adequate dietary calcium and phosphate intakes.

It is plausible that the actions of vitamin D on plasma calcium and phosphate homeostasis are dominant over its actions on bone mineral homeostasis. A recent report described a postmenopausal woman with very high bone turnover despite use of adequate vitamin D supplements. She required calcium supplementation to lower bone turnover [100]. This report supports such a concept. Actions of vitamin D on the skeleton can enhance or decrease bone mineral volume by modulating bone cell activities based on the physiological context of plasma calcium and phosphate homeostasis. Such actions include stimulation of bone resorption, inhibition of bone formation, inhibition of bone resorption, and stimulation of bone formation.

Many aspects of the interactions of calcium and possibly phosphate signaling and the other calciotropic hormones, particularly PTH, remain to be elucidated. More knowledge of these molecular mechanisms will provide further insight as to the levels of vitamin D metabolites required for bone health and how VDR activities may be harnessed to improve bone mineral status.

REFERENCES

1. Mellanby E. 1919. An experimental investigation on rickets. *Lancet* 193: 407–412.
2. Ross AC et al. 2010. Committee to review dietary reference intakes for vitamin D and calcium. Institute of Medicine.
3. Holick MF et al. 2012. Guidelines for preventing and treating vitamin D deficiency and insufficiency revisited. *J Clin Endocrinol Metabol* 97: 1153–1158.
4. DeLuca HF and Schnoes HK. 1976. Metabolism and mechanism of action of vitamin D. *Annu Rev Biochem* 45: 631–666.
5. Morris HA and Anderson PH. 2010. Autocrine and paracrine actions of vitamin D. *Clin Biochem Rev* 31: 129–138.
6. Bischoff-Ferrari HA. 2012. Vitamin D: why does it matter? Defining vitamin D deficiency and its prevalence. *Scand J Clin Lab Invest Suppl* 243: 3–6.
7. Hendrix I et al. 2005. Response of the 5′-flanking region of the human 25-hydroxyvitamin D 1α-hydroxylase gene to physiological stimuli using a transgenic mouse model. *J Mol Endocrinol* 34: 237–245.
8. Anderson PH et al. 2005. Modulation of CYP27B1 and CYP24 mRNA expression in bone is independent of circulating 1,25(OH)$_2$D3 levels. *Bone* 36: 654–662.
9. Malloy PJ et al. 2011. Hereditary 1,25-dihydroxyvitamin D-resistant rickets. in *Vitamin D*, Feldman, D et al., Eds. Academic Press: San Diego, pp. 1197–1232.
10. Brooks MH et al. 1978. Vitamin-D-dependent rickets type II: resistance of target organs to 1,25-dihydroxyvitamin D. *New Engl J Med* 298: 996–999.
11. Marx SJ et al. 1978. A familial syndrome of decrease in sensitivity to 1,25-dihydroxyvitamin D. *J Clin Endocrinol Metabol* 47: 1303–1310.
12. Malloy PJ et al. 1999. The vitamin D receptor and the syndrome of hereditary 1,25-dihydroxyvitamin D-resistant rickets. *Endocr Rev* 20: 156–188.
13. Stumpf WE et al. 1979. Target cells for 1,25-dihydroxyvitamin D3 in intestinal tract, stomach, kidney, skin, pituitary, and parathyroid. *Science* 206: 1188–1190.
14. Li YC et al. 1997. Targeted ablation of the vitamin D receptor: an animal model of vitamin D-dependent rickets type II with alopecia. *Proc Natl Acad Sci USA* 94: 9831–9835.
15. Yoshizawa T et al. 1997. Mice lacking the vitamin D receptor exhibit impaired bone formation, uterine hypoplasia and growth retardation after weaning. *Nat Genet* 16: 391–396.
16. Erben RG et al. 2002. Deletion of deoxyribonucleic acid binding domain of the vitamin D receptor abrogates genomic and nongenomic functions of vitamin D. *Mol Endocrinol* 16: 1524–1537.
17. Li YC et al. 1998. Normalization of mineral ion homeostasis by dietary means prevents hyperparathyroidism, rickets, and osteomalacia, but not alopecia in vitamin D receptor-ablated mice. *Endocrinology* 139: 4391–4396.
18. Amling M et al. 1999. Rescue of the skeletal phenotype of vitamin D receptor-ablated mice in the setting of normal mineral ion homeostasis: formal histomorphometric and biomechanical analyses. *Endocrinology* 140: 4982–4987.
19. Panda DK et al. 2004. Inactivation of the 25-hydroxyvitamin D 1α-hydroxylase and vitamin D receptor demonstrates independent and interdependent effects of calcium and vitamin D on skeletal and mineral homeostasis. *J Biol Chem* 279: 16754–16766.
20. Fraser D et al. 1973. Pathogenesis of hereditary vitamin-D-dependent rickets: an inborn error of vitamin D metabolism involving defective conversion of 25-hydroxyvitamin D to 1α,25-dihydroxyvitamin D. *New Engl J Med* 289: 817–822.
21. Glorieux FH et al. 2011. Pseudo-vitamin D deficiency. In *Vitamin D*, Feldman D et al., Eds. Academic Press: San Diego, pp. 1187–1195.
22. Fu GK et al. 1997. Cloning of human 25-hydroxyvitamin D-1 α-hydroxylase and mutations causing vitamin D-dependent rickets type 1. *Mol Endocrinol* 11: 1961–1970.

23. Wang JT et al. 1998. Genetics of vitamin D 1α-hydroxylase deficiency in 17 families. *Am J Hum Genet* 63: 1694–1702.

24. Dardenne O et al. 2001. Targeted inactivation of the 25-hydroxyvitamin D(3)-1(α)-hydroxylase gene (CYP27B1) creates an animal model of pseudovitamin D-deficiency rickets. *Endocrinology* 142: 3135–3141.

25. Need AG et al. 2008. Vitamin D metabolites and calcium absorption in severe vitamin D deficiency. *J Bone Miner Res* 23: 1859–1863.

26. Anderson PH et al. 2008. Vitamin D depletion induces RANKL-mediated osteoclastogenesis and bone loss in a rodent model. *J Bone Miner Res* 23: 1789–1797.

27. Baker MR et al. 1979. Plasma 25-hydroxy vitamin D concentrations in patients with fractures of the femoral neck. *Br Med J* 1: 589.

28. Morris HA et al. 1984. Vitamin D and femoral neck fractures in elderly South Australian women. *Med J Austral* 140: 519–521.

29. Lai JKC et al. 2010. Hip fracture risk in relation to vitamin D supplementation and serum 25-hydroxyvitamin D levels: a systematic review and meta-analysis of randomised controlled trials and observational studies. *BMC Publ Health* 10.

30. Lidor C et al. 1993. Decrease in bone levels of 1,25-dihydroxyvitamin D in women with subcapital fracture of the femur. *Calcif Tiss Intl* 52: 146–148.

31. Ray D et al. 2009. Predisposition to vitamin D deficiency osteomalacia and rickets in females is linked to their 25(OH)D and calcium intake rather than vitamin D receptor gene polymorphism. *Clin Endocrinol (Oxf)* 71: 334–340.

32. Chapuy MC et al. 1992. Vitamin D3 and calcium to prevent hip fractures in the elderly women. *New Engl J Med* 327: 1637–1642.

33. Bischoff-Ferrari HA et al. 2012. A pooled analysis of vitamin D dose requirements for fracture prevention. *New Engl J Med* 367: 40–49.

34. Prentice RL et al. 2013. Health risks and benefits from calcium and vitamin D supplementation: Women's Health Initiative clinical trial and cohort study. *Osteoporosis Intl* 24: 567–580.

35. Avenell A et al. 2009. Vitamin D and vitamin D analogues for preventing fractures associated with involutional and post-menopausal osteoporosis. *Cochrane Database Syst Rev* CD000227.

36. Nordin BE et al. 2004. Radiocalcium absorption is reduced in postmenopausal women with vertebral and most types of peripheral fractures. *Osteoporosis Intl* 15: 27–31.

37. Need AG et al. 1997. The response to calcitriol therapy in postmenopausal osteoporotic women is a function of initial calcium absorptive status. *Calcif Tiss Intl* 61: 6–9.

38. Aaron JE et al. 1974. Frequency of osteomalacia and osteoporosis in fractures of the proximal femur. *Lancet* 1: 229–233.

39. Wicks M et al. 1982. Absence of metabolic bone disease in the proximal femur in patients with fracture of the femoral neck. *J Bone Joint Surg Br* 64: 319–322.

40. Arnala I et al. 1997. Analysis of 245 consecutive hip fracture patients with special reference to bone metabolism. *Ann Chir Gynaecol* 86: 343–347.

41. Bell KL et al. 1999. Intracapsular hip fracture: increased cortical remodeling in the thinned and porous anterior region of the femoral neck. *Osteoporosis Intl* 10: 248–257.

42. Omdahl JL et al. 2002. Hydroxylase enzymes of the vitamin D pathway: expression, function, and regulation. *Annu Rev Nutr* 22: 139–166.

43. Cheng JB et al. 2004. Genetic evidence that the human CYP2R1 enzyme is a key vitamin D 25-hydroxylase. *Proc Natl Acad Sci USA* 101: 7711–7715.

44. Cheng JB et al. 2003. De-orphanization of cytochrome P450 2R1: a microsomal vitamin D 25-hydroxylase. *J Biol Chem* 278: 38084–38093.

45. Bieche I et al. 2007. Reverse transcriptase-PCR quantification of mRNA levels from cytochrome (CYP)1, CYP2 and CYP3 families in 22 different human tissues. *Pharmacogenet Genom* 17: 731–742.

46. Bikle DD et al. 1986. Assessment of the free fraction of 25-hydroxyvitamin D in serum and its regulation by albumin and the vitamin D-binding protein. *J Clin Endocrinol Metabol* 63: 954–949.

47. Fraser DR and Kodicek E. 1970. Unique biosynthesis by kidney of a biological active vitamin D metabolite. *Nature* 228: 764–766.

48. Salle BL et al. 2000. Perinatal metabolism of vitamin D. *Am J Clin Nutr* 71: 1317S–1324S.

49. Kallas M et al. 2010. Rare causes of calcitriol-mediated hypercalcemia: a case report and literature review. *J Clin Endocrinol Metabol* 95: 3111–3117.

50. Anderson PH et al. 2008. Co-expression of CYP27B1 enzyme with the 1.5 kb CYP27B1 promoter-luciferase transgene in the mouse. *Mol Cell Endocrinol* 285: 1–9.

51. St-Arnaud R and Naja RP. 2011. Vitamin D metabolism, cartilage and bone fracture repair. *Mol Cell Endocrinol* 347: 48–54.

52. Murayama A et al. 1998. The promoter of the human 25-hydroxyvitamin D3 1α-hydroxylase gene confers positive and negative responsiveness to PTH, calcitonin, and 1α,25(OH)₂D3. *Biochem Biophys Res Commun* 249: 11–16.

53. Gao XH et al. 2002. Basal and parathyroid hormone induced expression of the human 25-hydroxyvitamin D 1α-hydroxylase gene promoter in kidney AOK-B50 cells: role of Sp1, Ets, and CCAAT box protein binding sites. *Int J Biochem Cell Biol* 34: 921–930.

54. Zhong Y et al. 2009. Calcitonin, a regulator of the 25-hydroxyvitamin D3 1α-hydroxylase gene. *J Biol Chem* 284: 11059–11069.

55. Masuda S et al. 2005. Altered pharmacokinetics of 1a,25-dihydroxyvitamin D3 and 25-hydroxyvitamin D3 in the blood and tissues of the 25-hydroxyvitamin D-24-hydroxylase (Cyp24a1)-null mouse. *Endocrinology* 146: 825–834.

56. Kerry DM et al. 1996. Transcriptional synergism between vitamin D-responsive elements in the rat 25-hydroxyvitamin D3 24-hydroxylase (CYP24) promoter. *J Biol Chem* 271: 29715–29721.

57. Kumar R et al. 2010. Systematic characterisation of the rat and human CYP24A1 promoter. *Mol Cell Endocrinol* 325: 46–53.

58. Dwivedi PP et al. 2002. Role of MAP kinases in the 1,25-dihydroxyvitamin D3-induced transactivation of the rat cytochrome P450c24 (CYP24) promoter: specific functions for ERK1/ERK2 and ERK5. *J Biol Chem* M204561200.

59. Zierold C et al. 2003. Regulation of 25-hydroxyvitamin D3-24-hydroxylase mRNA by 1,25-dihydroxyvitamin D3 and parathyroid hormone. *J Cell Biochem* 88: 234–237.

60. Gao XH et al. 2004. Calcitonin stimulates expression of the rat 25-hydroxyvitamin D3-24-hydroxylase (CYP24) promoter in HEK-293 cells expressing calcitonin receptor: identification of signaling pathways. *J Mol Endocrinol* 32: 87–98.

61. Haussler MR et al. 2008. Vitamin D receptor: molecular signaling and actions of nutritional ligands in disease prevention. *Nutr Rev* 66: S98–S112.

62. Engel KB and Yamamoto KR. 2011. The glucocorticoid receptor and the coregulator Brm selectively modulate each other's occupancy and activity in a gene-specific manner. *Mol Cell Biol* 31: 3267–3276.

63. Boland RL. 2011. VDR activation of intracellular signaling pathways in skeletal muscle. *Mol Cell Endocrinol* 347: 11–16.

64. Khanal R and Nemere I. 2007. Membrane receptors for vitamin D metabolites. *Crit Rev Eukaryot Gene Expr* 17: 31–47.

65. Nemere I et al. 2004. Ribozyme knockdown functionally links a 1,25(OH)2D3 membrane binding protein (1,25D3-MARRS) and phosphate uptake in intestinal cells. *Proc Natl Acad Sci USA* 101: 7392–7397.

66. Bravo S et al. 2006. The classic receptor for 1α,25-dihydroxy vitamin D3 is required for non-genomic actions of 1α,25-dihydroxy vitamin D3 in osteosarcoma cells. *J Cell Biochem* 99: 995–1000.

67. Wali RK et al. 2003. Vitamin D receptor is not required for the rapid actions of 1,25-dihydroxyvitamin D3 to increase intracellular calcium and activate protein kinase C in mouse osteoblasts. *J Cell Biochem* 88: 794–801.

68. Bikle DD. 2012. Vitamin D and the skin: physiology and pathophysiology. *Rev Endocr Metabol Disord* 13: 3–19.

69. Mulholland DJ et al. 2005. Interaction of nuclear receptors with the Wnt/β-catenin/Tcf signaling axis: Wnt you like to know? *Endocr Rev* 26: 898–915.

70. Rawadi G and Roman-Roman S. 2005. Wnt signalling pathway: a new target for the treatment of osteoporosis. *Expert Opin Ther Targets* 9: 1063–1077.

71. Haussler MR et al. 2010. The nuclear vitamin D receptor controls the expression of genes encoding factors which feed the "Fountain of Youth" to mediate healthful aging. *J Steroid Biochem Mol Biol* 121: 88–97.

72. Shah S et al. 2006. The molecular basis of vitamin D receptor and β-catenin cross-regulation. *Mol Cell* 21: 799–809.

73. Malloy PJ et al. 2002. A novel mutation in helix 12 of the vitamin D receptor impairs coactivator interaction and causes hereditary 1,25-dihydroxyvitamin D-resistant rickets without alopecia. *Mol Endocrinol* 16: 2538–2546.

74. Anderson PH and Atkins GJ. 2008. The skeleton as an intracrine organ for vitamin D metabolism. *Mol Aspects Med* 29: 397–406.

75. Suda T et al. 1995. Modulation of osteoclast differentiation by local factors. *Bone* 17: 87S–91S.

76. Takeda S et al. 1999. Stimulation of osteoclast formation by 1,25-dihydroxyvitamin D requires its binding to vitamin D receptor (VDR) in osteoblastic cells: studies using VDR knockout mice. *Endocrinology* 140: 1005–1008.

77. Anderson PH et al. 2011. Target genes: bone proteins. In *Vitamin D*, Feldman D et al., Eds. Elsevier Academic Press: San Diego, pp. 711–720.

78. Kogawa M et al. 2010. The metabolism of 25(OH)-vitamin D3 by osteoclasts and their precursors regulates the differentiation of osteoclasts. *J Ster Biochem Mol Biol* 121: 277–280.

79. Kogawa M et al. 2010. Osteoclastic metabolism of 25(OH)-vitamin D3: a potential mechanism for optimization of bone resorption. *Endocrinology* 151: 4613–4625.

80. Kogawa M et al. 2013. Modulation of osteoclastic migration by metabolism of 25OH-vitamin D3. *J Steroid Biochem Mol Biol* 136: 59–61.

81. Owen TA et al. 1991. Pleiotropic effects of vitamin D on osteoblast gene expression are related to the proliferative and differentiated state of the bone cell phenotype: dependency upon basal levels of gene expression, duration of exposure, and bone matrix competency in normal rat osteoblast cultures. *Endocrinology* 128: 1499–1504.

82. Atkins GJ et al. 2007. Metabolism of vitamin D3 in human osteoblasts: evidence for autocrine and paracrine activities of 1 α,25-dihydroxyvitamin D3. *Bone* 40: 1517–1528.

83. Atkins GJ et al. 2003. RANKL expression is related to the differentiation state of human osteoblasts. *J Bone Miner Res* 18: 1088–1098.

84. Yang D et al. 2013. Differential effects of 1,25-dihydroxyvitamin D on mineralisation and differentiation in two different types of osteoblast-like cultures. *J Steroid Biochem Mol Biol* 136: 166–170.

85. Morris HA et al. 1991. Calcium absorption in normal and osteoporotic postmenopausal women. *Calc Tiss Intl* 49: 240–243.

86. Larik R et al. 2007. Determination of vitamin D-dependent calcium absorption by [45]Ca gavage in the rat. *J Steroid Biochem Mol Biol* 103: 517–520.

87. Cochran M et al. 2005. The effect of calcitriol on fasting urine calcium loss and renal tubular reabsorption of calcium in patients with mild renal failure: actions of a permissive hormone. *Clin Nephrol* 64: 98–102.

88. Armbrecht HJ et al. 1989. Expression of calbindin-D decreases with age in intestine and kidney. *Endocrinology* 125: 2950–2956.
89. DeLuca HF. 2004. Overview of general physiologic features and functions of vitamin D. *Am J Clin Nutr* 80: 1689S–1696S.
90. Yamamoto Y et al. 2013. Vitamin D receptor in osteoblasts is a negative regulator of bone mass control. *Endocrinology* 154: 1008–1020.
91. Lieben L et al. 2012. Normocalcemia is maintained in mice under conditions of calcium malabsorption by vitamin D-induced inhibition of bone mineralization. *J Clin Invest* 122: 1803–1815.
92. Gardiner EM et al. 2000. Increased formation and decreased resorption of bone in mice with elevated vitamin D receptor in mature cells of the osteoblastic lineage. *FASEB J* 14: 1908–1916.
93. Baldock PA et al. 2006. Vitamin D action and regulation of bone remodeling: suppression of osteoclastogenesis by the mature osteoblast. *J Bone Miner Res* 21: 1618–1626.
94. Anderson PH et al. 2011. Vitamin D metabolism within bone cells: effects on bone structure and strength. *Mol Cell Endocr* 347: 42–47.
95. Atkins GJ et al. 2007. Metabolism of vitamin D(3) in human osteoblasts: evidence for autocrine and paracrine activities of 1α,25-dihydroxyvitamin D(3). *Bone* 40: 1517–1528.
96. Hendrix I et al. 2004. Regulation of gene expression by the CYP27B1 promoter study of a transgenic mouse model. *J Ster Biochem Mol Biol* 89–90: 139–142.
97. Anderson PH et al. 2010. The effect of dietary calcium on 1,25(OH)2D3 synthesis and sparing of serum 25(OH)D3 levels. *J Ster Biochem Mol Biol* 121: 288–292.
98. Turner AG et al. 2011. Increased bone volume in the bone-specific CYP27B1 transgenic mouse. *Osteoporosis Intl* 22: S590–S591.
99. Anderson PH et al. 2011. Enhanced vitamin D synthesis in osteoblasts protects against age-related bone loss. *J Bone Miner Res* 26: S151.
100. Lafage-Proust MH et al. 2013. High bone turnover persisting after vitamin D repletion: beware of calcium deficiency. *Osteoporosis Intl* 24: 2359–2363.

8 Physiological Actions of Calcitonin

Rachel A. Davey and David M. Findlay

CONTENTS

8.1 MECHANISMS AND REGULATION OF SYNTHESIS AND SECRETION

Calcitonin (CT) is a 32-amino acid polypeptide hormone produced by C-cells found predominantly, but not exclusively, within the thyroid gland. CT is a hypocalcemic hormone secreted in response to a rise in serum calcium level [1]. The CT peptide family also includes the structurally-related molecules: CT gene-related peptide (CGRP), amylin, adrenomedullin, and adrenomedullin 2 (or intermedin). This chapter focuses on CT physiology.

Although increased serum calcium is an important secretagogue for CT, the exact mechanisms by which calcium provokes release of CT from C-cells have not been fully elucidated. The same extracellular calcium-sensing receptor that mediates decreased parathyroid hormone (PTH) secretion from parathyroid cells [2] is also found in C-cells and is likely to represent the primary molecular entity through which C-cells detect changes in extracellular calcium and control CT release.

Interestingly, while some calcimimetics equally suppress PTH secretion and increase CT secretion, others have been shown to produce differential effects on the two hormones [3]. It is also worth noting that mice, in which the gene for the calcitonin receptor (CTR) is deleted in all tissues (global CTRKO), show marked increases in serum CT levels [4] while animals with the CTR gene deleted specifically in osteoclasts (OCL-CTRKO) do not [5]. This suggests that the regulation of CT synthesis and/or secretion involves CTR-mediated actions directly in the thyroid and/or in other target tissues such as the brain.

Other CT secretagogues are gastrin and other gastrointestinal hormones including glucagon, cholecystokinin, and secretin, suggesting that CT may have a postprandial physiological role. The pentagastrin analogue can be used clinically as a provocative test for CT secretion in patients with medullary carcinoma of the thyroid. Other hormones that influence calcium homeostasis may also directly or indirectly influence CT secretion. For example, 1,25-dihydroxyvitamin D_3 (1,25D) administration has been reported to increase plasma CT levels [6]. Both CT and 1,25D levels are raised in pregnancy and lactation, leading to the suggestion that CT may act to protect the skeleton in the face of increased calcium demand by the fetus.

CT is synthesized as a larger precursor molecule, which is post-translationally cleaved and amidated C-terminally before secretion. The CT gene transcript also encodes CT gene-related peptide (CGRP) produced by tissue-specific alternative splicing of the same transcribed mRNA. CGRP and CT share sequence identity in the amino terminal regions but share little homology of nucleotide sequence at the carboxy terminal region. The CT/CGRP gene is transcribed largely as CT mRNA in the thyroid, while CGRP mRNA is found primarily in the nervous system [7]. Processing of the pre-mRNA to the CT mRNA transcript involves usage of exon 4 as a 3'-terminal exon with concomitant polyadenylation at the end of exon 4. Processing of the pre-mRNA to produce the CGRP mRNA involves the exclusion of exon 4 and direct ligation of exon 3 to exon 5 with polyadenylation at the end of exon 6.

8.2   SITES AND MECHANISMS OF ACTION

Calcitonin receptors are widely distributed although actions of CT have not yet been described in all situations. This may be due to the molecular context of the CTR. It can associate with additional molecules, giving it conformational characteristics to bind additional ligands of the CT family. Thus, the CTR has been demonstrated by radioactive isotope-labeled ligand binding studies and by expression of mRNA at sites as diverse as osteoclasts in bone [8], discrete regions of the brain [9], the testes [10], the kidney [11], the mammary glands [12], and a range of cancer cell types [13].

Receptor cloning showed that the CTR is a class B-type G protein-coupled receptor and that it exists in a number of species- and tissue-specific isoforms that display different ligand binding and signaling characteristics. The physiological significance of the splice variants remains unclear. The human receptor has at least five splice variants, with the most common hCTR splice variant generating a 16-amino acid insert in the first putative intracellular domain of the 7-transmembrane structure [14–16]. Other splice variants have been identified in other species, with alternate splicing in rodents yielding two receptor isoforms (denoted a and b) that differ by the presence or absence of an additional 37 amino acids in the second extracellular domain [17].

Activation by CT of its receptor can result in coupling to multiple signaling pathways via G_s, $G_{q/11}$, and G_i [18]. Signaling via Gs stimulates intracellular cAMP production and activation of protein kinase A-mediated pathways [19]. CT signals in osteoclasts through several pathways including Gs/cAMP-mediated and Gq-linked protein kinase C-dependent mechanisms. The latter are linked to dramatic morphological changes involving components of the cell skeleton including filamin A, talin, and Pyk2 [20].

As noted, the CTR can associate with additional molecules known as receptor activity-modifying proteins (RAMPs) that modulate its ability to bind other members of the CT peptide family. The CTR without RAMP appears to be sufficient for CT binding with no apparent requirement of RAMPs for cell surface expression of this receptor. Association of the CTR with RAMP1, 2, or 3 yields three subtypes of high-affinity receptors for the amylin peptide [21].

8.3   ACTION IN OSTEOCLASTS

The best understood action of CT is the inhibition of bone resorption by osteoclasts. These cells express abundant CTRs [8] and are exquisitely sensitive to the inhibitory action of CT, reflected as cessation of motility and contraction of the cells [22]. Early experiments in rats showed that CT lowered serum calcium levels. The effect was observed equally in control and nephrectomized animals and was therefore ascribed to a reduction in bone resorption [23]. CT substantially lowered urinary excretion of hydroxyproline in young rats, which suggested diminished collagen breakdown, again by inhibition of bone resorption [24]. Likewise, CT caused a striking reduction in the rate of resorption of pieces of rat bone in culture, as determined by release of hydroxyproline [25].

Chambers and Magnus [26] examined isolated osteoclasts on a glass slide and showed that these cells "were actively motile, the cytoplasm advancing behind broad pseudopodial (lamellipodial) processes which showed intense ruffling activity." CT treatment resulted in osteoclast quiescence with rapid (within minutes) cessation of lamellipodial activity. This effect was abrogated by prior treatment of osteoclasts with trypsin, suggesting that it was mediated by a trypsin-sensitive CTR present on the plasma membranes of the cells.

8.4   ACTION IN KIDNEY

In 1967, Robinson et al. [23] concluded that CT acted in both the bone and the kidney. They produced evidence that the effect of CT on bone resorption is usually dominant but when bone turnover is low, the skeletal action of CT is overshadowed by its phosphaturic effect. It is not clear whether this latter effect is of major physiological significance. CTRs are present in the kidney [11] and CT activates adenylate cyclase in the medullary and cortical portions of the thick ascending limb and in the early portion of the distal convoluted tubule [27].

A possible role for CT in the kidney is to regulate 1,25D levels since CT was reported to stimulate expression of the gene coding for 25-hydroxyvitamin D 1α-hydroxylase (CYP27B1) in the proximal straight tubules of the kidney [28]. On the other hand, CT has also been reported to stimulate expression of the gene coding for the 25-hydroxyvitamin D-24- hydroxylase (CYP24) in CTR-transfected HEK-293 cells [29], acting synergistically with 1,25D, possibly suggesting that CT may partly regulate serum calcium by controlling renal production of 1,25D.

8.5 EFFECTS ON APPETITE AND PAIN

Intraventricular administration of CT has potent effects on appetite [30], most likely by binding to amylin receptors [31]. It has been well documented that central amylin or sCT injection potently reduces food intake [31,32]. In addition, intramuscular injection of salmon CT (sCT) into adult male rhesus monkeys resulted in a dose-dependent suppression of food intake that persisted after termination of treatment [31]. This finding, which replicates in primates, data previously described from rodent studies, suggests that sCT is a potent anorexigenic peptide with lasting effects on feeding behavior.

Like its effects on appetite, central administration of CT also has amylinergic effects on pain reduction. Systemic treatment with CT has also been reported to produce analgesic effects on bone pain, which are probably mediated centrally [33]. Subcutaneous injection of CT for the treatment of Paget's disease provided relief of pain concurrently with its effect of decreasing bone turnover. In a systematic review of randomized controlled trials, Knopp et al. [34] found that CT appears effective in the management of acute pain associated with acute osteoporotic vertebral compression fractures. CT may also exert indirect effects on osteoarthritis pain; a number of studies suggested the potential benefit of CT for this condition [35,36]. By providing chondroprotection and reducing the progression of osteoarthritis, the pain associated with degenerative changes may also be reduced.

8.6 CONTRIBUTIONS TO PLASMA CALCIUM AND PHOSPHATE HOMEOSTASIS

CT acts to regulate the serum levels of calcium and phosphate, predominantly via its actions on osteoclasts and in the kidney. As stated above, CT potently inhibits osteoclastic bone resorption, thereby decreasing the release of calcium and phosphate from the bone matrix into the circulation. The action of CT in the kidney to regulate serum calcium is two-fold, first acting directly to decrease the tubular reabsorption of calcium and thereby increasing urinary calcium excretion [37]. Second, CT acts indirectly to increase intestinal calcium absorption by stimulating the renal conversion of 25-hydroxyvitamin D_3 (25D) to 1,25D by increasing CYP27B1 expression in the kidney [28]. CT, but not parathyroid hormone (PTH), has been shown to be the major regulator of renal CYP27B1 in normocalcemic states, at least in rodents [38].

CT may also play a role in the maintenance of phosphate homeostasis via its actions on the kidney to promote renal phosphate excretion [39,40]. A study in hypoparathyroid patients showed that these phosphaturic actions following infusion of CT are independent of parathyroid hormone [41]. Studies in rats have shown that CT acts directly on the kidney to decrease the proximal tubular reabsorption of phosphate [42,43].

8.7   CONTRIBUTIONS TO METABOLIC BONE DISEASE

Patients with very low levels of serum CT after thyroidectomy have no documented abnormalities in calcium and phosphate homeostasis or show any evidence of bone disease [44]. Conversely, patients with medullary thyroid carcinoma and high levels of serum CT do not appear to have any greater propensity for developing osteopetrosis than individuals with normal serum levels of CT [44].

While the pharmacological actions of CT are well accepted, the absence of any obvious pathophysiology in individuals with both deficient and excess levels of serum CT led to much debate about whether CT and/or its receptor fill physiological roles. To counter this concept that CT may be a largely vestigial hormone, an increasing body of literature indicates physiological roles for CT. CT acting via the CTR appears to regulate bone formation, in addition to regulating calcium and conserving bone during times of greatly increased bone resorption such as in states of high calcium demand including pregnancy and lactation and skeletal malignancy-related osteolysis, which can generate high serum calcium levels.

8.7.1   BONE FORMATION

In addition to the well-established role of CT acting via the CTR to inhibit osteoclastic bone resorption, recent studies utilizing genetically modified mouse models uncovered a possible role for CT and its receptor in regulating bone formation. The first mouse model was a global CT/CT gene-related peptide knockout (CT/CGRP KO) [45]. Unexpectedly, CT/CGRP-deficient mice were found to have increased trabecular bone compared to controls due to increased bone formation, while bone resorption and calcium homeostasis were unaffected [45]. These intriguing data provided the first evidence for an inhibitory effect of CT and/or CGRP on bone formation.

However, interpretation of the physiological actions of CT from CT/CGRP KO mice is confounded by potential effects arising from deletion of CGRP, which exerts documented effects on osteoclasts and osteoblasts [46,47] and potent vasodilatory effects on peripheral vasculature [48]. To elucidate whether the absence of CT or CGRP is responsible for the increased bone mass phenotype of the CT/CGRP KO mice, Schinke et al. [49] generated mice deficient only in α-CGRP. These mice had normal levels of serum CT, PTH, calcium, and phosphate but most interestingly displayed a mild osteopenic phenotype characterized by reduced trabecular bone volume due to decreased bone formation [49]. The absence of increased bone formation in the α-CGRP KO mice suggests that the high bone mass phenotype observed in the CT/CGRP KO mice is a result of the absence of CT, not α-CGRP. It may be important however, that the initial characterization of the CT/CGRP KO mice was carried out on mice of mixed genetic backgrounds [45].

Bone mineral density differs markedly among various inbred strains of mice [50] and characterization of genetically modified mice of mixed genetic backgrounds can be highly variable and difficult to interpret [51,52]. This effect of genetic background for mouse model studies is highlighted by a subsequent report by Gagel et al. [53] stating that the bone phenotype of increased bone formation was no longer evident in CT/CGRP KO mice following their back-crossing to a homogeneous C57BL/6 background. The homogeneous C57BL/6 CT/CGRP KO mice showed an age-related phenotype characterized predominantly by an increase in cortical porosity [53]. This report is in contrast to the findings of Schinke et al. [49] who included the CT/CGRP KO mice back-crossed to a C57BL/6 background for direct comparison with the α-CGRP KO mice. The CT/CGRPKO mice in this study displayed increased bone formation compared to controls. The reason for the differences in phenotypes among the CT/CGRP KO mice of different genetic backgrounds noted in several studies is difficult to ascertain.

Another approach to determining the physiological role of CT in regulating bone cell metabolism is generating genetically modified mice in which the cellular target for CT, the CTR, has been removed. Haplo-insufficient CTR mice with deletion of one copy of the CTR gene (CTR$^{-/+}$) demonstrated a 50% reduction in CTR mRNA expression and exhibited increased trabecular bone formation but no effect on bone resorption [54]. These data support the concept that the inhibitory action of CT on bone formation is mediated by the CTR.

Further use of the haplo-insufficient CTR mice to elucidate the role of the CTR in bone formation is limited because CTR$^{-/-}$ mice die before initiation of skeletal formation—in addition to the complication of their mixed genetic backgrounds. To further clarify the physiological role of the CTR in regulating bone formation, we generated a viable global CTRKO mouse model on a homogeneous C57BL/6 background using the Cre/loxP by mating floxed CTR mice with CMV-Cre mice. The CTR was deleted in all tissues of these mice by more than 94% but less than 100%, which abolished the inhibitory effects of CT on osteoclasts [4].

Global CTRKO mice also displayed increased bone formation, but this was only evident in males, was of smaller magnitude than in haplo-insufficient CTR mice, and was not reflected as an increase in trabecular bone volume [4]. These data suggest a modest physiological role for the CTR in regulating bone turnover in the basal state. The difference in magnitude between the haplo-insufficient CTR$^{-/+}$ and global CTRKO mouse models is difficult to reconcile. However, it is most likely attributable to a number of factors including differences in the technology used to generate the genetically modified mice, the region of the CTR targeted for deletion, and the genetic backgrounds of the mice.

Furthermore, potential environmental factors arising from generating and characterizing the mice in different laboratories may also have influenced the phenotypes of these models. Nonetheless, taken together, these studies utilizing gene knockout mouse models of CT or the CTR provide intriguing evidence for a physiological role of CT acting via the CTR to inhibit bone formation.

The mechanism by which CT activation of the CTR inhibits bone formation remains to be elucidated. Evidence from Cre/loxP mice in which the CTR was deleted specifically in osteoclasts expressing cathepsin K (OCL-CTRKO) suggests that the inhibitory effects of CTR are not mediated by its actions on osteoclasts since OCL-CTRKO mice do not exhibit changes in bone formation [5]. A study by Gooi et al. [55] suggests that CT may exert its inhibitory action on bone formation, at least in part, by regulating production of sclerostin, an osteocyte-derived inhibitor of bone formation (Figure 8.1a).

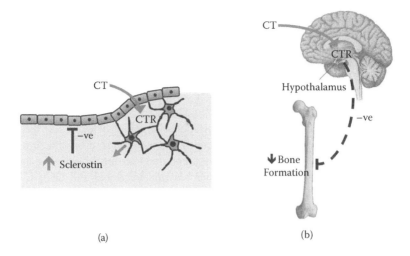

(a)   (b)

FIGURE 8.1 Possible mechanisms of calcitonin (CT) action to inhibit bone formation. (A) CT action via the calcitonin receptor (CTR) in osteocytes stimulates the production of sclerostin by the osteocytes, resulting in a subsequent reduction in osteoblastic bone formation. (B) CT acting via the CTR in the arcuate nucleus of the hypothalamus to activate a yet unidentified efferent neural pathway to inhibit bone formation.

Osteocytes are the most abundant bone cells and are embedded within the bone where they sense and regulate bone tissue adaption to changes in mechanical strain by signaling to osteoblasts and osteoclasts. Both systemic and local injections of CT in young rodents were shown to produce a rapid increase in gene expression and protein levels of sclerostin, which in turn decreased bone formation [56], presumably by inhibiting the Wnt signaling pathway [57]. We have recently shown that sclerostin targets pre-osteocytes and osteocytes and acts as a master regulator of bone mineralization [58].

Although speculative, another mechanism by which CTR may exert its inhibitory effects on bone formation is by central actions within the brain (Figure 8.1b). The rationale for this hypothesis is that the CTR is expressed at high levels within the arcuate nucleus of the hypothalamus [9,59,60].

Other hormones, such as neuropeptide Y and leptin, which are also expressed at high levels within the arcuate nucleus, regulate bone remodeling by acting via efferent neural pathways originating from hypothalamic nuclei [61]. This notion of a central action of CT via the CTR is supported by recent studies demonstrating that CT and CGRP act via the CNS to inhibit appetite and gastric acid secretion, modulate hormone secretion, exert analgesic effects, and control prolactin secretion [62–65]. The precise mechanism by which CT and the CTR inhibit bone formation remains unclear and warrants further investigation.

8.7.2 HYPERCALCEMIA

The first evidence for a biological role of CT to regulate calcium homeostasis in hypercalcemic states was provided by clinical studies performed in the 1960s. In thyroidectomized patients with very low levels of serum CT, serum calcium levels remained elevated for an extended period after challenge with an intravenous calcium infusion [66,67]. The ability of CT to reduce serum calcium levels is dependent on the rate of bone turnover. CT rapidly decreases serum calcium in states of high bone turnover, such as during childhood or in patients with malignancy-induced hypercalcemia. In contrast, little effect of CT was observed in adults with lower rates of bone turnover [68,69].

We have shown that global and osteoclast-specific deletion of the CTR (OCL-CTRKO) in mice results in significantly elevated peak serum calcium levels following calcitriol-induced hypercalcemia, compared to controls [4,5]. The increase in serum calcium following induced hypercalcemia in global and OCL-CTRKO mouse models was accompanied by an increase in bone resorption evidenced by increased osteoclast surface and serum carboxy-telopeptide (CTx; a biochemical marker of bone resorption) [5].

Taken together, these data suggest that the protective effect of the CTR is conferred predominantly by its expression in osteoclasts to acutely inhibit bone resorption. In addition, we showed that peak serum calcium levels following induced hypercalcemia were higher in global CTRKO versus OCL-CTRKO mice, suggesting a possible, additional hypocalcemic action mediated by the CTR at a site or sites other than osteoclasts, such as a hypercalciuric action in the kidney.

Consistent with this theory, TmCa, the calcium concentration at which renal tubular reabsorption is maximal, was significantly higher in global CTRKO mice following induced hypercalcemia, while it was unaffected in OCL-CTRKO mice [5]. These data are consistent with the CTR in renal cells conferring some protection against induced hypercalcemia, most likely by promoting calcium excretion via its action to inhibit calcium reabsorption, as reviewed by Sexton et al. [70].

8.7.3 Pregnancy and Lactation

CT acting via the CTR may also play a physiological role in embryonic development and in protecting the skeleton during pregnancy and lactation. As discussed previously, homozygous deletion of the CTR results in embryonic lethality [54] and transient expression of CT in the uterus is required for implantation of the blastocyst [71]. Interestingly, data from the CT/CGRP KO mice suggest that, while CT and CGRP are not required for the fetal regulation of calcium homeostasis, they are necessary for normal regulation of fetal magnesium metabolism [72].

The calcium and phosphorus requirements for fetal skeletal growth during the third trimester and during lactation increase dramatically. These demands for calcium are met from maternal sources, primarily via the breakdown of bone. In addition, rodents exhibit an increase in vitamin D-mediated intestinal calcium absorption that does not occur in humans. For instance, women lose 5 to 10% of trabecular bone mineral content during lactation, while mice lose 20 to 25% [73,74]. It has been proposed that the mobilization of calcium from the skeleton during lactation is mediated by PTHrP released from the lactating breast [75]. The increased serum PTHrP levels also increase the tubular reabsorption of calcium in the kidney and decrease serum PTH levels [73].

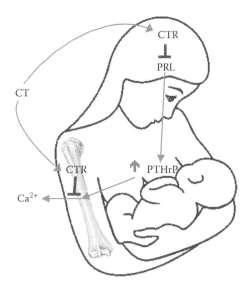

FIGURE 8.2   Actions of calcitonin (CT) to protect the skeleton during lactation. (1) Circulating CT derived from thyroid and mammary tissues acts via the calcitonin receptor (CTR) in the pituitary to decrease prolactin secretion, which in turn decreases the production of PTHrP by the breast. (2) CT acting via the CTR on osteoclasts (and potentially osteocytes) within bone opposes the actions of PTHrP to limit the amount of calcium released from the bone matrix.

Previous studies have also shown serum CT to be increased during pregnancy and lactation in both humans and mice [76,77], consistent with the view that CT, via its inhibitory actions mediated by the CTR on osteoclasts, plays a protective role to prevent excessive resorption of the maternal skeleton at these times of high calcium demand by opposing the actions of PTHrP (Figure 8.2) [73,76,77].

Interestingly, the source of serum CT during lactation may be the breast rather than the thyroid, as serum CT levels remain elevated in thyroidectomized women during lactation [78]. Data to support a protective role of CT during pregnancy and lactation have, until recently, been difficult to obtain due to the lack of an appropriate experimental model. Previous studies using thyroidectomy in rodents as a CT-deficient model for testing this hypothesis did not account for the production of CT at extrathyroidal sites including the breast and placenta during pregnancy [73].

A recent significant advance in determining the role of CT during pregnancy was made by Woodrow et al. [74], who demonstrated that the loss of bone at the spine during lactation doubled in CT-deficient CT/CGRP KO mice compared to littermate controls. This increase in bone loss in lactating CT/CGRP KO mice was associated with increased levels of serum PTH and mammary expression of PTHrP, and increased bone resorption while intestinal calcium absorption remained normal. Daily treatment with salmon CT, but not CGRP, normalized the bone loss in CT/CGRP KO mice during lactation [74].

It appears from this study, that the action of CT is short-term. CT acts during lactation to prevent excessive bone resorption and the release of calcium from the skeleton.

Interestingly, in both CT/CGRP KO and wild type mice, the skeleton recovered fully postweaning, showing that CT was redundant for bone recovery. It has also been shown that maternal serum levels of CT are increased 1 day postweaning in mice, which is associated with the loss of osteoclast function and the initiation of apoptosis [77].

Evidence suggests that osteocytes may express the CTR [56]. These cells have been shown recently by Qing and colleagues [79] to play an important role during lactation by mobilizing calcium from their surrounding mineralized matrix within lacunae. These remodeling actions of osteocytes are dependent on the PTHR1 receptor and thus likely to be mediated via the actions of PTHrP, the serum levels of which are elevated during lactation. It is tempting to speculate that CT may also exert its protective effect to limit the bone lost during lactation by acting on osteocytes to oppose the resorptive effects of PTHrP. To date, a possible role for the CTR in regulating osteocyte-mediated bone resorption during pregnancy and lactation has not been investigated.

CT via the CTR may also exert its protective actions on the skeleton during pregnancy and lactation indirectly via its central inhibitory activity of prolactin secretion, a key hormone in controlling lactation [80] (Figure 8.2). It has been proposed that this action of CT is mediated by enhancement of hypothalamic inhibitory pathways controlling prolactin secretion [64,65], most likely involving dopaminergic neurons [80]. In addition, CT has also been shown to inhibit the proliferation of prolactin-producing lactotrophs within the anterior pituitary [81]. Whether these actions of CT in the regulation of prolactin secretion within the CNS are mediated by the CTR or another CT-related receptor is yet to be determined.

8.8 CONCLUSIONS

The physiological roles of calcitonin and its receptor (CTR) have long been debated, with many suggesting that CT is no more than a vestigial hormone. Significant advances have been made recently in identifying possible physiological roles for CT and the CTR in bone and calcium metabolism by the use of genetically modified mouse models. Data from these studies utilizing global and tissue-specific gene knockout mouse models for calcitonin and the CTR provided evidence for two distinct functions of the CTR: (1) to inhibit bone formation and (2) to protect the skeleton in times of calcium stress. Given the localization of CTRs in other tissues, actions of CT at these other sites remain to be elucidated. Future studies utilizing genetically modified mouse models in which CT or the CTR is deleted in a developmental- and/or tissue-specific manner are required to provide further insights into the physiological roles of CT and the CTR.

REFERENCES

1. Foster GV et al. 1964. Thyroid origin of calcitonin. *Nature* 202: 1303–1305.
2. Brown EM et al. 1993. Cloning and characterization of an extracellular Ca^{2+}-sensing receptor from bovine parathyroid. *Nature* 366: 575–580.
3. Henley C III et al. 2011. Discovery of a calcimimetic with differential effects on parathyroid hormone and calcitonin secretion. *J Pharmacol Exp Ther* 337: 681–691.

4. Davey RA et al. 2008. The calcitonin receptor plays a physiological role to protect against hypercalcemia in mice. *J Bone Miner Res* 23: 1182–1193.
5. Turner AG et al. 2011. The role of the calcitonin receptor in protecting against induced hypercalcemia is mediated via its actions in osteoclasts to inhibit bone resorption. *Bone* 48: 354–361.
6. Freake HC and MacIntyre I. 1982. Specific binding of 1,25-dihydroxycholecalciferol in human medullary thyroid carcinoma. *Biochem J* 206: 181–184.
7. Zaidi M et al. 1987. Biology of peptides from the calcitonin genes. *Q J Exper Physiol* 72: 371–408.
8. Nicholson GC et al. 1986. Abundant calcitonin receptors in isolated rat osteoclasts: biochemical and autoradiographic characterization. *J Clin Invest* 78: 355–360.
9. Sexton PM. 1991. Central nervous system binding sites for calcitonin and calcitonin gene-related peptide. *Mol Neurobiol* 5: 251–273.
10. Chausmer A et al. 1980. Identification of testicular cell plasma membrane receptors for calcitonin. *J Lab Clin Med* 96: 933–938.
11. Sexton PM et al. 1987. Localization and characterization of renal calcitonin receptors by in vitro autoradiography. *Kidney Intl* 32: 862–868.
12. Ismail PM et al. 2004. Progesterone induction of calcitonin expression in the murine mammary gland. *J Endocrinol* 180: 287–295.
13. Findlay DM. 2006. Regulation of cell growth mediated by the calcitonin receptor. *Cell Mol Biol* 52: 3–8.
14. Gorn AH et al. 1992. Cloning, characterization, and expression of a human calcitonin receptor from an ovarian carcinoma cell line. *J Clin Invest* 90: 1726–1735.
15. Moore EE et al. 1995. Functionally different isoforms of the human calcitonin receptor result from alternative splicing of the gene transcript. *Mol Endocrinol* 9: 959–968.
16. Albrandt K et al. 1995. Molecular cloning and functional expression of a third isoform of the human calcitonin receptor and partial characterization of the calcitonin receptor gene. *Endocrinology* 136: 5377–5384.
17. Sexton PM et al. 1993. Identification of brain isoforms of the rat calcitonin receptor. *Mol Endocrinol* 7: 815–821.
18. Horne WC et al. 1994. Signal transduction by calcitonin: multiple ligands, receptors, and signaling pathways. *Trends Endocrinol Metabol* 5: 395–401.
19. Ng KW et al. 1983. Calcitonin effects on growth and on selective activation of type II isoenzyme of cyclic adenosine 3′:5′-monophosphate-dependent protein kinase in T 47D human breast cancer cells. *Cancer Res* 43: 794–800.
20. Marzia M et al. 2006. Calpain is required for normal osteoclast function and is down-regulated by calcitonin. *J Biol Chem* 281: 9745–97454.
21. Sexton PM et al. 2012. RAMPs as drug targets. *Adv Exp Med Biol* 744: 61–74.
22. Wada S et al. 1996. Physiological levels of calcitonin regulate the mouse osteoclast calcitonin receptor by a protein kinase α-mediated mechanism. *Endocrinology* 137: 312–320.
23. Robinson CJ et al. 1967. Mode of action of thyrocalcitonin. *J Endocrinol* 39: 71–79.
24. Martin TJ et al. 1966. The mode of action of thyrocalcitonin. *Lancet* 1: 900–902.
25. Flanagan B and Nichols G Jr. 1969. Bone matrix turnover and balance in vitro. I. The effects of parathyroid hormone and thyrocalcitonin. *J Clin Invest* 48: 595–606.
26. Chambers TJ and Magnus CJ. 1982. Calcitonin alters behaviour of isolated osteoclasts. *J Pathol* 136: 27–39.
27. Chabardes D et al. 1976. Distribution of calcitonin-sensitive adenylate cyclase activity along the rabbit kidney tubule. *Proc Natl Acad Sci USA* 73: 3608–3612.
28. Kawashima H et al. 1981. Calcitonin selectively stimulates 25-hydroxyvitamin D3-1 α-hydroxylase in proximal straight tubule of rat kidney. *Nature* 291: 327–329.

29. Gao XH et al. 2004. Calcitonin stimulates expression of the rat 25-hydroxyvitamin D3-24-hydroxylase (CYP24) promoter in HEK-293 cells expressing calcitonin receptor: identification of signaling pathways. *J Mol Endocrinol* 32: 87–98.

30. Yamamoto Y et al. 1982. Calcitonin-induced anorexia in rats: a structure–activity study by intraventricular injections. *Jpn J Pharmacol* 32: 1013–1017.

31. Baldo BA and Kelley AE. 2001. Amylin infusion into rat nucleus accumbens potently depresses motor activity and ingestive behavior. *Am J Physiol Reg Integr Comp Physiol* 281: R1232–R1242.

32. Freed WJ et al. 1979. Calcitonin: inhibitory effect on eating in rats. *Science* 206: 850–852.

33. Chesnut CH, 3rd et al. 2008. Salmon calcitonin: a review of current and future therapeutic indications. *Osteoporosis Intl* 19: 479–491.

34. Knopp JA et al. 2005. Calcitonin for treating acute pain of osteoporotic vertebral compression fractures: a systematic review of randomized, controlled trials. *Osteoporosis Intl* 16: 1281–1290.

35. Behets C et al. 2004. Effects of calcitonin on subchondral trabecular bone changes and on osteoarthritic cartilage lesions after acute anterior cruciate ligament deficiency. *J Bone Miner Res* 19: 1821–1826.

36. Sondergaard BC et al. 2007. The effect of oral calcitonin on cartilage turnover and surface erosion in an ovariectomized rat model. *Arthr Rheumat* 56: 2674–2678.

37. Friedman PA and Gesek FA. 1995. Cellular calcium transport in renal epithelia: measurement, mechanisms, and regulation. *Physiol Rev* 75: 429–471.

38. Shinki T et al. 1999. Calcitonin is a major regulator for the expression of renal 25-hydroxyvitamin D3-1α-hydroxylase gene in normocalcemic rats. *Proc Natl Acad Sci USA* 96: 8253–8258.

39. Kenny AD and Heiskell CA. 1965. Effect of crude thyrocalcitonin on calcium and phosphorus metabolism in rats. *Proc Soc Exp Biol Med* 120: 269–271.

40. Robinson CJ et al. 1966. Phosphaturic effect of thyrocalcitonin. *Lancet* 2: 83–84.

41. Haas HG et al. 1971. Renal effects of calcitonin and parathyroid extract in man: studies in hypoparathyroidism. *J Clin Invest* 50: 2689–2702.

42. Berndt TJ and Knox FG. 1984. Proximal tubule site of inhibition of phosphate reabsorption by calcitonin. *Am J Physiol* 246: F927–F930.

43. Yusufi AN et al. 1987. Calcitonin inhibits Na+ gradient-dependent phosphate uptake across renal brush border membranes. *Am J Physiol* 252: F598–F604.

44. Zaidi M et al. 2002. Calcitonin and bone formation: a knockout full of surprises. *J Clin Invest* 110: 1769–1771.

45. Hoff AO et al. 2002. Increased bone mass is an unexpected phenotype associated with deletion of the calcitonin gene. *J Clin Invest* 110: 1849–1857.

46. Cornish J et al. 2001. Effects of calcitonin, amylin, and calcitonin gene-related peptide on osteoclast development. *Bone* 29: 162–168.

47. Cornish J et al. 1999. Comparison of the effects of calcitonin gene-related peptide and amylin on osteoblasts. *J Bone Miner Res* 14: 1302–1309.

48. Brain SD and Grant AD. 2004. Vascular actions of calcitonin gene-related peptide and adrenomedullin. *Physiol Rev* 84: 903–934.

49. Schinke T et al. 2004. Decreased bone formation and osteopenia in mice lacking α-calcitonin gene-related peptide. *J Bone Miner Res* 19: 2049–2056.

50. Beamer WG et al. 1996. Genetic variability in adult bone density among inbred strains of mice. *Bone* 18: 397–403.

51. Davey RA and MacLean HE. 2006. Current and future approaches using genetically modified mice in endocrine research. *Am J Physiol Endocrinol Metabol* 291: E429–E438.

52. Davey RA et al. 2004. Genetically modified animal models as tools for studying bone and mineral metabolism. *J Bone Miner Res* 19: 882–892.

53. Gagel RF et al. 2007. Deletion of calcitonin/CGRP gene causes a profound cortical resorption phenotype in mice. *J Bone Miner Res* 22: S35.
54. Dacquin R et al. 2004. Amylin inhibits bone resorption while the calcitonin receptor controls bone formation in vivo. *J Cell Biol* 164: 509–514.
55. Winkler DG et al. 2003. Osteocyte control of bone formation via sclerostin, a novel BMP antagonist. *EMBO J* 22: 6267–6276.
56. Gooi JH et al. 2010. Calcitonin impairs the anabolic effect of PTH in young rats and stimulates expression of sclerostin by osteocytes. *Bone* 46: 1486–1497.
57. van Bezooijen RL et al. 2007. Wnt but not BMP signaling is involved in the inhibitory action of sclerostin on BMP-stimulated bone formation. *J Bone Miner Res* 22: 19–28.
58. Atkins GJ et al. 2011. Sclerostin is a locally acting regulator of late-osteoblast/preosteocyte differentiation and regulates mineralization through a MEPE-ASARM-dependent mechanism. *J Bone Miner Res* 26: 1425–1436.
59. Kuestner RE et al. 1994. Cloning and characterization of an abundant subtype of the human calcitonin receptor. *Mol Pharmacol* 46: 246–255.
60. Sheward WJ et al. 1994. The expression of the calcitonin receptor gene in the brain and pituitary gland of the rat. *Neurosci Lett* 181: 31–34.
61. Baldock PA et al. 2005. Hypothalamic control of bone formation: distinct actions of leptin and y2 receptor pathways. *J Bone Miner Res* 20: 1851–1857.
62. Wimalawansa SJ. 1997. Amylin, calcitonin gene-related peptide, calcitonin, and adrenomedullin: a peptide superfamily. *Crit Rev Neurobiol* 11: 167–239.
63. Tache Y et al. 1990. Central nervous system action of peptides to influence gastrointestinal motor function. *Gastroenterology* 98: 517–528.
64. Netti C et al. 1989. Evidence of a central inhibition of growth hormone secretion by calcitonin gene-related peptide. *Neuroendocrinology* 49: 242–247.
65. Sibilia V et al. 1990. Inhibitory effects of centrally administered/ASU1-7/eel calcitonin on basal and stimulated prolactin release in rats. *J Endocrinol Invest* 13: 507–511.
66. Hirsch PF and Munson PL. 1969. Thyrocalcitonin. *Physiol Rev* 49: 548–622.
67. Williams GA et al. 1966. Evidence for thyrocalcitonin in man. *Proc Soc Exp Biol Med* 122: 1273–1276.
68. Martin TJ and Melick RA. 1969. The acute effects of porcine calcitonin in man. *Australas Ann Med* 18: 258–263.
69. Cooper CW et al. 1967. An improved method for the biological assay of thyrocalcitonin. *Endocrinology* 81: 610–616.
70. Sexton PM et al. 1999. Calcitonin. *Curr Med Chem* 6: 1067–1093.
71. Zhu LJ et al. 1998. Attenuation of calcitonin gene expression in pregnant rat uterus leads to a block in embryonic implantation. *Endocrinology*. 139: 330–339.
72. McDonald KR et al. 2004. Ablation of calcitonin/calcitonin gene-related peptide-α impairs fetal magnesium but not calcium homeostasis. *Am J Physiol Endocrinol Metabol* 287: E218–E226.
73. Kovacs CS and Kronenberg HM. 1997. Maternal–fetal calcium and bone metabolism during pregnancy, puerperium, and lactation. *Endocr Rev* 18: 832–872.
74. Woodrow JP et al. 2006. Calcitonin plays a critical role in regulating skeletal mineral metabolism during lactation. *Endocrinology* 147: 4010–4021.
75. Yamamoto M et al. 1992. Concentrations of parathyroid hormone-related protein in rat milk change with duration of lactation and interval from previous suckling, but not with milk calcium. *Endocrinology* 130: 741–747.
76. Stevenson JC et al. 1979. A physiological role for calcitonin: protection of the maternal skeleton. *Lancet* 2: 769–770.
77. Bowman BM, Miller, S.C. 2005. Rapid osteoclast apoptosis at the end of lactation in the maternal skeleton. *J Bone Miner Res* 20: S258.

78. Bucht E et al. 1986. Immunoextracted calcitonin in milk and plasma from totally thyroidectomized women: evidence of monomeric calcitonin in plasma during pregnancy and lactation. *Acta Endocrinol* 113: 529–535.
79. Qing H et al. 2012. Demonstration of osteocytic perilacunar/canalicular remodeling in mice during lactation. *J Bone Miner Res* 28.
80. Tohei A et al. 2000. Calcitonin inhibition of prolactin secretion in lactating rats: mechanism of action. *Neuroendocrinology* 71: 327–332.
81. Shah GV et al. 1999. Calcitonin inhibits anterior pituitary cell proliferation in the adult female rats. *Endocrinology* 140: 4281–4291.

9 Definition, Diagnosis, and Significance of Osteoporosis

B.E. Christopher Nordin and Richard L. Prince

CONTENTS

9.1 INTRODUCTION

Osteoporosis is an important health problem, particularly in the elderly, because it increases the risk of and significantly contributes to fractures in women after menopause and in men from after age 60. As women age, the main fracture locations are the wrists in their 50s, the spine in their 60s, and their hips in their 70s and 80s. The condition carries very significant morbidity and mortality and costs the healthcare system billions of dollars yearly. However, impaired bone status is not the only factor predisposing to fracture. Other factors are the frequency and force involved in falls [1]; these factors are not discussed in this chapter.

Bone is a connective tissue composed of about 40% protein known as osteoid, which provides its tensile strength, and 60% mineral (calcium phosphate), which gives it compressive strength [2]. The mineral, known as hydroxyapatite, is a particular crystal form of calcium phosphate and water that precipitates on osteoid. Bone formation proceeds by the production of bone proteins within the osteoblasts. The proteins are exported to the osteoid matrix following which mineral crystals are deposited on this extracellular matrix. Thus, in normal bone formation, under-mineralized osteoid that is about to be mineralized can be detected by light microscopy.

This compartment is assessed by measurement of osteoid surface, thickness, and volume. Normally mineralized bone has an osteoid volume of 1.5% of total bone volume or less. Clinical osteomalacia is associated with an osteoid volume of 10% or more. A more complex definition includes the concept of mineralization lag time in combination with increased osteoid thickness [3]. Mineralization lag time is the time required for newly formed osteoid to mineralize and should be 30 days or less.

These parameters are calculated from bone biopsies made after exposure to two separate pulses of compounds that are deposited in bone only at the new mineralization front. Tetracycline is commonly used to mark newly mineralized bone and can be detected in histological sections under the application of ultraviolet (UV) light as bright yellow lines. If two pulses are given 2 weeks apart and a biopsy taken, the amount of osteoid deposited and mineralized during this period can be calculated. The distance between the lines and their lengths allow calculation of the rate of normally mineralized bone formation and can detect excess osteoid or increases in mineralization lag time [2].

9.2   DEFINITION

As explained above, under-mineralized bone may have the same volume as normal bone but will exhibit lower mass on bone densitometry because of the deficiency of the mineral component. This caused many to question the widely quoted definition of osteoporosis developed by a World Health Organization (WHO) study group [4] in turn taken from an earlier Consensus Development Conference [5]: "A disease characterized by low bone mass and microarchitectural deterioration of bone tissue, leading to enhanced bone fragility and a consequent increase in fracture risk."

The problem is that this definition can apply to bone disorders other than osteoporosis; it could apply to osteomalacia. The definition of a disorder needs to be specific to that disorder and exclude all others. The only valid definition of osteoporosis in our opinion is "too little bone in the bone" as illustrated in Figure 9.1. Because osteoporosis can be induced in vertebrate species including humans by a diet low in calcium, osteoporosis can be considered as the "index disease" of calcium deficiency [6]. Osteoporosis weakens bone because of reduced calcium quantity in bony tissue. Osteomalacia weakens bone because of its reduced mineral content and resulting reduced mechanical resistance to bending. The two conditions can coexist as may occur in patients with hip fractures [7] who commonly suffer from hypovitaminosis D [8].

9.3   DUAL ENERGY X-RAY ABSORPTIOMETRY (DXA)

The current standard test for the diagnosis of osteoporosis is the measurement of areal bone mineral density (BMD) by dual energy x-ray absorptiometry (DXA). This technology assesses the mass of bone mineral by its ability to absorb photons from an x-ray source within a defined two-dimensional bone projection area. The mineral mass is then divided by the area to produce a composite areal BMD score. Because the mass is corrected for area but not volume, the result is not a true density value but is a widely used measure of osteoporosis.

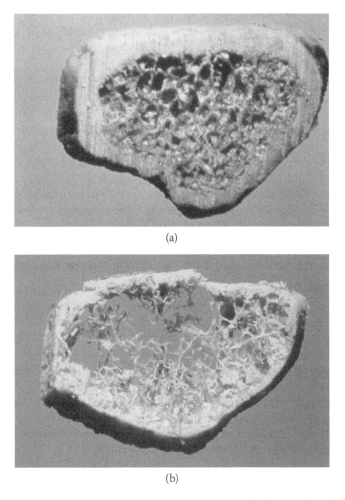

(a)

(b)

FIGURE 9.1 Sections of ulna from normal (a) and osteoporotic (b) bone show that osteoporosis involves less bone tissue within bone as an organ.

9.3.1 Cube Square Law

The area of a three-dimensional object increases by the square of the length and the volume increases by the cube of the length. Because the mass of a scanned three-dimensional bone is determined by its external size and internal structure, the mass increases as the cube of the length whereas the area increases only by the square of the length and thus only partially compensates for the varying bone size. Thus areal BMD is an inverse function of bone size and a positive function of bone mass, both of which influence fracture risk.

Areal DXA for osteoporosis and osteomalacia—The photon absorption and scatter used to determine bone mass is dependent only on the mineral phase of the bone, not the osteoid. The mineral phase is determined by a pre-determined cut-off value for absorption and scatter of photons; it does not quantify the degree of mineralization of the bony tissue. Thus, this technique cannot determine the difference between low bone mass caused by insufficient mineralized bone within the bone (osteoporosis) and under-mineralized bone due to rickets or osteomalacia.

9.3.2   VARIATION OF AREAL BMD CAUSED BY VARIATION ON BONE PROJECTION AREA

Because bones are irregular in outline, variations in the two-dimensional bone projection area within which the measurement of mineral mass is made may contribute to variations in the measured bone mass. Areal BMD is the mass per unit area and therefore depends on the two-dimensional bone projection used to measure it. Thus, any variation in the positioning of a patient from one BMD measurement to the next will result in variation of the two-dimensional bone projection areas and alter the areal BMD measurement without actual change in bone status.

9.3.3   INTERPRETATION OF AREAL BMD VALUES AND USE OF REFERENCE RANGES

Reference ranges are generally based on measurements in young healthy adult volunteers. The BMD is actually a measure of bone mineral. The standard deviation (SD) around the young normal mean at the same site in the same sex is the T score. The normal range for most clinical measurements is a T score from –2 to +2 SD and therefore the diagnosis of osteoporosis should probably be based on a T score below –2 [9,10]. However, current practice follows a WHO report that defines T scores between –1 and –2.5 as osteopenic and those below –2.5 as osteoporotic for reasons that are not entirely clear [4]. Our proposal that osteoporosis should be defined as a BMD T score below –2 has recently been vindicated since a BMD with a T score below –2 separates patients who experienced minimal trauma fractures from non-fracture subjects better than a T score of –1.5 or –2.5 [11].

9.3.4   SENSITIVITY AND SPECIFICITY OF AREAL BMD FOR DIAGNOSIS OF OSTEOPOROSIS

Sensitivity and specificity for the diagnosis of osteoporosis by BMD measurement cannot be calculated in the conventional way because in practice the only way to diagnose osteoporosis short of a bone biopsy is by DXA. However, since the only significance of osteoporosis is that it increases fracture risk, positive and negative predictive values can be calculated from prospective studies relating initial areal BMD to subsequent fracture rate.

These studies show that the predictive power of areal BMD is comparable to the predictive ability of blood cholesterol in respect to heart attack and blood pressure measurement in relation to stroke [12]. As shown in Figures 9.2 and 9.3, the decrease in BMD with age is associated with a progressive rise in fractures of all kinds. This does not mean that all minimal trauma fracture cases are osteoporotic. The true figure is about 30% [13].

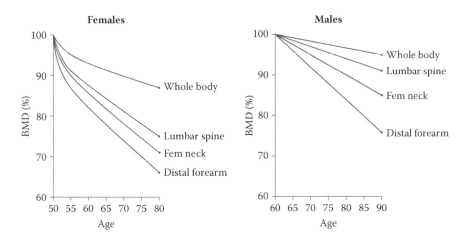

FIGURE 9.2 Declines in bone mass density with age at four skeletal sites in both sexes.

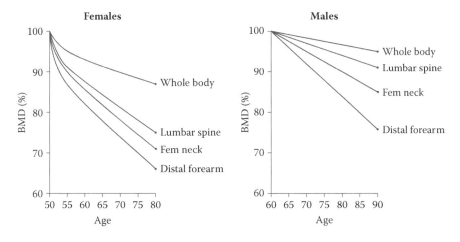

FIGURE 9.3 Total fracture incidence in both sexes. (a) Rates cited by Donaldson et al. [27] refer to all fractures. (b) Rates of Knowelden et al. [28] refer to all fractures. (c) Garraway et al. [29] rates refer to all limb fractures including hips; Geelong, Australia [21] rates refer to all non-spine fractures. *Source:* Sanders KM et al. 1999. Age- and gender-specific rate of fractures in Australia: a population-based study. *Osteoporosis Intl* 10: 240–247. With permission.

The fracture risk in women as a function of age and hip BMD is shown in Figure 9.4 [14]. The 6-year risk rises from about 2% at a T score of 0 at age 51 to 55 years to some 60% at a T score of −4 at 81 to 85 years, partly due to more frequent falls over time [15]. Each unit decrease in T score increases fracture risk by about the same degree as a 5-year increase in age. The dataset used to derive Figure 9.4 indicates that the risk derived from a prevalent fracture after age 50 was equivalent to a 5-year increase in age.

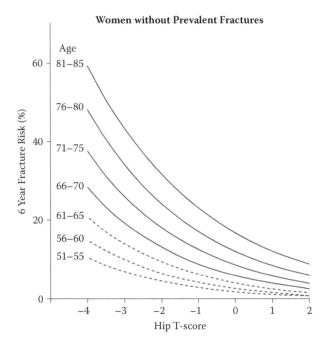

FIGURE 9.4   The relation of total hip bone mass density and 6-year fracture risk calculated from a prospective study in 1,098 female volunteers over age 70 [14]. The interrupted lines are extrapolations. *Source:* Tucker G et al. 2007. The importance of calculating absolute rather than relative fracture risk. *Bone* 41: 937–941. With permission.

Other studies report a somewhat greater effect of prevalent fracture on fracture risk calculated in a different way [16]. Figure 9.4 can also be used to calculate fracture risk in men if one unit is added to a man's T score because men and women fracture at similar BMD values but not at the same T scores [17]. Keep in mind, however, that the *immediate* cause of fracture is trauma; low BMD simply increases the risk of fracture from any given trauma. A third risk factor of comparable importance is bone turnover [18], which will not be considered further because its measurement has not yet been standardized.

9.3.5   Effects of Menopause and Age on Bone Mineral Density

As long as children and adolescents receive sufficient calcium in their diets and sufficient vitamin D from sunlight, their skeletons will grow in parallel with the rest of their organs and tissues until they reach peak size and peak bone mass in their late teens or early twenties. After adulthood is reached, the BMD remains relatively stable until menopause in women and about age 60 in men, and then declines in both sexes—more rapidly in women than in men (Figure 9.2).

In postmenopausal women, the loss of bone is predominantly due to increased bone breakdown due to the negative calcium balance from estrogen deficiency and an associated relative deficit in bone formation. In men, a reduction in bone formation

[19] possibly arises from a decline in serum testosterone and a decrease in intestinal calcium absorption [20] after about age 60. In both sexes, the fracture rate rises as the BMD declines, more rapidly in women than in men (Figures 9.2 and 9.3) [12]. In the early stages, the main fracture site is the distal forearm; after age 70, the much more disabling hip fracture assumes major importance in both sexes [21].

All measured physiological variables are subject to differences between individuals (inter-individual variations) and to changes within an individual (intra-individual variations). The tendency for an individual with high normal values to remain in the high normal range and for those with low normal values to remain in the low normal range is called tracking and is a feature of many physiological variables. Height is a good example; children who are tall for their age generally grow into tall adults. Tracking within the normal range is seen in many blood variables such as calcium levels [22] and is particularly obvious in relation to bone density.

Although postmenopausal women lose bone at different rates, the differences between the rates of loss are small compared with the differences between the initial BMD values. Thus, women whose bone density is in the upper part of the normal range at menopause will tend to be in the upper part of the range 10 years later and probably much longer [23]. The implication that BMD in later life is significantly related to BMD at menopause is borne out by the power of BMD to predict fracture risk for up to 25 years [24].

In a Danish trial of estrogen treatment that started with women at menopause and lasted 10 years, the initial BMD in the 872 controls was a strong predictor of osteoporosis and/or fracture 10 years later [23]. Using a T score threshold of 0, the sensitivity of spine BMD in relation to osteoporosis or fracture (mainly of the wrist) was 89.7% (95% confidence interval 84.7 to 93.1) and the specificity was 39.3% (35.6 to 43.1).

In the Düppe study [24], 410 of 1076 women aged 20 to 78 years were observed for 20 to 25 years, by which time they suffered 213 fractures of wrist, proximal humerus, hip, or spine. The relative risk of hip fracture associated with a 1 SD decrease in the initial forearm BMD was 1.66 (1.13 to 2.46) and of vertebral fracture 1.79 (1.22 to 2.62). These data demonstrate the potential value of determining a woman's bone status at menopause before she has osteoporosis rather than waiting until she reaches age 65 [25] or 70 [26] or has a fracture. The menopause is the main risk factor for minimal trauma fracture in women. In men, the main risk factor is probably age over 60 years.

9.4   CONCLUSION

Osteoporosis is defined by a low mass of normally mineralized bone within the external surfaces of bone and is generally diagnosed by the DXA measurement of areal BMD. Despite the limitations of DXA technology including the measurement of areal bone density as opposed to volumetric bone density, variation as a result of differences in positioning of patients at each BMD measurement episode and interpretation of measurements utilizing normal reference ranges, this technique is highly useful in clinical practice.

Areal BMD provides sensitivity and specificity for the diagnosis of osteoporosis and risk of fracture comparable to the sensitivity and specificity of blood cholesterol measurement for predicting heart attacks and blood pressure levels in predicting strokes. BMD demonstrates tracking of individuals within a population and indicates that postmenopausal women at the high end of the normal distribution remain at the high end for at least 10 years. More importantly, measurement of BMD in postmenopausal women predicts the risks of fracture for 20 to 25 years.

Such data demonstrate the potential value of determining a woman's bone status at menopause rather than waiting until she reaches age 65 or 70 years of age or incurs a fracture. As discussed elsewhere in this volume, women with negative T scores at menopause should be advised to adopt lifestyle measures such as high dietary calcium intake, adequate vitamin D status, and exercise regimens that have been demonstrated to reduce the rate of bone loss.

REFERENCES

1. Zhu K et al. 2011 "Timed up-and-go test" and bone mineral density measurement for fracture prediction. *Arch Int Med* 171: 1655–1661.
2. Revell PA. 1986. *Pathology of Bone*. Springer-Verlag: Heidelberg.
3. Parfitt AM et al. 2004. The mineralization index: a new approach to the histomorphometric appraisal of osteomalacia. *Bone* 35: 320–325.
4. World Health Organization. 1994. Assessment of fracture risk and its application to screening for postmenopausal osteoporosis. Technical Report Series 843. Geneva.
5. Consensus Development Conference. 1993. Diagnosis, prophylaxis, and treatment of osteoporosis. *Am J Med* 94: 646–650.
6. Heaney RP. 2003 Long-latency deficiency disease: insights from calcium and vitamin D. *Am J Clin Nutr* 78: 912–919.
7. Aaron JE et al. 1974. Frequency of osteomalacia and osteoporosis in fractures of the proximal femur. *Lancet* 1: 229–233.
8. Morris HA et al. 1984. Vitamin D and femoral neck fractures in elderly South Australian women. *Med J Austral* 140: 519–521.
9. Nordin BEC. 1987. The definition and diagnosis of osteoporosis. *Calcif Tiss Intl* 40: 57–58.
10. Nordin BEC. 2008. Redefining osteoporosis. *Calcif Tiss Intl* 83: 365–367.
11. Wu Q et al. 2010. Does using lower limit of normal values enhance the ability of a single bone mineral density measure to predict fractures? *Osteoporosis Intl* 21: 1881–1888.
12. Marshall D et al. 1996. Meta-analysis of how well measures of bone mineral density predict occurrence of osteoporotic fracture. *Brit Med J* 312: 1254–1259.
13. Stone KL et al. 2003. BMD at multiple sites and risk of fracture of multiple types: long-term results from the Study of Osteoporotic Fractures. *J Bone Miner Res* 18: 1947–1954.
14. Tucker G et al. 2007. The importance of calculating absolute rather than relative fracture risk. *Bone* 41: 937–941.
15. Graafmans WC et al. 1996. Falls in the elderly: a prospective study of risk factors and risk profiles. *Am J Epidemiol* 143: 1129–1136.
16. Nguyen ND et al. 2008. Development of prognostic nomograms for individualizing 5-year and 10-year fracture risks. *Osteoporosis Intl* 19: 1431–1444.
17. Selby PL et al. 2000. Is a calculated total hip BMD of clinical use? *Osteoporosis Intl* 11: 368–371.
18. Heaney RP. 2003. Is the paradigm shifting? *Bone* 33: 457–465.
19. Aaron JE et al. 1985. The microanatomy of trabecular bone loss in normal aging men and women. *Clin Orthop Rel Res* 215: 260–271.

20. Nordin BEC et al. 2011. Recalculation of the calcium requirement of adult men. *Am J Clin Nutr* 93: 442–445.
21. Sanders KM et al. 1999. Age- and gender-specific rate of fractures in Australia: a population-based study. *Osteoporosis Intl* 10: 240–247.
22. Morris HA et al. 1995. The 5-year reproducibility of calcium-related biochemical variables in postmenopausal women. *Scan J Clin Lab Invest* 55: 383–389.
23. Abrahamsen B et al. 2006. Ten-year prediction of osteoporosis from baseline bone mineral density: development of prognostic thresholds in healthy postmenopausal women: the Danish Osteoporosis Prevention Study. *Osteoporosis Intl* 17: 245–251.
24. Düppe H et al. 1997. A single bone density measurement can predict fractures over 25 years. *Calcif Tiss Intl* 60: 171–174.
25. Doherty DA et al. 2001. Lifetime and 5-year age-specific risks of first and subsequent osteoporotic fractures in postmenopausal women. *Osteoporosis Intl* 12: 16–23.
26. Lips P. 1997. Epidemiology and predictors of fractures associated with osteoporosis. *Am J Med* 103(2A): 3S–11S.
27. Donaldson LJ et al. 1990 Incidence of fractures in a geographically defined population. *J Epidemiol Community Health* 44: 241–245.
28. Knowelden J et al. 1964. Incidence of fractures in persons over 35 years of age: a working party on fractures in the elderly. *Br J Prev Soc Med* 18: 130–141.
29. Garraway WM et al. 1979. Limb fractures in a defined population I. Frequency and distribution. *Mayo Clin Proc* 54: 701–707.

Index